Sport and International Understanding

Proceedings of the Congress
Held in Helsinki, Finland, July 7–10, 1982

Edited by
Maaret Ilmarinen

Editorial Board:
P.V. Komi A. Koskela P. Seppänen R. Telama P. Vuolle

With 7 Figures and 32 Tables

Springer-Verlag
Berlin Heidelberg New York Tokyo 1984

Editor:

Maaret Ilmarinen
Secretary for Information and International Affairs, The Finnish Society for Research in Sport and Physical Education, Annankatu 4B, SF-00120 Helsinki 12

ISBN 978-3-642-49963-0 ISBN 978-3-642-49961-6 (eBook)
DOI 10.1007/978-3-642-49961-6

Library of Congress Cataloging in Publication Data
Main entry under title:
Sport and international understanding.
Papers from the Congress on Sport and International Understanding organized by the Finnish Society for Research in Sport and Physical Education, Finnish Central Sport Federation, and the Worker's Sport Federation
Bibliography: p. Includes index. 1. Sports and state - Congresses. 2. Sports - International cooperation - Congresses. I. Ilmarinen, Maaret. II. Congress on Sport and International Understanding (1982: Helsinki, Finland). III. Liikuntatieteellinen Seura. IV. Suomen Valtakunnan Urheiluliitto. V. Työväen Urheiluliitto (Helsinki, Finland) GV706.8.S64 1984 796 84-23526
ISBN 978-3-642-49963-0

Softcover reprint of the hardcover 1st edition 1984

Typesetting: Druckservice K. Teichmann, D-6901 Mauer

2119/3140-543210

Preface

In recent years concern has been growing about the preservation of world peace, while over the past few decades there has been a vast increase in the amount of international sporting activity and hence more opportunities to advance international understanding and peace. It is this situation which caused the Congress on Sport and International Understanding to be convened, the idea for it first having arisen after the Helsinki Conference on Security and Co-operation in Europe in 1975. The venue for the Congress was, as for the Conference on Security and Co-operation, Finlandia Hall. It was held under the auspices of the International Council of Sport and Physical Education (ICSPE) and was organised by the Finnish member organisations, the Finnish Society for Research in Sport and Physical Education (organising association), Finnish Central Sport Federation (SVUL) and the Workers' Sport Federation (TUL).

The aim of the Congress was to analyse the role of sport in advancing international understanding and to promote research in this field. In addition, the Congress wished to offer researchers and those involved in sporting activities an opportunity to exchange ideas about the themes under discussion. The aim of the Congress was to find the answers to the following questions:

1. What forms does international co-operation take in present-day competitive and top-level sport, sports for all and other forms of physical culture? What is its historical background and future?
2. What is the role of sport in international political, social, cultural and scientific co-operation? Does it promote international coexistence and understanding in these fields?
3. By what means can international sport advance co-operation and understanding?

A total of 300 research workers and persons engaged in various tasks in organisations for sports and physical education participated in the Congress, representing 27 countries. Seventy-eight lectures and introductory lectures were given.

As this was the first large international congress in this field, the number of lectures fulfilling strict scientific criteria was rather small. Instead, the Congress provided a lot of material for developing a scientific approach to the problems discussed and will hopefully make it possible to find practical solutions to the various difficulties that exist with regard to international co-operation in sport and physical culture.

The role of sport in advancing or weakening international coexistence and understanding was analysed most thoroughly in the lectures given at the Congress. The final outcome of the sociological, political and organisational research, especially in respect of international top-level sports, was that sport affords a vast potential which, when guided along the rigth lines, may contribute to promoting international co-operation and peace. Although this conclusion could not be directly confirmed by scientific research, a variety of in-depth analyses based on scientific literature and practical experience backed it up. In this respect, the lectures at the Congress emphasised the importance of the international mass media, the Olympic movement and other international organisations. In addition to these analyses, some detailed reports were delivered on the extent and content of international sport and on measures to promote international co-operation, such as education for internationalism and co-operation with developing countries. However, further attention needs to be focused on these areas in the future.

The organisation of this volume does not follow exactly the proceedings of the Congress: The content was re-arranged partly on scientific and partly on theme-related criteria. All lecturers were given the possibility of having their papers published, but in cases where there was no response to the request for alterations, the paper had perforce to be left aside. Of the 78 lectures given, 58 are published here.

We hope that this volume will fulfil its purpose as a review of the connection between sport and international understanding at the beginning of the 1980s and serve as a basis for and promoter of further research in the field.

We wish to thank wholeheartedly the representatives of ICSPE for their help and support in preparing for and during the Congress. The Congress was financed by the Ministry of Education, to whom we wish to extend our warmest gratitude. Expression of thanks belongs also to Oy Veikkaus Ab, to the Aura General Mutual Insurance Company and to the City of Helsinki for their support in arranging social events during the Congress. Finally, thanks are due to the Organising Committee, who at all times lent the Congress their benevolent support; to the contributors to these Proceedings for preparing their manuscripts and for responding to the deadline dates so well; and to the speakers, chairmen and participants, who made it possible to carry through the Congress so successfully.

The Scientific Committee

Pauli Vuolle (Chairman)
Paavo V. Komi
Aarni Koskela
Paavo Seppänen
Risto Telama

The Editor

Maaret Ilmarinen

Contents

I. Opening Ceremony

II. The Role of International Sport in Advancing or Weakening International Co-existence and Understanding

1. The Role of Sport in International Cultural and Social Co-operation

2. The Role of Sport in International Politics

3. The Role of the Olympic Games

4. The Role of International Organisations

III. The Extent and Content of International Co-operation in Sport

1. Competitive and Top-Level Sport

2. Sport for All

3. Sport for Special Groups

IV. Measures Related to International Co-operation in Sport

1. Mass Media and International Understanding

2. Co-operation with Developing Countries

Organising Committee of the Congress

Chairman

Juhani Perttunen	Secretary General to the President of the Republic, Chairman of the Finnish Society for Research in Sport and Physical Education, Annankatu 4B, SF-00120 Helsinki 12

Members

Kaarlo Hartiala	Professor and Chancellor of the University of Turku, SF-20500 Turku
Heikki Klemola	Director, Department for Sports and Youth Affairs, Ministry of Education, Aleksanterinkatu 15B, SF-00100 Helsinki 10
Aarni Koskela	Director, Department of Physiology, Institute of Occupational Health, Laajaniityntie 1, SF-01620 Vantaa 62
Mauri Oksanen	Secretary General, Finnish Central Sport Federation, Topeliuksenkatu 41a, SF-00250 Helsinki 25
Raimo Railo	Deputy Secretary General, Workers' Sport Federation, Paasivuorenkatu 4–6, SF-00530 Helsinki 53
Ossi Sjöman	Secretary General, Workers' Sport Federation, Paavisuorenkatu 4–6, SF-00530 Helsinki 53
Reijo Vartia	Head of Bureau, Department for Sports and Youth Affairs, Ministry of Education, Aleksanterinkatu 15B, SF-00100 Helsinki 10
Pauli Vuolle	Assistant Professor, Department of Sociology and Planning for Physical Culture, University of Jyväskylä, SF-40100 Jyväskylä 10
Marcel Hebbelinck	Professor, Vrije Universiteit, Brussels, Chairman of the Research Committee of the ICSPE, Pleinlaan 2, B-1050 Brussels

Secretariat

Joel Juppi	Secretary General of the Congress, Secretary General of the Finnish Society for Research in Sport and Physical Education, Annankatu 4B, SF-00120 Helsinki 12
Raija Mattila	Secretary for International Affairs, Department for Sports and Youth Affairs, Ministry of Education, Aleksanterinkatu 15B, SF-00100 Helsinki 10
Maaret Veistola (Ilmarinen)	Secretary of the Scientific Committee of the Congress, Secretary for Information and International Affairs of the Finnish Society for Research in Sport and Physical Education, Annankatu 4B, SF-00120 Helsinki 12
Bibi Korsström	Congress Secretary (ex officio)
Address of the Secretariat:	The Finnish Society for Research in Sport and Physical Education, Annankatu 4B, SF-00120 Helsinki 12, Telephone 0-640306

Referees

Pauli Vuolle	Assistant Professor, Department of Sociology and Planning for Physical Culture, University of Jyväskylä, SF-40100 Jyväskylä 10
Paavo V. Komi	Professor, Department of Biology of Physical Activity, University of Jyväskylä, SF-40100 Jyväskylä 10
Aarni Koskela	Departmental Director, Department of Physiology of the Institute of Occupational Health, Laajaniityntie 1, SF-01620 Vantaa 62
Paavo Seppänen	Dean, Faculty of Social Sciences, University of Helsinki, Franzeninkatu 13, SF-00500 Helsinki 50
Risto Telama	Dean, Faculty of Physical and Health Education, University of Jyväskylä, SF-40100 Jyväskylä 10

Contributors

Ahde M.	Workers' Sport Federation, Paasivuorenkatu 4–6 A, SF-00530 Helsinki 53
Ajisafe M.	Department of Physical and Health Education, University of Benin, Benin City, Nigeria
Bannister Sir Roger	c/o The Sports Council, 70 Brompton Road, GB-London SW3 1EX
Bedecki T.	Capher, 333 River Road, Vanier, Ontario K1L 8B9, Canada
Booth B. F.	School of Human Kinetics, University of Ottawa, 35 MacDougal, Ontario K1N 6N5, Canada
Buggel E.	State Secretariat for Physical Culture and Sport, Mohrenstrasse 6, DDR-1080 Berlin
Caldwell J. E.	5324 Keuka Court, Anchorage, Alaska 99504, USA
Cantelon H.	Centre for the Study of Sport and Leisure, Queen's University, Kingston, Ontario K7L 3N6, Canada
Daly N.	Health Education Bureau, 34 Upper Mount St., Dublin 2, Ireland
de Wachter F.	Hoger Instituut voor Wijsbegeerte, Kard. Mercierplein 2, B-3000 Leuven
Diem L.	Deutsche Sportschule Köln, Blumenallee 24, D-5000 Köln 40
Drowatzky J.	The University of Toledo, Toledo, OH 43606, USA
Erbach G.	State Secretariat for Physical Culture and Sport, Mohrenstrasse 6, DDR-1080 Berlin
Galtung J.	Wissenschaftskolleg zu Berlin, Wallotstrasse 19, D-1000 Berlin 33
Gitter W.	German Sports and Gymnastics Union, Storkower Str. 118, DDR-1055 Berlin
Han Y. S.	Yonsei University, Suh Dae Moon Ku, Seoul, Korea
Happel D.	Ministry of Culture, Recreation and Social Work, P. O. Box 5406, NL-2280 Hk Rijswijk
Hebbelinck M.	Vrije Universiteit Brussel, Pleinlaan 2, B-1050 Brussels
Heikinnen E.	Department of Health Science, University of Jyväskylä, SF-40100 Jyväskylä 10
Heinilä K.	Department of Sociology and Planning for Physical Culture, University of Jyväskylä, SF-40100 Jyväskylä 10
Heinilä L.	Department of Physical Education, University of Jyväskylä, SF-40100 Jyväskylä 10
Hietanen A.	Tampere Peace Research Institute, Hämeenkatu 13 b A, SF-33100 Tampere 10
Jääskeläinen M.	The Finnish Society for Research in Sport and Physical Education, Annankatu 4B, SF-00120 Helsinki 12
Jimenez-Ottalengo R.	Instituto de Investigaciones Sociales, Torre de Humanidades 2–7° Piso, Ciudad Universitaria, Coyacan 20, D. F., Republica Mexicana
Jochheim K.-A.	Institut für Rehabilitation und Behindertensport an der Universität zu Köln, Rehabilitationszentrum der Universität, D-5000 Köln-Lindenthal
Karvonen M. J.	World Health Organization, CH-1211 Geneva, 27
Kirsch A.	Federal Institute for Sports Science, Hertzstrasse 1, D-5000 Cologne
Kirsch K.	Deutsche Sporthochschule Köln, Holbeinstrasse 59, D-5020 Frechen 4
Kirvesniemi H.	Department of Biology of Physical Activity, University of Jyväskylä, SF-40100 Jyväskylä 10
Kivistö K.	Ministry of Education, Rauhankatu 4, SF-00170 Helsinki 17
Klemola H.	Ministry of Education, Aleksanterinkatu 15 B, SF-00100 Helsinki 10
Koivumäki K.	The Finnish Society for Research in Sport and Physical Education, Annankatu 4 B, SF-00120 Helsinki 12

Koivusalo I. (†)	Department of Physical Education, University of Jyväskylä, Seminaarinkatu 15, SF-40100 Jyväskylä 10
Koskela A.	Institute of Occupational Health, Laajaniityntie 1, SF-01620 Vantaa 62
Kramer R.	Ministry of Cultural Affairs, Recreation and Social Welfare, Steenvoordelaan, 370, NL-2280 Rijswijk (Z. H.)
Krüger A.	Institut für Sportwissenschaften, Georg-August-Universität, Sprangerweg 2, D-3400 Göttingen
Lahtinen U.	Department of Physical Education, University of Jyväskylä, SF-40100 Jyväskylä 10
Laitinen A.	Department of Sociology and Planning for Physical Culture, University of Jyväskylä, SF-40100 Jyväskylä 10
Lüschen G.	Institut für Sportwissenschaft, Technische Hochschule, D-5100 Aachen
Mäki-Reinikka H.	Finnish Student Sport Federation, Kalevankatu 26 A7, SF-00100 Helsinki 10
Marcal H.	The University of Lodrina, 86.100 Parana, Brazil
McIntosh P.	West London Institute of Higher Education, 16 Upper Woburn Place, GB-London WC1H OQP
Milshtein O.	USSR Committee for Physical Culture and Sport, Skaternyi Pereulek 4, Moscow, USSR
Niwa T.	Department of Physical Education, Faculty of Letters, Nara Women's University, Nara, Japan
Olafson G.	Faculty of Human Kinetics, University of Windsor, Windsor, Ontario N9B 3P4, Canada
Olin K.	Department of Sociology and Planning for Physical Culture, University of Jyväskylä, SF-40100 Jyväskylä 10
Paulín-Siade G.	Instituto de Investigaciones Sociales, Universidad Nacional Autónoma de México, Torre 2 de Humanidades 9, Piso, Mexico
Perttunen J.	The Finnish Society for Research in Sport and Physical Education, Annankatu 4 B, SF-00120 Helsinki 12
Petrov R.	Higher Institute of Physical Culture, 96 Angel Gergov Street, bl. III, vh. A, Sofia 1407, Bulgaria
Petrova N.	Higher Institute of Physical Culture, 96 Angel Gergov Street, bl. III, vh. A, Sofia 1407, Bulgaria
Preising W.	Bundesinstitut für Sportwissenschaft, Hertzstrasse 1, Postfach 400109/110, D-5000 Köln 40
Puputti V.	The Rehabilitation and Motion Center Peurunka, SF-41350 Laukaa
Riordan J.	University of Bradford, 15 Bankfield Drive, Shipley, GB-W. Yorks BD18 4AD
Sanadze L.	The Central Scientific Research Institute of Physical Education, Skaternyj Pereulek 4, Moscow, USSR
Saram P.	Department of Sociology, University of Alberta, Edmonton T6G 2H4, Canada
Sastamala A.	Finnish Schools' Sports Association, Mariankatu 26 B 23, SF-00170 Helsinki 17
Schüssler I.	Deutsche Sporthochschule Köln, Philosophie-Seminar, Carl-Diem-Weg 2, D-5000 Köln 41
Seppänen P.	Department of Sociology, University of Helsinki, Franzeninkatu 13, SF-00500 Helsinki 50
Ståhlberg M.	Finlands Svenska Centralidrottsförbund, Temppelikatu 19 D 37, SF-00100 Helsinki 10
Šugman R.	Faculty for Physical Culture, University of Edvard Kardelj, Livarska 14, 61000 Ljubljana, Yugoslavia
Sýkora F.	Faculty of Physical Education and Sport, Comenius University, Bratislava 81106, Czechoslovakia
Tallberg P.	Aleksanterinkatu 21, SF-00100 Helsinki 10
Uunila J.	Finnish Central Sport Federation, Topeliuksenkatu 41 A, SF-00250 Helsinki 25
Varis T.	Tampere Peace Research Institute, Hämeenkatu 13 b A, SF-33100 Tampere 10
Väyrynen R.	Department of Political Science, University of Helsinki, Aleksanterinkatu 7, SF-00100 Helsinki 10

Vriessen C. Lopez von	Department of Physical Education, Catholic University of Valparaiso, Casilla 4059, Valparaiso, Chile
Vuolle P.	Department of Sociology and Planning for Physical Culture, University of Jyväskylä, SF-40100 Jyväskylä 10
Walker G.	Council of Europe, BP 431 R6, F-67006 Strasbourg cedex
Wohl A.	Institute of Philosophy and Sociology, Academy of Physical Education in Warsaw, Dluga 19 m. 28, Warsaw, Poland
Wolańska T.	Academy of Physical Education, Marymoncka, 34, 01-813 Warsaw, Poland
Zachariev Z.	Section of Structures, Content and Methods of Education, United Nations Educational Scientific and Cultural Organization, 7. place de Fontanoy, F-75700 Paris
Žvan M.	Univerza Edvarda Kardelja V Ljubljani, Visoka Skola za T lesno Kulturo, Gortanova 22, 61000 Ljubljana, Yugoslavia

Chairmen

Bierstedt H.	State Secretary for Physical Culture and Sport, Mohrenstrasse 6, DDR-1080 Berlin
Buggel E.	State Secretary for Physical Culture and Sport, Mohrenstrasse 6, DDR-1080 Berlin
Coghlan J. F.	ICSPE, 16 Upper Woburn Place, GB-London WC1H OQP
Diem L.	Deutsche Sportschule Köln, Blumenallee 24, D-5000 Köln 40
Ghibu E.	Consiliul National Pentru, Educatie Fizica si Sport, Str. Vasile Conta 16, Bucuresti, Rumania
Hebbelinck M.	Vrije Universiteit Brussel, Pleinlaan 2, B-1050 Brussels
Jääskeläinen M.	The Finnish Society for Research in Sport and Physical Education, Annankatu 4 B, SF-00120 Helsinki 12
Jokl E.	University of Kentucky, Medical Center, 340 Kingsway, Lexington, KY 50502, USA
Juppi J.	The Finnish Society for Research in Sport and Physical Education, Annankatu 4 B, SF-00120 Helsinki 12
Karvonen M. S.	World Health Organization, CH-1211 Geneve 27
Kirsch A.	Federal Institute for Sport Science, Hertzstrasse 1, D-5000 Cologne
Komi P. V.	Department of Biology of Physical Activity, University of Jyväskylä, SF-40100 Jyväskylä 10
Koskela A.	Institute of Occupational Health, Laajaniityntie 1, SF-01620 Vantaa 62
Laitinen A.	Department of Sociology and Planning for Physical Culture, University of Jyväskylä, SF-40100 Jyväskylä 10
Landry F.	1235 Allard Ste-Foy, Quebec G1W 3G2, Canada
Mickwitz M.	Ministry of Ecudation, Rauhankatu 4, SF-00170 Helsinki 17
Milshtein O. A.	USSR Committee for Physical Culture and Sport, Skaternyi Pereulek 4, Moscow, USSR
Muthiah C. M.	Special Organising Committee IX Asian Games, Hall No 1, Pragati Maidan, Mathura Road, New Delhi 110 001, India
Niemelä O.	Finnish Central Sport Federation, Topeliuksenkatu 41 a, SF-00250 Helsinki 25
Oja P.	UKK-Instituutti, Kaupinpuistokatu 1, SF-33500 Tampere
Olsen M. A.	c/o Norges Idrettshøgskole, P. O. Box 40 Kringskå, Oslo 8, Norway
Riondet J.	Ministére de la Jeunesse, des Sports et des Loisirs, 118 Avenue de President Kennedy, F-75016 Paris
Ruiz R. A.	Inder Ciudad Deportiva, Havana, Cuba
Sevelius B.	Sveriges Riksidrottsförbund, Idrottens Hus, S-12387 Farsta
Stensaasen S.	Institute for Educational Research, University of Oslo, Blindern, Oslo 3, Norway
Svensson N.-E.	Riksbankens Jubileumsfond, P. O. Box 1649, S-111 86 Stockholm
Telama R.	Department of Physical Education, University of Jyväskylä, SF-40100 Jyväskylä 10
Tiainen J. (†)	Department of Physical Education, University of Jyväskylä, SF-40100 Jyväskylä 10
Tuomioja E.	City of Helsinki, Pohjoisesplanadi 11–13, SF-00100 Helsinki 10
Vartia R.	Ministry of Education, Aleksanterinkatu 15 B, SF-00100 Helsinki 10
Vuolle P.	Department of Sociology and Planning for Physical Culture, University of Jyväskylä, SF-40100 Jyväskylä 10
Walker G.	Council of Europe, F-67006 Strasbourg

Participants

(excluding contributors and chairmen)

Austria

Tollich H.
Brünnerstrasse 1, A-1210 Vienna

Valkievicz R.
Bacherplatz 14, A-1000 Vienna

Belgium

Remans A.
Galerie Ravenstein 4-27, B-1000 Brussels

van Lierde A.
Kolonienstraat 29, B-1000 Brussels

Wielki C.
Institut d'Education Physique, Place de Coubertin 1, B-1348 Louvain-La-Neuve

Bulgaria

Tochokova L.
Bulgarian Sports Council, Boul. Tolbuchin 18, 1000 Sofia

Canada

Finlay J.
365 Laurier Ave., W., Ottawa, Ontario K1A OX6

Lucas G.
University of Calgary, Calgary, Alta T2N 1N4

Lund R.
School of Physical and Health Education, Queen's University, Kingston, Ontario K7L 3N6

Sequin G.
3460 Linton app. 404, Montreal, P. Quebec H3S 1T2

Cuba

Hernández R. C.
Higher Institute of Physical Culture, Ave. Sta. Catalina Y Boyeros, Havana

Czechoslovakia

Macák I.
Mabr. arm. generale, L. Svobodu, Bratislava

Denmark

Kristensen P.
Parkbo 8, DK-2500 Valby, Copenhagen

Nordam A.
Dansk Idræts Forbund, Idrættens Hus, Brøndby Station 20, DK-2600 Glostrup

Egypt

Abdel K.
8 Ahmed Mohammed el Adham, San Stefano Alexandia, Hans 1

Abdel R. A.
Faculty of Physical Education, Cairo

Fadali M. M.
33 Haroun St. Doikki - 612A

Kandil I.
Golf, Cairo - Maadi

Federal Republic of Germany

Dohrmann R.
Eisenbacherweg 35, D-6392 Neu-Anspach 1

Grupe O.
Wilhelmstrasse 124, D-7400 Tübingen

Pfister G.
Hans-Böhm-Zeile 5, D-1000 Berlin 37

Willmans B.
Marienburgerstrasse 70, D-8000 München 81

Finland

Aalto A.
Topeliuksenkatu 41 a, SF-00250 Helsinki 25

Ahala M.
Löylykatu 10A12, SF-40700 Jyväskylä 70

Avellan L.
Gengatan 4D24, SF-00170 Helsinki 17

Bärlund T.
Workers Association for Physical Exercise, Siltasaarenkatu 3-5B, SF-00530 Helsinki 53

Bergholm T.
Finnish Student Sport Federation, Kalevankatu 26A7, SF-00100 Helsinki 10

Elo M.
Myllärintie 11, SF-28600 Pori

Eloranta O.
Sammonkatu 26, SF-45100 Kouvola 10

Eräkare P.
Topeliuksenkatu 41 A, SF-00250 Helsinki 25

Ervasti E.
Vaajakoskentie 1-5 C 32, SF-40320 Jyväskylä 32

Hakala E.
Pellonpääntie 3 B 11, SF-40820 Haapaniemi

Halme M.
Kulottajantie 4 E 71, SF-44100 Äänekoski

Häggman P.
Kuusikallionkatu 3 C 47, SF-02210 Espoo 21

Hänninin M.
EMT 10 N 805, SF-40740 Jyväskylä 74

Hautamäki E.
Vuokatin Urheiluopisto, SF-88615 Vuokatti

Heikkinen E.
SF 31500 Koski T. I.

Heikura M.
Keskiyöntie 19 A 4, SF-02210 Espoo 21

Heinonen K.
Hämeen läänin urheilulautakunta, PL 150,
SF-13101 Hämeenlinna 10

Haiska T.
Kynnystie 1 F 7, SF-40630 Jyväskylä 63

Hellman S.
Poroholmankatu 1, SF-26100 Rauma 10

Helminen H.
Sammakkolammentie 1 A 1,
SF-70200 Kuopio 20

Hentilä S.
Sunankalliontie 60, SF-02760 Espoo 76

Hietanan R.
Finnish Student Sport Federation,
Kalevankatu 26 A 7, SF-00100 Helsinki 10

Huhtamäki E.
University of Jyväskylä, SF-40100 Jyväskylä 10

Hurme H.
Workers' Association for Physical Exercise,
Siltasaarenkatu 4–6, SF-00530 Helsinki 53

Ilmarinen J.
Institute of Occupational Health,
Laajaniityntie 1, SF-01620 Vantaa 62

Järvinen A.
Workers' Sport Federation,
Haapaniemenkatu 14, SF-00530 Helsinki 53

Jääskeläinen L.
Kiiltokalliontie 13 B, SF-02180 Espoo 18

Juntto P.
Finnish Student Sport Federation,
Kalevankatu 26 A 7, SF-00100 Helsinki 10

Juvonen A.
Koivukyläntie 9 D 135, SF-01350 Vantaa 35

Kalaja S.
Löylykatu 10 A 12, SF-40700 Jyväskylä 70

Karjalainen P.
Hämeentie 152 E 114, SF-00560 Helsinik 56

Kattelus E.
Vellamonkatu 8 C 13, SF-40700 Jyväskylä 70

Kautto A.
Finnish Swimming Association,
Topeliuksenkatu 41 A, SF 00250 Helsinki 25

Kempas M.
Workers' Sport Federation, P. O. Box 315,
SF-00531 Helsinki 53

Kinnunun K.
Yliopistonkatu 10 A 15, SF-40100 Jyväskylä 10

Kivi L.
Matinlahdentie 2 E 24, SF-02230 Espoo 23

Kivimäki A.-M.
Humalistonkatu 1 A 19, SF-00250 Helsinki 25

Kolsi L.
Lukionahde 5 B 13, SF-02710 Espoo 71

Komsi T.
TNT 9 A 501, SF-40740 Jyväskylä 74

Kukkonen J.
Vaajakoskentie 1-5 C 32, SF-40300 Jyväskylä 30

Kuusela K.
Kerttulinkatu 14 B 23, SF-20500 Turku 50

Lähdesmäki M.
Urheiluopisto, SF-63170 Kuortane

Laiho I.
Workers' Sport Federation, P. O. Box 315,
SF-00531 Helsinki 53

Laine P.
Kiljanderinkatu 2 A 1, SF-40600 Jyväskylä 60

Launonen P.
Salmelaisenkatu 5, SF-70500 Kuopio 50

Lehtinen A.
Hannikaisenkatu 7, SF-40100 Jyväskylä 10

Lehtovirta E.
Tuulimyllyntie 8 B, SF-14200 Turenki

Leino E.
Workers' Sport Federation,
Haapaniemenkatu 4–6, SF-00530 Helsinki 53

Lindholm H.
Viitatie 16, SF-01640 Vantaa 64

Lindroos J.
Finnish Student Sport Federation,
Kalevankatu 26A7, SF-00100 Helsinki 10

Miettinen M.
Eduskuntatalo, SF-00102 Helsinki 10

Mikkelsson L.
Pitkäkatu 35A11, SF-40700 Jyväskylä 70

Mikkola K.
Topeliuksenkatu 41A, SF-00250 Helsinki 25

Mikkonen O.
Kärsämöntie 26, SF-45120 Kouvola 12

Moisio P.
Vaajakoskentie 1-5C32, SF-40300 Jyväskylä 30

Mononen H.
Ahdinkatu 15A10, SF-40100 Jyväskylä 10

Myllyaho I.
Taitoniekantie 9D805, SF-40740 Jyväskylä 74

Nieminen R.
Mekaniikanpolku 20B, SF-33720 Tampere 72

Nieminen R.
The Finnish Sport Museum, Stadion,
SF-00250 Helsinki 25

Ojakangas A.
Workers' Sport Federation,
Haapaniemenkatu 4-6A, SF-00530 Helsinki 53

Ollikainen P.
Workers' Sport Federation,
Haapaniemenkatu 4-6A, SF-00530 Helsinki 53

Oksanen M.
Finnish Central Sport Federation,
Topeliuksenkatu 41A, SF-00250 Helsinki 25

Oksanen T.
Kehäkatu 5, SF-44100 Äänekoski

Paakkari J.
TNT 9A501, SF-40740 Jyväskylä 74

Paakkinen P.
Mahlamäentie, SF-04310 Tuusula kk

Pääkkö T.
Workers' Sport Federation,
Paasivuorenkatu 4-6, SF-00530 Helsinki 53

Paavola S.
Haavikatu 8B17, SF-50170 Mikkeli 17

Palvalin K.
Porslahdentie 10D5, SF-00980 Helsinki 98

Pekkanen O.
Finnish Central Sport Federation,
Topeliuksenkatu 41A, SF-00250 Helsinki 25

Pekkanen P.
Finnish Central Sport Federation,
Topeliuksenkatu 41A, SF-00250 Helsinki 25

Perälä A.-M.
TNT 9E804, SF-40740 Jyväskylä 74

Piispanen A.
Kauppakatu 10A11, SF-40100 Jyväskylä 10

Portman H.
Fleminginkatu 15B33, SF-00500 Helsinki 50

Pullinen M.
Topeliuksenkatu 41A, SF-00250 Helsinki 25

Puronaho K.
TNT 9C11, SF-40740 Jyväskylä 74

Purontakanen J.
Finnish Central Sport Federation,
Topeliuksenkatu 41A, SF-00250 Helsinki 25

Putkonen M.
TNT 9E409, SF-40740 Jyväskylä 74

Railo R.
Workers' Sport Federation,
Paasivuorenkatu 4-6, SF-00530 Helsinki 53

Raivio M.
Runeberginkatu 56B2, SF-00260 Helsinki 26

Rantanen T.
Puomikatu 2, SF-33410 Tampere 41

Rasinperä K.
Finnish Olympic Committee,
Topeliuksenkatu 41A, SF-00250 Helsinki 25

Römpötti K.
Lähderanta 3A, SF-02720 Espoo 72

Ruokonen M.
Hannikaisenkatu 29A19,
SF-40100 Jyväskylä 10

Saarinen P.
Kasarmintie 4, SF-90100 Oulu 10

Saits-Kesti K.
Tammitie 5, SF-02270 Espoo 27

Salmenkylä M.
Kotipolku 1, SF-00600 Helsinki 60

Sandström H.
Finnish Student Sport Federation,
Kalevankatu 26A7, SF-00100 Helsinki 10

Santavuo T.
Finnish Student Sport Federation,
Kalevankatu 26A6, SF-00100 Helsinki 10

Sarkama R.
Lehmusti 1C, SF-00780 Helsinki 78

Savolainen J.
Finnish Student Sport Federation,
Kalevankatu 26A7, SF-00100 Helsinki 10

Selin A.
Rakuunantie 18A14, SF-00330 Helsinki 33

Seppälä K.
Pitkäkalliontie 5B19, SF-02170 Espoo 17

Sevon K.
Finnish Student Sport Federation,
Kalevankatu 26A7, SF-00100 Helsinki 10

Siltavuori S.
Finnish Student Sport Federation,
Kalevankatu 26 A 7, SF-00100 Helsinki 10

Sinkkilä J.
Ministry of Education, Aleksanterinkatu 15 B,
SF-00100 Helsinki 10

Sjöman O.
Workers' Sport Federation,
Paavisuorenkatu 4–6, SF-00530 Helsinki 53

Soininen V.
Takametsäntie 15 C, SF-00620 Helsinki 62

Suhonen L.
Voionmaankatu 15 B 47, SF-40700 Jyväskylä 70

Suikki S.
Cygnauksenkatu 5 A 20, SF-40100 Jyväskylä 10

Suomi K.
Haperontie 6-8 E 46, SF-40640 Jyväskylä 64

Suortti K.
Finnish Central Sport Federation,
Topeliuksenkatu 41 A, SF-00250 Helsinki 25

Syväsalmi H.
Finnish Student Sport Federation,
Kalevankatu 26 A 7, SF-00100 Helsinki 10

Tammilehto E.
Rasikatu 2 A 5, SF-40320 Jyväskylä 32

Terho A.-K.
Dosentintie 1 A 9, SF-00330 Helsinki 33

Trygge H.
Iirislahdentie 37 C 2, SF-02230 Espoo 23

Tuominen K.
Finnish Olympic Committee,
Topeliuksenkatu 41 A, SF-00250 Helsinki 25

Vehniäinen M.
Finnish Ski Track, Fabianinkatu 7,
SF-00130 Helsinki 13

Viitasalo J.
Jyväskylä University, SF-40100 Jyväskylä 10

Yli-Hemmo A.
Finnish Central Sport Federation,
Topeliuksenkatu 41 A, SF-00250 Helsinki 25

France

Moustrad B.
Avenue Calude-Vellefaux, F-75010 Paris

German Democratic Republic

Oehmigen G.
Friedrich-Ludwig-Jahn-Allee 59,
DDR-7010 Leipzig

Schfrik J.
Mohrenstrasse 6, DDR-1080 Berlin

Great Britain

Bisset C.
23 Bonlay Rise, Edinburgh, Scotland

Collins M.
35 Elvendon Rd., London N13 4SH

Needham J.
Crewe and Alsager College of Health
Education, Alsager, Cheshire

Roberts I.
Crewe and Alsager College of Health
Education, Alsager, Cheshire

Slater B.
University of Birmingham,
P. O. Box 366, Birmingham B15 2TT

Slater W.
55 Green Meadow Rd., Birmingham B29 4DD

Hungary

Cal T.
Rosenberg hp. u. l., Budapest

Italy

Ristori U.
Foro Italico, 00194 Roma

Standoli M.
Foro Italiaco, 00194 Roma

Japan

Meshizuka T.
1.22.9, Nishiki, Nerima-ku, Tokyo

Netherlands

Bertels H.
Burg van Karnebeeklaan 6–8,
NL-2508 GN Den Haag

de Heer W.
Burg van Karnebeeklaan 6–8,
NL-2508 GN Den Haag

Nigeria

Fabunmi T.
P. M. B. 12100, Lagos

Fagbemi O.
National Sport Comission, Lagos

Fatile A.
Ahmadu Bello University, Zaria

Norway

Halvari H.
4 b 1066 Kringsjå studentby, Oslo 8

Jacobsen T.
State Office for Youth and Sports,
P. O. Box 8172 Dep., Oslo 1

Mellegaard B.
Norges Idrettsforbund, Hauger Skolevein 1, N-1346 Gjettum

Nilsen M.
State Office for Youth and Sport, P.O. Box 8172 Dep., Oslo 1

Skaset H.
Norges Idrottshögskole, Songvein 220, Oslo 8

Skirstad B.
Sognsc. 220, Oslo 8

Thorsen R.
Muthesgt. 20, Oslo 2

Tronvik H.
Norges Idrottsforbund, Hauger Skolevein 1, N-1346 Gjettum

Wickstrand K.
Norges Idrottsforbund, Hauger Skolevein 1, N-1346 Gjettum

Poland

Tryhus W.
Wilcza 51 m. 12, Warsaw

Saudi Arabia

Bassiouni M.
King Saud University, College of Education, P.O. Box 2458, Riadh

Taha A.
King Saud University, P.O. Box 2458, Riadh

Sweden

Aggestedt B.
Idrottshögskolan, S-70230 Örebro

Eriksson S.
P.O. Box 3057, S-44802 Floda

Höglund P.
Göran Perssons Väg 19, S-17155 Solan

Jägnemys O.
Glomman 116, S-70230 Örebro

Leppänen E.-K.
Fridhemsgatan 61 C, S-85242 Sundsvall

Lyberg W.
Valhallavägen 112, 4, S-11441 Stockholm

Patriksson G.
Rävekärrsgatan 163, S-43133 Mölndal

Rörs I.
Skutskärsvägen 19, S-12243 Enskede

Switzerland

Burgener L.
Gesellschaft 81, CH-3012 Berne

Feuz H.
Université de Neuchatel, Avenue de ler Mars 26, CH-2000 Neuchatel

Schori B.
Bahnhofstrasse 83, CH-3613 Steffisburg

Spain

Inaki U. G.
Guadalupe Jauregizar Garcia, Lagua, Vitoria

Unites States of America

Goodman A.
60 Temple Street, New Haven, CT 06150, USA

Jacobson P.
Brigham Young University, 294 Richards Building, Provo, UT 84602, USA

Kasch F.
4882 Edgeware Rd., San Diego, CA 92116, USA

Knutten H.
Boston University, 1 University Road, Boston, MA 02215, USA

Lucas J.
The Pennsylvania State University, 101 White Building, University Park, Pennsylvania, USA

Union of Soviet Socialist Republics

Aslanjan S.
5/7 Zhdanova Str., Moscow 103031

Kazimina V.
USSR Committee for Physical Culture and Sport, Skatenyj Pereulek 4, Moscow

Morozova E.
USSR Committee for Physical Culture and Sport, Skaternyj Pereulek 4, Moscow

Yugoslavia

Stajkovic D.
Fédération Yugoslave de Culture Physique, Terazije 35/II, Beograd

Vujovic V.
Fédération Yugoslave de Culture Physique, Terazije 35/II, Beograd

I

Opening Ceremony

Opening of the Congress by the Minister of Education

K. Kivistö

On behalf of the Government of Finland, I have the great honour of welcoming the distinguished delegates of the Congress on Sport and International Understanding to Helsinki, capital of Finland, and to the Finlandia Hall, where the Conference on Security and Co-operation in Europe was concluded in 1975. That conference, which is of major importance to our country, to our continent and to the whole world, was held under entirely different international political circumstances than those which dominate the international relations of today. Seven years ago the High Representatives of 35 participating states agreed upon, among other things, the development of international sporting relations in the following way: "In order to expand existing links and co-operation in the field of sport the participating states will encourage contacts and exchanges of this kind, including sports meetings and competitions of all sorts, on the basis of the established international rules, regulations and practice."

In recent years, however, the development of relations between the participating states had not followed the spirit of the Final Act; rather the increasing international tension and the arms race threaten to undermine the results already achieved. In addition to this, the fundamental problems of the developing countries, which are becoming increasingly critical, and devastating wars threaten all healthy and human exchanges between people.

Therefore we have every reason to greet with joy the theme of this congress, as well as the broad basis of its organisers. The peoples of the world want neither war nor armaments but peace and peaceful exchange with each other. The programme of this congress is scientific and aimed at professionals in the field, but I believe that it will also become an expression of the will of peoples in favour of peace and co-operation and against all forms of discrimination, racialism and the use of force in international relations.

As early as 1959 the Government of Finland organised a conference where one theme was "sports and international understanding". One of the recommendations made by the conference reflected serious concern about the political tensions in the world and the destruction brought about by modern armament. The Conference called upon the sportsmen of the world to live heroically on the playing fields as ambassadors of the peoples they represent, to fight courageously the fight for peace and to propagate the true brotherhood of all mankind. This noble goal is today ever more timely for sportsmen who act as ambassadors of their people.

Sport and international understanding has also been a topic of other European sports conferences at which Finland has expressed her position. We are aware that today sport is a world-wide sociopolitical and cultural phenomenon which extends its influence to various spheres of life, including international relations. We are also aware that international sport has never taken place in a vacuum but that the existing socio-political reality has always been reflected in it. We can only state that the importance of sport and other cultural relations is given more emphasis in the international climate of today.

We believe that sport may become a very positive factor in international relations because of the fact that through sport masses of people are able to get in touch with the people and life of other countries. In a world of tensions and radical changes, sporting relations may become a stabilising factor in international relations, provided that they are consistent and pursued in a determined fashion.

Recent developments have shown that public opinion and the citizens' activity may have an impact on governments and international relations. The rise of the peace movement is convincing evidence of this, but the organisation and the carring through of such major sporting events as the Olympic games at the time of a tense international situation also supports the idea that international sport is a vital element in the peace movement between peoples.

We have to bear in mind that when the Constitution of UNESCO was written after the experiences of the Second World War, the aim was to build peace in the minds of men and to eradicate ignorance and prejudice. It was stated that "...the great and terrible war which has now ended was a war made possible by the denial of the democratic principles of dignity, equality and mutual respect of men, and by the propagation, in their place, through ignorance and prejudice of the doctrine of the inequality of men and races." These words sound very timely even today! As the number of independent countries has increased rapidly during recent decades, the problem of democracy in international sporting relations, as well as that of democratic responsibility and control, has become a central issue. Because of this, President Urho Kekkonen expressed in 1971 his strong support for UNESCO in its endeavours to develop international sporting relations. The Government of Finland has actively supported UNESCO in this field.

It is a great honour for the Finnish organisers, the Finnish Society for Research in Sport and Physical Education, th Finnish Central Sport Federation and the Workers' Sport Federation, to have the pleasure of organising this congress under the auspices and with the co-operation of the International Council of Sport and Physical Education (ICSPE), which has a consultative status with UNESCO. One of the principal aims of these organisations is the promotion of the physical, moral, social, civic and international education of youth. At the present, youth needs belief in the future and a strong will to struggle for a better life and for peace. We should do our utmost to shift sports on to an entirely new level in international relations and in the activities of youth. We should always bear in mind that the vast majority of the world's youth is still living in inhuman conditions and poverty. Brotherhood and development should concern the whole world, not just one part of it.

While we support the work of UNESCO with all governmental means, we also subscribe to the idea expressed in the preamble to the UNESCO Constitution which states that "... a peace based exclusively upon the political and economic arrangements of governments would not be a peace which could secure the unanimous, lasting and sincere support of the peoples of the world, and that the peace must therefore be founded, if it is not to fail, upon the intellectual and moral solidarity of mankind" Therefore it is of major importance to co-operate with independent international sports federations and national associations devoted to the ideals of sport. It has even been claimed that if the world governments would show the same seriousness in their co-operation in the United Nations as the representatives of sports federations and associations show in their organisations, the world would be on its way to a lasting peace.

Sports organisations as well as governments continuously face new tasks and a new reality. Although the theme of this congress is of such significance and concerns us all, scientific research into the problem has been relatively meagre. In the organising country we have investigated these problems, and with the support of Finnish organisations, the Tampere Peace Research Institute (TAPRI) has carried out a study which will be presented at this congress. The study indicates that in practically all countries the role of the state has increased in sports, especially in the form of financing. Therefore we have to discuss to a greater extent socio-political aspects of sports. We also have to recognise that international sporting relations are an essential element of international politics. It was the idea of the founder of the modern Olympic games, Baron Pierre de Coubertain, that co-operation in sports between peoples can promote world peace and improve the relations beetween states.

To conclude, I want to stress that it is extremely important to discover concrete means through which international sporting relations can extend their impact on international political relations in order to stabilise them. From this point of view, your congress is of vital importance and I wish you all success and a constructive spirit of co-operation.

Statement by the Official Representative from UNESCO

Z. Zachariev

Mr. Minister,
Mr. President of the International Council of Sport and Physical Education,
Mr. Chairman of the Organizing Committee,
Ladies and Gentlemen,

It is my privilege to represent the Director-General of UNESCO at this opening session of the congress on Sport and International Understanding and to speak on his behalf.

First of all, I should like to express the Director-General's thanks for your kind invitation and to express his deep regret that he could not be present in person at this ceremony, due to a prior engagement. Mr. Amadou Mahtar M'Bow has asked me to convey his very best wishes for the success of the conference, which will no doubt realise the aims designated by its organisers.

It is indeed an honour to be with you and to meet again these eminent personalities in the world of sport and physical education with whom we have established a strong tradition of co-operation and understanding for the benefit of UNESCO and the international community.

All research and efforts which are undertaken in the world to promote mutual respect and understanding between men, whether sportsmen or spectators, and between peoples and nations, are considered to be particularly important not only for our Organisation but also for today's society, where individuals are so close to each other and yet so quick to confront each other in a world in which man's capacity to annihilate himself surpasses all imagination.

The major themes of this congress are very similar to those which have been promoted by UNESCO in its efforts, since its creation, to strengthen the bonds between men and between Member States as well as their co-operation and understanding through education, science, culture and communication. In a climate of friendship, peace and mutual respect it is easier to assume the development of physical education and sport, which are recognised as fundamental rights for every human being and which contribute to the destiny of mankind. In the words of the Director-General, Mr. Amadou Mahtar M'Bow, in his speech to the Second Special Extraordinary Session of the United Nations General Assembly devoted to Disarmament in June 1982, "...this responsibility must transcend the frontiers of selfish interest and narrow calculations and scale the heights of human solidarity. The solidarity is possible because, despite all their differences, people share similar anxieties, confront similar dilemmas and cherish similar hopes, which are expressed in a thousand ways but which all converge in the moral foundation of our being".

UNESCO has participated in this congress with the greatest interest. Like the organisers, it wishes to see the identification of new strategies to overcome known obstacles and to strengthen the favourable aspects of international sporting competitions and events. Through discussion and the exchange of ideas and experience, the solutions to existing problems will be found more easily. Thus, international understanding and co-operation, in all their various forms which are so necessary for the continued promotion of physical education and sport for all, may be strengthened.

A great effort has yet to be made to overcome all obstacles. It is true that this effort must be made in several domains: educational, financial, material, technical and methodological. I shall not dwell upon these now. However, I can only repeat yet again that in the realisation of this effort and in the challenge to be met, UNESCO supports and will continue to support the contribution of the non-governmental organisations.

Over the past few years in a great number of countries there has been an ever-increasing awareness of the essential challenge now facing human societies and the international community itself: namely, the imperative choice between rupture and renewal, a renewal based on the regeneration of the deepest cultural, aesthetic and moral values.

Today, the peoples of the world seem closer than ever before and humanity has at its disposal immense possibilities for bringing them still closer together and for eliminating the numerous disparities, obstacles, risks and dangers. Certain global challenges such as the arms race, world hunger, which afflicts millions of people, the non-respect of human rights and the freedom of peoples now seem to be considered in terms of human survival. Since the different peoples of the world are united in a network of vital relations and even multidimensional and mutual dependency, the perspective open should be that of united world community permanently reconciled, where everyone would have the means to live better and in peace and where greater freedom and creativity could flourish. Because we have the intellectual and technical means, because the will to act in this way exists and because our survival is at stake, I am sure that our era will be able to formulate our mutual hopes in a language common to all mankind.

To conclude, I should like to express the conviction that the spirit of collaboration and faith in the future, which unite us today in this town, the name of which has become a symbol of co-operation and understanding, constitute the best wager for the success of your work and our common future. The complexity and difficulty of your noble task are such that I can only wish you the best of luck in surmounting the obstacles with the wisdom, lucidity and mutual understanding which are your customary qualities.

Statement by the President of ICSPE

Sir Roger Bannister

Mr. Minister,
Mr. Zachariev,
Ladies and Gentlemen,

I greatly welcome your invitation to me as president of ICSPE to be so closely associated with your World Congress. How appropriate it is to hold this congress in Finnland! Your country is respected around the world for top sportsmen, and as a former athlete myself I think of the runners from Paavo Nurmi to Lasse Viren, as well as for a love of participation in "sport for all" that is as high as anywhere in the world.

It has been rightly said that there are three great problems that the world (that is the developed and developing world) faces: (1) preservation of peace, (2) realisation of health and (3) integration of work and leisure. I believe this congress can make some progress on all these problems.

The international council, ICSPE, is the only world body which co-ordinates sports sciences and so this will be my theme in my remarks. There are several different approaches at a conference of this kind. For some there is the pursuit of knowledge for its own sake, as the exchange of ideas itself produces new ideas. Such a congress provides a fertile chance for the greatest human talent for co-operation. This is the right moment to remind ourselves that the fruits of scientific research belong not to one country but are truly international.

It is also the time to reflect that despite the appalling misunderstandings this century that have led to war and loss of life of millions, medical science has led to even more millions being saved from disease and starvation. In Finland we have a particular lesson to learn from the example of the population of North Karelia province, which has had one of the highest rates of heart attack in the world. Now as a result of positive health advice, of which sport is a part, that rate is falling. There is no doubt that sport is one of the most powerful forces for good in the world this century. A philosopher once said that the majority of people lead lives of quiet desperation. If this is true, sport provides an outlet for a craving for individual freedom in many lives that have become artificial and restricted. Sometimes the effort of sport brings discomfort or even pain, and strange, even mystical experiences have been described by those who attempt to extend their physical powers to the limit and beyond. Science and medicine cannot yet explain why the urge to struggle gives us satisfaction, perhaps the most real satisfaction we ever have in life. But I feel confident that in the next ten years we shall come much closer to understanding this paradox. As a neurologist it seems that the release of mysterious chemicals called endorphins in the brain plays a major part.

But it is a reflection that should shame the consciences of us all that two-thirds of the world's population suffers from malnutrition and has no chance to take part in sports under any circumstances. The General Assembly of ICSPE yesterday agreed to give a high priority to a working group of members from Latin America, Africa and India, and I hope that the needs of developing countries will be carefully considered at this congress too. Sport in developing countries needs the right facilities. But, just as important, sport needs the right ethical values, including "fair play". Without these it loses its moral and educational force, which is as important as its physical value.

At this congress I expect there will be many different attitudes towards sports science. Some look upon man as a machine, a thinking machine, on the path to absolute breaking point. Some look upon sports as an acceptable means of releasing man's aggressive instincts. Some look upon sports as a ritual drama, the interplay of good and bad, watched by millions on television and fulfilling a human need for pageantry and excitement.

However, we cannot speak only in glowing and optimistic terms of sport. Behind the progress in record breaking and participation there are some unhealthy aspects we cannot ignore; for example, drug abuse. Two-thirds of the heavy event athletes questioned anonymously at the Munich Olympics admitted using anabolic steroids in their training. Science brings not only aid to the athletes diet, training and injuries but dangerous knowledge too. So science must now, through international understanding, find ways to detect those athletes' and their coaches and doctors who cheat in this way, at the same time running risks of injuring the athletes physically. There are also reports that the physique of gymnasts has been medically distorted in order to keep the "elfin" shape needed for successful competition. It is a grotesque misuse of science when taking part in sport risks damaging the body and mind instead of making young people healthier and more capable than others of leading a normal life when their short top-level career is over. In this field of drug control the price of success will be high, testing centres and random testing needing international understanding and eternal vigilance.

At present there is too great a gap between sport on the one side and sports sciences and physical education on the other. This congress will serve to bridge that gap. In reality all the different people in sport live in a single world: the man, the woman, the child, the young, the old, the recreational football player, the dancer we have seen this morning, the highly skilled athlete, the humble teacher in the school or club, the famous national team coach. All are working towards the same end - releasing a sense of power and beauty that lies in the human body.

Each world sports congress adds to our knowledge, standing as it were on the shoulders of its predecessors to offer a broader perspective than the last. Sports science is no longer in its infancy but it has not yet become adult. It has vitality and enthusiasm but not yet the self-criticism of a mature science. Often it is still in the descriptive phase without the experiments needed to test validity.

We all owe a debt of gratitude to the Organising Committee of this Conference for the programme they have arranged and for the working conditions we enjoy here.

On behalf of ICSPE/CIEPS I welcome everyone; to you, Mr. Minister, and your colleagues my renewed thanks, and to Mr. Zachariev, the representative of the Director-General of UNESCO, my gratitude for giving us his time to be here.

Welcoming Address by the Chairman of the Organising Committee

J. Perttunen

Honourable Minister of Education,
Esteemed UNESCO and ICSPE Delegates,
Ladies and Gentlemen,

Concern over the preservation of peace in the world is, at present, more tangible than ever. For this reason it is necessary to encourage all measures that further the positive communication between the nations of the world.

The premise of sport in increasing mutual interaction between the nations of the world as well as widening their knowledge of each other could be based on the wide popularity of sport all over the world. With the aid of modern communications, sporting events are transmitted directly to the living-rooms of spectator sport's enthusiasts in every continent in the world. The basic ideology behind sport has alsways embraced the notion of promoting peace, and sport has even been regarded as the world's first peace movement.

The main purpose of this congress is to study the possibilities which sport can offer to promote international understanding. For the present, surprisingly little light has been shed on this aspect. Modern research can only provide partial answers to the main questions of the themes of our congress: "What is international co-operation in sport in the modern world?", "Who is taking part in it and how?", and "How did it get it's start?".

An even more problematic task is to determine whether the communication in sports promotes a spirit of togetherness and peace between people in a sufficiently concrete manner and to establish what the challenges to co-operation in sport will be in the future. In order to answer these questions it will be necessary to develop further research work in this area.

Equally important to gathering information is the ability to put this knowledge to good use, and for this reason the co-operation between research workers and the decision-makers, who have the power to implement their objectives, is of central significance. One of the purposes of this congress is to create the opportunities for this kind of co-operation. As the research work in this area is still in its early stages, it may be an advantage for those who are concerned with the more practical affairs in sport to air their views first and then to focus research workers' attention on the central problems.

Both research workers and representatives from various sports sectors have taken part in the planning and organisation of this congress. As far as Finland is concerned, the Finnish society for Research in Sport and Physical Education, the Finnish Central Sport Federation, the Workers' Sport Federation and the Ministry of Education have taken part in this work. I would like to extend my tanks to these organisations for the work they have done in preparing this congress.

At the same time I would like to thank ICSPE and all the other international organisations that have given their support. These are the Association Internationale des Ecoles Superieures d'Education Physique (AIESEP), the Federation Internationale d'Education Physique (FIEP), the International Association of Physical Education and Sports for Girls and Women, the International Council of Health, Physical Education and Recreation (ICHPER) and the International Society of Sports Psychology (ISSP).

All in all, 300 representatives from 27 different countries are represented at the congress and we will hear about 80 presentations. This clearly indicates the real interest that the themes of the congress have stirred amongst researchers, scientists and those working in the field. As the nature of this congress is research and inquiry, and not to issue public statements, it affords an excellent opportunity for far-ranging and varied exchanges of opinion on these themes.

I sincerely hope that the work carried out here is fruitful, promotes common understanding and provides new impulses.

On behalf of the Organising Committee, I would like to extend to all delegates a warm welcome to Finland.

II

The Role of International Sport in Advancing or Weakening International Co-existence and Understanding

1. The Role of Sport in International Cultural and Social Co-operation

Sport and International Understanding: Sport as a Carrier of Deep Culture and Structure

J. Galtung

„Wer immer strebend sich bemüht, den können wir erlösen" says Goethe in *Faust*. I start with this quotation since the paper itself takes a relatively definite stand against competitive sport, and particularly against competitive sport at the international level. So let it be said from the beginning: this is not an argumentation against individual achievement, or collective achievement for that matter, against people doing their best, trying to achieve what has not been achieved before. The problem is whether the method of achievement should be through competition or through the individual, and the group, working with and on itself – in the field of sports as well as in the arts.

Competitive Sport – an Expression of Western Culture

Why, then, this negative attitude towards competitive sport? Is it not merely an expression of the envy of the intellectual, himself certainly not good at competitive sport although personally enjoying various forms of bodily exercise such as cycling, swimming and hiking? Is it not simply an expression of distance from what happens, from the co-operation in competition, the delight at sharing rules, at fair play? And when this even happens across international borders does is not also cement friendships, and even constitute a bulwark against war? More particularly, would this not also apply not only to the participants themselves, but to the other two important categories in institutionalised sport: the organisers and the spectators? Will not fine threads of mutual respect be spun, a web of interrelations, so dense that it may have a protective effect against some of the dangers in our present world?

The position taken is that while there may be something to the kind of argumentation referred to above, there is another argument, in the opposite direction, that to my mind carries much more weight. The argument is this: Competitive sport in general and international competitive sport in particular carries a message through its very structure, and that message is more important than anything else. It is a clear expression of basic apsects of Western culture, precisely in being competitive, in rating nations, teams and individuals. Western deep structure and culture is a set of firmly entrenched patterns and beliefs, usually unconsciously held and rarely challenged, except from those outside that civilisation. Even though the striving for mastery has many good aspects, it also underlies a striving for world domination in political, economic, military and other fields. In team sport, individualism is overcome in favour of collective and often relatively horizontal (egalitarian) co-operation; but competitiveness comes in again in the competition between the teams. At the same time there is an isomorphism between the competitive sport system and the world system, carried by the notion of national teams.

This will now be spelt out in the following, using an analytical framework of six dimensions for analysing civilisations in general, and Western civilisations in particular (see Galtung 1980). The dimensions will be given below, and their implications in the field of sport, or rather translation to the field of sport, are entered upon.

Main Characteristics of Western Civilisation

1. *The Conception of Space.* The Western conception of space is highly centre-periphery oriented, with the West in the centre. The West, in its Christian, liberal and Marxist versions, and incidentally also in its Islamic conceptualisation (but then the word "Occident," somewhat broader than, "the West," should be used), sees itself as the origin of all that is valid. That which is outside is archaic, to be overcome. The causal force of the social universe is highly concentrated in the West and radiates outwards. So also with sport: the sports currently serving as a basis for competition are mainly Western sports, to a considerable degree with Greek and English origins. The social conditions for the emergence of sports must have been the existence of a leisure class, with time; and at the same time some structural/cultural element that makes high status in society combinable with bodily exercise, even outside the field of military prowess. In short, the radiation of patterns from the West to the rest of the world also holds in the field of sport, and no doubt this has been one factor in the tendency for the winners to come from the West. To take a somewhat contrived example: if sitting in the Buddha position, practically speaking without moving, in front of a wall, were a sport, then in all likelihood cultures with hundreds or even thousands of years of experience with meditation might have provided most of the winners. It does matter to what extent the peculiar and particular type of behaviour involved in a acompetitive sport is internal or external to the local structure and culture. The existence of blacks who gained gold medals in the Berlin Olympics of 1936 changes nothing of this: a black American is also a part of the West, only a suppressed part.

It may be objected that some of this is now changing: that a New International Football Order (NIFO) is even emerging. But this is not entirely true. First, the new football nations may not belong to the core of the West, but they certainly belong to the Occident - with South America as a major part of the Occident. Second, to the extent that this is the case, it is obviously a part of Western colonialism, with people in the former British colonies now competing quite well with their former mastern - even to the point of beating them. At the same time Western sports as an institution have penetrated and will also stand in the way of more indigenous pursuits.

2. *The Conception of Time.* The Western conception of time ist highly dramatic: there is a point of origin; there is progress, linear or even, if possible, exponential; there is crisis (in the Greek sense of movement, dramatic movement) and after that there is one of two things: catharsis, or fall. Western life is dramatic life. Sports are dramatic: everything hangs on the moment of competition. Heaven or hell, win or fail. To this may be objected that in sport there is always a second chance, there is the same competition repeated next year, or every 4 years - it is not as "unique" (einmalig) as is here

portrayed. But this applies to Western life in general: a series of small crises, capped by the big drama – will I make it or not? In the spiritual career of an individual in Christianity and Islam this becomes the overriding question of making it to paradise. In the occupational career of more secular systems this becomes the overriding question of making it to a top job in sight during one's own lifetime. And in these two major dramas there is certainly *Einmaligkeit.* And here there seems to be a carry-over to sports: there are many small competitions, repetitive or not, but in the life of a sportsman or sportswoman there also seems to be something called the competition, the big event for which one has prepared oneself. Then it is up or out, as in certain university systems which are also very competitive: the basic point is whether one gets tenure or not.

3. *The Conception of Knowledge.* Western knowledge is atomistic rather than holistic; it focuses on few but on the other hand very well-defined dimensions, many of them even quantitative in the stricter sense of measurement. So also in sport: human achievement, even top achievement, is operationalised exactly as in physics to dimensions of time, distance and weight and a couple of others; simple, quantitative and divisible into the most minute fractions so that ranking even of individuals and teams that are practically speaking equal in achievement becomes possible. If not unidimensional it is certainly not multidimensional. The dimensions are somatic, there is a cult of the body. The mental, the spiritual dimensions do not count except for tenacity and the ability to abide by the rules of the game. Aesthetics and ethics beyond that are out. Through competitive sport and its measurement people, men and women, are rated exactly the same way as machines. Actually, machines can also be made to compete, gradually reducing th human element, substituting computers. The logical conclusion of this is a full-scale war, e.g. in outer space. Boxing looks rather similar to this.

4. *The Conception of Relations to Nature.* Western relations to nature have been characterised by mastery and domination rather than by partnership. Nature is there to be controlled, to be used – with "abused" being just around the corner. The consequence of this is highly visible in the ecological crises of the world today: the decrease of maturity in ecosystems; depletion and pollution. In this field sport plays a minor role, but the inclination is in the same direction. Sporting events decreasingly take place in natural surroundings, and increasingly in special places made for the purpose, with an overwhelming amount of concrete rather than just pure, uncontaminated, unmanipulated nature. The sports palace and the stadium, Olympic or not, are anti-nature and have to be so because they are near-laboratory settings in which the unidimensionality of competitive sports can unfold itself under controlled conditions. Pure nature has too much variation in it, too much "noise." This may favour one or the other. Strict, intersubjective evaluation of the achievement becomes impossible with so many unmeasurable, unknown and even unknowable factors intervening. Although the human body is nature and nature also is the human body, the distance between sport and nature in itself seems to be ever increasing. Again, this is not a major factor in the destruction of nature going on today, but as a process it is located in the same general direction.

5. *The Conception of Interpersonal Relations.* Typically, the Western conception is vertical in terms of above and below, combined with being individualistic, seeing the

individual human being as the social atom, the ultimate unit, out of which social molecules are made. The combination of verticalism and individualism is found in competition. The ultimate form of competition is social Darwinism, survival of the fittest. But between competition in general and social Darwinism in particular there is a continuum described in terms of the number of constraints, or rules, that have to be respected in the competitive process. The more circumscribed a competition, the less free it is, the further removed from social Darwinism; the fewer rules, the more is the individual given a green light in exercising all that is in him and her to beat others. (I am talking about restraining rules, not rules encouraging ruthlessness, e.g. like those which there must have been among certain SS soldiers in concentration camps). Rules of fair play, of fair competition, are basic to the competitive sports institution; they are, in fact, what makes it an institution. But the same also applies to rules about arms races; arms control is to arms races what fair play is to sport. In both cases achievement, build-up unlimited, is encouraged. There is no such thing as a stop signal, as saying "this is enough, there is no reason why human beings should run faster than this, throw a spear even further, lift more weights." The rules define the process, and the process then goes on without limits.

6. *The Conception of GOD.* GOD is a three-letter-word; competitive sports are secular, the victories are in this world, the medals are even made of the sort of stuff that is highly perishable according to the Bible, e.g. gold. But the exercise is steered by another three-letter word, WIN. Gods are usually arranged in a hierarchy, and so are "wins." The ultimate WIN is the Olympic one; its priesthood, assuring that the approach is the correct one, is the International Olympic Committee. It is a stingy God, appearing only every 4 years as opposed to the more generous Christian God, which appears twice a year, in the mysteries of the birth of Christ and the Easter Passion. But a God it is, with a clear position in the total configuration: above and in the centre.

Competitive Sport as a Message of Western Social Cosmology

The basic point to be made is that these six dimensions, together with their interpretation in competitive sport, constitute a configuration. As such they carry a message, the message of Western social cosmology. Each competitive sporting event is a reinforcement of that message. It is an almost ideal-typical presentation of what the West is about. As such it is very hard to believe that it does not serve a major socio-psychological and psycho-political function: that of reinforcing and legitimising the West as an ongoing enterprise. Most important in this connection ist the legitimacy given to the idea of beating others; competition rather than co-operation. The softer side of human life, foregoing personal victory in order to help others - or simply being unconcerned with victory over others - is tantamount to non-participation. It is like economic competition: one generally does not slow down in order to give one's major competitor a better chance; one may do so for the smaller competitors, but then probably with alliance formation in mind. And the same is true of political and military competition, the latter usually referred to as war: the game may be played according to the laws of war - also in the class of rules of "fair play" - but within those constraints the game goes on with no holds barred. It is you or me. With teams that are national in their composition and compete against other national teams, the configuration even becomes isomorphic to economic, political and military competition between nations, states and nation-states.

Thus, one may say that competitive sport is liberalism in a very clear, almost undiluted form. Society is seen not even as a social system but as a social set of free-moving social atoms, individuals or social molecules, teams. They bounce against each other; that bouncing may be regulated and stimulated in certain directions, circumscribed and used to arrive at evaluations. This can be done at regular or irregular intervals, preferably the former. Participation in one such institution may serve as preparation for the other - hence the strong linkage between high-level competitive sport and business enterprise (golf, tennis) or military organisation (more demanding, less elegant sports without upper-class connotations). For a queer but funny expression of this type of mentality, see the *Guinness Book of Records,* the records almost all being held by Westerners. It is an institution crying for rules, "sans fair play le sportn'est plus le sport". For a less funny expression of the same basic principle, see the *Fortune List* of the top 500 transnational corporations of *Jane's Book of Fighting Ships,* not to mention the various yearbooks of military and strategic balances.

It is also a part of liberalism to make ranking multidimensional. The more complex the society, the more ranking ladders there are in vertical, individualist social systems. Multidimensional ranking systems do not reduce the total amount of climbing, rather they increase it because everybody is admonished to climb on many ladders, in fact on all of them. But they do introduce a new element into the competition: multidimensional ranking, the notion that a high rank on one dimension may compensate for a low rank on the other. Sport may be said to have that function: it is a ladder handed down to the lower classes form the leisure classes in which sports originated, with an invitation on it saying "here you may climb, and you may in fact come to the top - even if the major social ladders, those leading to economic and political elite positions, are blocked for you after a couple of rungs have been scaled." Whether the compensation is good as a psychological reward, or bad because it leads to rank disequilibrium with all kinds of problems, or bad because it mystifies society by giving people illusions about its penetrability, is a matter of political taste.

The same can be done for nations: international competitive sport is a corresponding ladder, handed down from the centre countries to the periphery, admonishing them to start climbing with the suggestion that perhaps they will make it. It is a ladder well utilised by centrally planned countries who use sporting elites to acquire a position in the sporting arenas of the world, possibly far above the positions attained in economic, political, military and cultural spheres. It is a way of arriving before arrival. But just as for the intra-societal aspect, it may be argued that rather than serving peace, understanding and co-operation this will mainly serve competition as a key institution, the idea of ascendancy over others. It will not foster co-operation except among the few organisers who have to agree on the rules and the settings within which this institution can unfold itself.

What Is the Alternative?

Any social institution can only be understood in terms of its negation. For comprehension it is not so important whether this negation exists empirically or only potentially, in our minds. The question should now be asked: what ist the alternative, what would be the type of sport (if that is a word we want to keep) that would deviate from the deep structure and culture of Western civilisation as here portrayed?

Space. To start with the dimension of space: a de-Westernisation of sport. This goes far beyond the periphery increasingly penetrating the ranks of the winners of sporting competitions. It is also a question of introducing non-Western sports and activities. The Japanese, for instance, have a number of those; why should not they, just as much as the Western ones, be in the limelight of international sporting attention? Decentralisation can also be achieved by regionalising sport, by having competition in regions with a lower level of Western participation - somewhat akin to south-south cooperation in economic affairs. This is already happening, and there will be more of it as economic, political and military regionalism gains more of a foothold in the present world structure. Structures in different institutional realms tend to be, even have to be to a large extent isomorphic with each other. Predictably this will make the West lose some of its interest in international sporting events. They will no longer be "as in the old days," they will be "unrealistic;" a little similar to the way in which the United Nations is seen when the West no longer dominates it (merely "propaganda").

Time. When it comes to time something might be gained by counteracting the notion of the sporting event. A step in that direction might be to abolish the Olympic Games. Arguments to that effect can be heard: they are often said to have outlived themselves. But there is also another approach, somewhat akin to the British way of abolishing aristocracy by bestowing knighthood on so many that nobility becomes almost meaningless: organising even more events, so many that nothing stands out any longer. A more Oriental/Buddhist and less Occcidental/Christian time perspective could be engendered if sporting events were organised in such a way that there really always was a "next time"; they go on and on. But to the extent that sports are so linked to precise and forceful mastery of the body, achievement is also correlated with youth. It is even institutionalised as a rank compensation for the young over the middle-aged and the old. Perhaps the latter two categories could become less marginalised if they received more encouragement ot compete in their own age classes, or with handicaps? Today this is being done in less competitive sports, in the mass events organised in so many countries - maybe this is something that could also be carried into more formalised competitive sports?

Knowledge. As to the dimension of knowledge, or actually epistemology: Perhaps unidimensional sports should be discouraged? In winter sports, skiing events, multidimensionality is institutionalised in various types of combinations, alpine and non-alpine; they may be all said to be snow-country versions of the Greek decathlon. In ski-jumping style plays a certain role: in skating it is an overriding dimension. Maybe the aesthetic dimension should also penetrate into other sports?

Nature. As to relations to nature: If sports are essentially well-guided exercises of the body, then lakes and oceans should be marvellous settings for swimming competitions of a much more imaginative nature than merely doing a certain straight distance in the shortest possible time. A much more imaginative form of sport is orienteering; running in the woods with a map and compass, finding or not finding the hidden treasures of the various posts. Sports organisations should be in the forefront of the ecological movements combatting the conquest of nature through overwhelming quantities of concrete to create laboratory conditions.

Co-operation and Fun Instead of Competition?

Crucial, however, is the aspect of competition itself. Whether on the individual, team or nation level, as long as so much emphasis is put on who is number one, number two or number three competitiveness will remain king. Sports journalism may accentuate this more than it is intended by the organisers and experienced by the participants and editors may in fact be the major culprits when they compose their headlines. Interviews with regular participants, how they experienced the whole thing, what was fun and what was not could be given much more attention. But it may also be argued that in doing what they do the sports jounalists have fully understood the nature of the game and the hunger with which their messages seem to be received bears some testimony to this.

Instead of focusing on who beats whom, one could also focus on how every individual, team or nation does relative to last time. Is there improvement? - regardless of how this is measured? The Buddhist idea, also known in Christianity, of improving oneself and not over and above others, and certainly not at the expense of others, could become a major part of the whole enterprise. Linked to this, then, would be co-operation: helping others perform, helping others improve themselves. Intra-personal and intra-team comparison rather than inter-personal and inter-team would be the order of the day. The debate is well-known from school pedagogy: should grading focus on how an individual does relative to others or relative to him/herself? The arguments are about the same: in a highly competitive social order it is how you do relative to others that counts, even more than how you do relative to yourself, because social organisation links many individuals together, not only one individual to itself, in splendid isolation like hermits. There is something to this but there is also something to the counter-argument: by introducing into society islands of restfulness from inter-personal competition one might make this into a social counterpoint and thereby direct the social order in a less competitive direction.

Tennis players co-operation in keeping the ball in the air rather than competing in making each other unable to hit it would be an exercise in co-operating - unless one pair of players starts competing with another pair of players as to who can keep the ball in the air for the longest period. The moment that happens we have actually merely witnessed a transformation from individual competitive sprots to team competitive sports.

Isomorphism between a world of nation-states and an arena of national teams can be broken down by a very simple method: by composing mixed teams. If there were sports on Mars or Venus, and they had been appropriately colonised by the Greeks and the British and their latter-day followers in defining what constitutes sports, such a mixed Earth team would become natural. The Earth Sports Committee would compose the team, and there would even be Soviet–US joint participation. But why not also try it before Mars and Venus are able to participate? One joint East–West team competing with another joint East–West team.... People would tend to disaggregate the results, would tend to focus on their own within those teams and try to imagine what it would have been had the teams been "pure." But that may also be merely a transitional phase. Later on the enjoyment of sports as such might gain the upper hand over national competition trying to pass innocently as a non-bloody substitute for more destructive pursuits (our thesis being that it may in fact reinforce the legitimacy of the world nation-state system and stimulate less than restrained competition among the nation-states). Within nation-states, e.g. in the field of football, this often happens even if it runs against local patriotism in some instances.

Finally, what would be the three-letter word that should be written on top of this entire exercise, this mix of co-operation and competition, individualism and collectivism, the purity of the team and the high-level entropy of the mixtures that could be envisaged, the improvement of oneself and the co-operation with others in helping them to improve themselves? Very simply: FUN. Is that not more important than winning? Look at the facial expressions of people who compete, look at the strain, the stress, not only the perspiration resulting from the strennuous exercise of the body but also the anxiety, the aggressiveness bordering on destructiveness: Is this really what we want? Think of the many nasty events associated with sport – doping, tricks of various types, violence and corruption – are these impurities in a system that only has to be purified, or are they actually constituent, natural components of the system? Could one not instead think in terms of some kind of festival of the body and of the mind, of people having fun doing strange things, running and jumping, throwing balls alone and together, sometimes measuring what they do to compare with oneself and with others, sometimes not? All over the world, in a random order, not pitting nation against nation on the assumption that the winners will mainly be from the centre of the world, thereby reconstituting again a detrimental and probably also moribund world order? In short, could we not through these events communicate a better image of what the world, international relations and inter-personal relations could be about than the image conveyed by deadly serious school competition known as individual sport, co-operate competition known as team sport and national competition known as international sport?

Conclusion

I actually think that competitive sport at the national level belongs to the 1648 Westphalian system of world order and that its decline and ultimate fall is overdue, like so many other aspects of that system. If it has led to mass non-serious sports, fine – I would like to see some evidence to be convinced that it was a sufficient condition; it was hardly ever a necessary condition. That it can serve to displace some national aggression may be true, but as with TV violence, the other hypotheses of reinforcement of aggressive inclinations seems more credible. And that leads me to the conclusion with which I started.

Reference

Galtung J (1980) Five cosmologies. Proceedings of the Norwegian Academy of Sciences, Oslo, pp 130–153

The Totalisation Process in International Sport

K. Heinilä

Introduction

One of the most fundamental premises in any scientific endeavour is that of problem-orientation. Without challenging conventional wisdom or conventional pratice, there is no need for studies or new knowledge nor any space for development.

No human activity can guarantee, per se, that its effects will be positive; they may also be problematic, and activities regarded as good may be accompanied by negative consequences and a potential for evil. In the light of national interests an actitivity may be positive but judged according to international interests it may appear negative. This applies equally well to sporting competition. Competition, too, has its border limits and exceeding these may cause problems or even serious disturbances and conflicts.

The Upgrading of the Level of Demands

The level of demands refers to the performance capacity of an athlete or team which guarantees the likelihood of success in competition. Statistics about the progress of records in different sporting disciplines clearly show this upgrading trend in the level of demands. In my opinion the upgrading of the level of demands is the most significant determinant in the development of top-level sport.

According to my chosen frame of reference (cf. Pfetsch et al. 1975), the determinants of the upgrading of the level of demands can, in their turn, be grouped, with a view to simplifying the matter, into three main categories: (1) the spiral of competition, (2) the increasing value placed on success ("overvaluation of success") and (3) the totalisation of competition (Fig. 1).

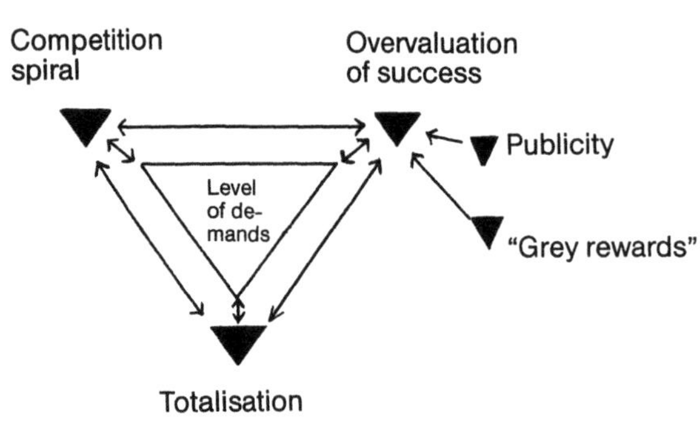

Fig. 1. The determinants of the level of demands

The Spiral of Competition

The basic idea of competition is simple: to establish who is the best or the order of superiority amongst the participants.

Thesis 1. Competition's inconclusiveness raises competition's level of demands.

The inconclusiveness of competition in sport creates a spiral phenomenon which raises the level of demands: the winner of today may very well be the loser of tomorrow and in order to avoid this fate the winner is continually forced to improve his performance capacity.

Thesis 2. In inconclusive competition the performance capacity of the winner dictates the target level of the other competitors, which in turn constitutes a threat to the winner, who then raises his performance capacity as well (= spiral of competition).

In inconclusive competition the performance capacity of the winner dictates the level of performance which the other competitors attain or preferably exceed if they want to be successful in the future. The winner, in his turn, must respond to this predicted threat of losing by raising his level of performance.

Thesis 3. The spiral of inconclusive competition raises the level of demands relatively more when the group of reference competing for success is large in number and even in its level of performance.

Observations indicate that the spiral of inconclusive competition is sharper the larger the number of participants in a certain discipline, the more even this group is in terms of performance and the bigger the group of reference is against whose level of performance the athlete/team compares his own level when setting his target.

The "Overevalution" of Success

Success in top-level sport today demands from the athletes increasing stakes and more total devotion to a sports career than ever before. Christopher Brasher (1968), gold medallist in Melbourne, thus talks about the "time professionals" by whom he means athletes who, contrary to the spirit of amateurism, "devote all their time and energy to their chosen sport". Whereas during the period of true amateur sport the practice of sport was adapted to normal life and, for instance, to the demands of studying, work and familiy life, nowadays it is increasingly common for normal life to be adapted to the demands made by the practice of sport, which is often regarded as a sacrifice for the sake of sport (Heinilä and Vuolle 1970). These experiences of sacrifice, in their turn, give rise to expectations, even demands, of compensation.

Thesis 4. The higher the level of demands, the stronger the incentives that are necessary and the greater the importance of the extrinsic means of placing value on success.

Although the practice of sport even at top-level possesses a good deal of sport's own intrinsic attraction, it is hardly sufficient in itself for anyone as an incentive for long-term, almost year-round training, let alone compensation for increasing "sacrifices". Thus the strongest incentives for the practice of top-level sport are nowadays external incentives for success.

Thesis 5. The more publicity and large-scale popularity top-level sport enjoys, the greater the overevaluation os success.

The factor which has perhaps most significantly influenced the value placed on success is today's mass media and its comprehensive and spectacular coverage of the most important national and above all international sporting events. The mass media make winners and record breakers into world celebrities and national heroes whose worship - hero worship - is so overwhelming that it overshadows achievements in, for example, the arts and sciences.

The widening of the publicity given to sporting events is in a reciprocal cause and effect relationship to the large-scale public interest in top-level sport. This large audience has become the most important interest group of top-level sport, as indicated by the way the needs of the public and mass media are given such great consideration in the organisation and services of large competitions. Whereas previously a competition was primarily intended for the athletes themselves, it is now increasingly aimed at the public.

In top-level sport the mass media and the public provide recognition whose power as an incentive is probably many times greater than the competition's official prizes. Top-level sport would not be what it is today, nor could its phenomena be understood or explained, without taking into consideration the public and the role of mass media serving its interests in the rewarding of success in competitions and the increasing value placed on it.

Thesis 6. The greater the financial benefit of success, the greater the value placed on it.

Public interest has brought commercialism with its associated businessmen and sponsors into top-level (see, e. g. Ewald 1981). Since the public's primary demand is success in competition, the producers of these moments of success - athletes/teams - naturally want to get their share of the increasing stream of money coming into sport. No rules or pool agreements can prevent this "grey" money from flowing into athletes' pockets. Even sports organisations increasingly use this financial incentive as a stimulus to succeed in competition, and employers and home towns (in some countries also the state) who share in the success reward the achievements of their heroes with certain material privileges.

"Grey money" and other financial benefits made available by success have likewise significantly increased the value placed on success. Whereas the immanent incentives of sport, publicity, fame and public worship, are likely to wear thin and lose their power to stimulate, financial incentives retain their value as a spur and even when "worn thin" - or perhaps exactly for that reason - stimulate the demand for more.

Thesis 7. The value placed on success works primarily to the benefit of winning and strengthens the overvaluation of winning.

The Totalisation of Top-Level Sport

The level of demands in top-level sport has risen tremendously since Paavo Nurmi ran Finland onto the world map. He created the myth of Finland's sporting reputation. This myth, I dare say, is still a burden to Finnish sports culture. Paavo Nurmi was phenomenal but largely only in the sense that he and other "Flying Finns" (Goodhart and Chataway 1968) who lived in difficult circumstances and were interested in sport took it seriously while other runners in other countries still took sport light-heartedly, in a game-like way. We in Finland did not learn to have fun in sport until the 1950s and 1960s, when our society reached its state of social welfare, and meanwhile elsewhere athletes had learned to take sport seriously as a result of the rising level of demands; thus Finland's "Golden Age" came to an end.

Thesis 8. "The Iron Law of Totalisation": As a consequence of continuous upgrading of demands in international sport, competition totalises into a competition between "systems".

In Paavo Nurmi's days top-level sport was simply a superiority contest between individuals and teams, i. e. success in a competition depended crucially on the athletes/teams themselves. The situation in top-level sport today is totally different. Although athletes still seemingly fight for superiority amongst themselves, success in top-level sport depends increasingly on the background forces in sport, the performance capacity of the system of which the athlete/team is a representative (see e. g. Neidhardt 1982). As a result of this international sport has become increasingly more total, a contest between systems of sport. This totalisation is the third determinant in the development of top-level sport in my frame of reference and at the same time it is a logical and rational response to the upgrading of the level of demands.

The totalisation of top-level sport implies that as a consequence of this upgrading the national systems responsible for representative sport try to mobilise and utilise all relevant national resources in order to guarantee success in international competitions. Table 1 depicts those processes and measures with the aid of which available resources are most commonly utilised in the leading sporting countries. It is obvious that this totalisation varies considerably with regard to the strength and comprehensiveness of the system in different countries (cf. Ojala and Pelttari 1980).

Thesis 9. Totalisation aims at covering all kinds of resources which affect the productive capacity of the system.

Since the system of sport has to take care of the utilisation of all relevant resources - in order to produce top-athletes - totalisation is not limited to one or two measures but tends to cover all relevant resources.

Thesis 10. The more total the utilisation of relevant resources, the greater the probability of international success.

The more total the manner in which this utilisation of relevant resources is arranged, the greater is the likelihood of success in international competition.

Table 1. Allocations of society's resources in sports culture and top-level sport in the leading sporting countries

Infrastructure	Sports culture	Top-level sport
1. *Human being*		
Size of population and well-being	Sporting population	Selection of talent
Stratification	Competitive athletes Hobby athletes Spectators	Top-class athletes Athletes in special training Migrant athletes Spectators
Education	Physical education in schools College and club courses	Special schools Training camps Guided training
National defence	Physical education in the defence forces	Sports companies
Social welfare and security	Sports clinics and medical centres	Sports clinics and Sports medical service Accident insurance Scholarship systems
2. *Know-how*		
Science	Sports sciences	Research promoting top-level sport
University education	Teacher training Training of sports doctors	Training of coaches Training of sports doctors
3. *Technology*		
Construction and equipment technology	Sports facilities Sports equipment Fitness technology	Special facilities Fitness technology Specialised equipment technology
4. *Administration*		
State administration Provincial administration Communal administration Private administration Business establishments Organisations Labour market unions	State Sports Council Provincial sports committees Communal sports committees Sports organisations	NOC Special federations Athletes' associations Special clubs "Stables"
5. *Finance*		
National income	State subsidy Communal subsidy Business income Income from membership fees Voluntary work	State support Gate money Pool agreements Advertising income Income from sponsors Support foundations Job arrangements

International statistics show that so-called socialist countries have recently achieved relatively greater success in major international competitions, which probably indicates that the totalisation of sport has also progressed furthest in these countries.

The totalisation of top-level sport is thus a logical and rational reaction to the rising level of demands in top-level sport but at the same time it is a new kind of reason for the continuation of this upgrading which, in its turn, nourishes the expansion of totalisation and more efficient utilisation of resources.

The Concomitant Developments and Consequences of Totalisation

The totalisation of top-level sport has many significant concomitant developments and consequences which on the one hand affect the nature of sport itself and on the other affect the system.

The Intervention of Society

Thesis 11. The totalisation of top-level sport and the upgrading of the level of demands increase state and other public sector intervention.

Totalisation has made the increasing intervention of society unavoidable, since only with the aid of state support and measures is it possible to utilise many relevant resources. These are, for example, pursuit of the sports sciences, scientific training of coaches and other specialists, special service for athletes in the army, training centres with large modern halls and state subsidies for training. Table 2 illustrates the distribution of private and public sector resources in Finland.

Table 2. Distribution of private and public sector resources in Finland

Resources	Private sector	Public sector (state and communes)
Special schools		++
Special service in the defence forces		++
Training of coaches	+	++
Training of sports doctors	+	++
Scientific research	+	++
Sports facilities	+	++
Sports clinics and centres	+	++
Social security	++	+
Finance	+	++
Administration	++	
Mass media	++	

\+ Minor role
++ Major role or total responsibility

With the upgrading of the level of demands, expectations of a more extensive and effective allocation of resources from the public sector seem to gain strength in the private sector of sport. The system thus increasingly relies on the state-supported conditions for activities, and an athlete taking advantage of these conditions is therefore more or less "a state amateur" regardless of the political order of a country.

Thesis 12. Totalisation and the increase in state intervention reinforce the politicisation of the system.

One result of the growing intervention of the state and other public sector bodies is the politicisation of top-level sport, in other words, the increasing legitimate participation of political parties in decision making affecting top-level sport. The autonomous system of top-level sport which preceded totalisation becomes, during the process of totalisation, increasingly bound to the will of political decision makers (see e.g. Governmental Responsibility for Sport 1978).

The Strengthening of National Interest

Thesis 13. Totalisation is likely to strengthen and enlarge the national interests in top-level sport.

Prior to totalisation, when the success of athletes/teams was primarily founded on their own terms, the national interests linked to top-level sport were mainly ideological in nature and based on a national feeling of solidarity and identification. As a consequence of totalisation and the increasing intervention of the public sector, the whole society is to an increasing extent involved in top-level sport and in international success or defeat. Thus totalisation reinforces both ideological and politico-economic national interests in sport.

Under the pressure of national interests in a situation of upgrading, the biggest cause of worry to the system is the guaranteeing of success. Only success satisfies national interests in totalising sport; Coubertin's idea of "participation and fair play" is no longer enough – if it ever was. And the price of success is going up. The late president of the International Olympic Committee, Avery Brundage, said at the 75th anniversary celebration of the Olympic movement in Helsinki in 1969: "An Olympic medal has to be won, it can't be bought." His argument is only true when taken literally, since as a result of the totalisation of top-level sport the price of a medal has multiplied even in the recent history of the Olympic Games and it will continue to increase and approach its absolute price limit. When this is exceeded it will be too high and demand will slacken!

The Position of the Athletes

Thesis 14. Totalisation increases the athlete's ties to the conditions and control of the system in top-level sport.

With the totalisation of sport the status of the athlete changes: whereas earlier he was free, a "private entrepreneur" practising sport on his own terms, nowadays the athlete is more or less bound to the conditions of the system and its regulation. The athlete is at the same time the object and the subject of the system's production machine. When the purpose of the system is realised in the achievements of the athlete it increasingly strives by means of different sanctions to control the athletes' behaviour and the adaptation of their lives to the demands of sport, in other words, to make sure that athletes make effective use of the services offered by the system.

Thesis 15. The binding of the athlete to the system causes conflicts of interests and leads to measures aimed at protecting individual interests.

When binding himself to the conditions and control of the system, the athlete's personal interests, e.g. professional, financial and family interests, easily come into conflict with the interests of the system (see, e.g. Neidhardt 1982). For these reasons the binding of the athlete to the system is gaining a contract-like nature and approaching the type of job contract common to the labour market. In the contracts between the system and the athlete the rights and duties of the athlete are defined for a certain contract period.

Competition on Unequal Terms

The whole point of competition is that it takes place on equal terms. In actual competition general and uniform rules, venues and equipment are responsible for the realisation of this principle. Competition loses its sense if a competitor exploits some special advantage and is successful for that reason (see, e.g. Szymiczek 1962).

Thesis 16. The unequal terms of the systems in totalising top-level sport increasingly regulate success.

As a result of totalisation the success of an athlete/team nowadays, however, depends increasingly on the performance capacity of the national system, on its effectiveness in utilising all relevant resources for the benefit of sport. The performance capacity of different national systems varies considerably in this respect.

It is significant that while we very carefuly try to ensure the realisation of the principle of equal terms in actual competition, at the same time in the systems we just as consistently try to gain advantages allowed by unequal terms in order to ensure success (see, e.g. Voigt 1975, 12).

The Ethos of Effectiveness

Thesis 17. The greater the pressure to succeed, the more prevalent the ethos of effectiveness in top-level sport becomes.

Upgrading, totalisation and the strengthening of national interests as a joint effect increases the pressure to succeed and is correspondingly likely to change the ethos of top-level sport, the spirit of the game. When "only one thing is important - victory", the humanistic norms of fair play are easily pushed aside by norms of effectiveness which permit and encourage, if not positively demand, the use of hardness, violence and tricks in order to achieve success (Heinilä 1974a, to be published; Lüschen 1976).

Thesis 18. The greater the pressure to succeed, the more likely the use of dubious means.

As a result of the growing pressure to succeed and the leniency of the moral of effectiveness, the use of various dubious means has spread in top-level sport, of which the misuse of pharmacological products with its associated health risks is the most alarming. This is also supported by Günther Lüschen's (1976) claim: "The rewards that are at stake in a contest will determine the amount and severity of cheating." Although comprehensive and expensive measures have been taken, they have remained, and perhaps will remain, insufficient or inadequate to eliminate misuse, let alone prevent it.

Thesis 19. The greater the national interests involved in success, the less strictly the systems control the use of dubious means.

The effectiveness of control is not so much dependent on international as on national measures and because of their national interests the systems seem to have neither sufficient desire nor sufficient practical means covering the athletes' training in particular to adopt effective measures. And if not all the national systems accept control, then some have to compete on worse terms - which is literally visible to the naked eye in the power disciplines for example! The misuse of pharmacological products in top-level sport is, however, only part of the more extensive use of dubious means, stemming from this pressure to succeed, in which by exploiting product development the intention is to ensure success through advantages in equipment. In many so-called equipment disciplines the rules surprisingly allow the utilisation of this kind of special advantage; in other disciplines this is forbidden or has been eliminated with the aid of strict standardisation. The special advantage provided by these dubious means is, particularly in an even competition with a high level of demands, a key factor in whether one achieves success or not. This is why it is strange that the use of dubious means is allowed, although it would be possible to prevent it with rules of standardisation.

The change-over from a humanistic ethos to an ethos of effectiveness in sport is a logical and rational consequence of upgrading, but in the form of dubious means it leads to conflict with the rules and/or with competition's vital principle of equal terms. Not only athletes are to blame for the use of dubious means; the other beneficiaries of success are also involved, including businesses which profit from product development and sports organisations that share the benefits with businesses via pool agreements.

Competition as a Test of Superiority

Competition is the way of measuring superiority. When applying the criteria of science to competition as a way of measuring we can lay down the requirements of validity and reliability. In this connection I will only concentrate on the validity problem in international competition (Callois 1961; Heinilä 1974b).

The validity requirement for competition can be reduced to these questions: what is competition supposed to measure and what does it in fact measure? If competition measures in reality what it is supposed to measure, it has perfect validity.

Thesis 20. Competition as a test of superiority is valid when competition takes place on equal terms, and invalid if superiority is determined by the special advantage gained by the use of dubious means.

True competition, if and when it takes place on equal terms, is a valid test of superiority. For then it measurues at least in the ordinal scale those sporting skills and abilities characteristic of each discipline and on the basis of these determines the order of superiority of the participants. Different disciplines can also contain a certain element of chance but that, too, has been accepted in the criteria of sporting superiority. If, on the other hand, superiority is determined by advantages in equipment, doping, blood-doping or the use of other dubious means, competition loses its sporting validity and easily becomes a measure, especially if the participants are even, of the fraudulent superiority achieved through equipment or tricks. In that case it is a competition between promoters of dubious means and product developers, rather than a competition between athletes. So much for the validity of true competition in the sports arena. But this is only part of the truth.

The validity of competition as a measure of superiority is shown in a totally different light when competition and the performance capacity of the athletes/teams it is measuring is considered as a function of the preceding training process, which is many times more extensive. While competition itself nowadays takes place in general on the participants'/teams' own terms - the significance of assistants in some disciplines such as ball games and skiing may often be considerable - the raising of the performance capacity during the training process takes place increasingly on the terms of the system. These terms are, as we have already seen, very unequal as a result of totalisation. As competition totalises into a competition between systems, it in fact increasingly measures the superiority of one system over another (see, e. g. Voigt 1975, pp 41–42).

The validity problem in international competition can now be expressed in one key question: What should international events or, for example, the Olympic Games, measure, or what are they supposed to measure? I will leave this question open. It is a matter of international sports policy and replying to it is the responsibility of international federations and the International Olympic Committee. The answer will decide the validity or invalidity of competition as a test of superiority - and possibly also the whole future of international sport.

Conclusion

As a professional in the field of sport and international understanding I believe in the potential of sport to promote international common good. The current trend, however, indicates rather an increase in conflicts and common bad. Co-operation between researchers and international organisations is badly needed for the promotion of common good in sport. A medical commission debating the narrow symptom complex of doping is by no means enough; the question of the problems and future of international sport is fundamentally a social one and in searching for the solution we need the expertise of sociologists, political scientists and other social scientists. A critical evaluation of the present state of top-level sport is also required, together with consideration of alternatives and scenarios for its future.

The academician and philosopher Oiva Ketonen recently said in reference to futurological research:

In my opinion we can know what the future can probably be and what it cannot be and the most important premise for gaining this knowledge is the analysis of the present, the identification of the factors presently affecting life.

This is what I have tried to do in my presentation.

References

Callois R (1961) Man, play and games. Free Press, Glencoe, Ill., pp 111–128
Ewald M (1981) Bulletin. National Olympic Committee of the DDR XXVII:12–14
Goodhart P, Chataway C (1968) War without weapons. W. H. Allen, London, p 10
Governmental Responsibility for Sport (1978) Resolutions. 2nd Conference of European Ministers, London, 4–7 Apr 1978
Heinilä K (1974a) Ethics of sport - junior football players as cross-national interpretes of the moral concepts of sport. Department of Sociology and Planning for Physical Culture. University of Jyväskylä 4
Heinilä K (1974b) Kilpailu paremmuustestinä (Competition as a test of superiority). In: Urheilu, ihminen, yhteiskunta (Sport-man-society). Gummerus, Jyväskylä, pp 28–31
Heinilä K (to be published) Ethics of sport; with reference to the regulation and humanization of competitive sport. Report presented in the World Scientific Congress, Tbilisi 10–16 July 1980
Heinilä K, Vuolle P (1970) Huippu-urheilijan karriääri (The career pattern of top athletes). Liikuntapedagogiikan laitos. Jyväskylän yliopisto 1, pp 17–21
Lüschen G (1976) Cheating in sport. In: Landers DM (ed) Social problems in athletics. University of Illinois Press, Urbana, pp 67–77
Neidhart F (1982) Soziale Bedingungen individuellen Handelns und einige Strukturprobleme im Hochleistungssport. Sportwissenschaft 12:9
Ojala T, Pelttari H (1980) Suomalaisen liikuntajärjestelmän julkinen ohjaus ja seuranta (The public regulation of Finnish sport system). Liikuntasuunnittelun laitos. Jyväskylän yliopisto. Opetusmoniste 8 (mimeograph. No 8)
Pfetsch FR, in cooperation with Beutel P, Stork H-M, Treutleim G (1975) Leistungssport und Gesellschaftssystem - Soziopolitische Faktoren im Leistungssport. Hofmann, Schorndorf
Szymiczek O (1962) Adhesion to the principles of the Olympic ideals. The International Olympic Academy. Second Session. Athens, p 115
Voigt D (1975) Soziologie in der DDR. Verlag Wissenschaft und Politik, Köln, pp 12, 41–42

On the Character and Contents of Sport and of International Sporting Activities at Present and in the Future

G. Erbach

The Maintenance of Peace

The main topic of the conference "Sport and International Understanding" is dedicated to an aim to which sport in the socialist German Democratic Republic feels deeply devoted. We regard this conference as a contribution to be highly appreciated, acting as it will in the interest of sporting relations in their functions of maintaining, strengthening and extending the progress achieved so far in the field of detente and of opposing the impending danger of a thermonuclear world war. There is a permanent challenge to sport throughout the world as its inherent political-moral and educational potential as well as its deeply humanistic basic aims, its function and its effectiveness directly depend on peaceful co-existence among peoples and nations.

This meeting in Helsinki reminds us that with the adoption of the Final Act of the Helsinki Conference on Security and Co-operation in Europe in 1975, an extraordinarily important step was taken towards maintaining peace on the European continent and all over the world. "Convinced by the necessity to undertake efforts in order to convert detente into a comprehensive process" (Final Act of the Helsinki Conference 1975), the highest representatives from 35 countries confirmed their pledge to peace, security and justice. In the following years many countries made efforts to bring the objectives of the conference into full effect. Consideration of the principles of peaceful co-existence brought many results in the co-operation of peoples and countries, and among these successes we can point out with good reason to the progress achieved in the field of international sporting relations and activities.

Peace is the basic precondition for the maintenance of human life and the solution of all the other economic, political, social and cultural problems of mankind - this means that the present increasing gravity of international relations caused by the policy of confrontation and enforced armament pursued by aggressive circles of certain imperialist countries is to be considered the biggest threat to the further international development of sport. With NATO calculating a nuclear first strike and the leading US representatives turning away from Salt II, and in view of the means of mass destruction already stock piled and being continuously produced and developed, the future of human life is being called in question. Mankind is inevitably faced with the question of whether to make use of all the opportunities available to maintain and consolide peace or to allow the risk of war to remain and even grow. "At present, there is no more substantial or more important question for any people than safeguarding peace, safeguarding the first and foremost right of every man - the right to live." (Breshnev 1981).

This most human of all rights cannot be maintained by a simple desire for peace, by a mere interest in peace, by an elementary feeling of attraction to the idea of peace;

as important as these may be, concrete action is needed. To be in accordance with the spirit of Helsinki, quoted so often when speaking of the responsibility for the maintenance of peace, today means to commit oneself to it and to work for it, to approach all controversial international questions by means of dialogue, understanding, negotiations and peaceful co-operation, to stop the arms race and to take concrete measures towards disarmament on the basis of equality and equal security. Such positions and steps as those included in the programme for peace of the Soviet Union and the other socialist countries will give fresh impulses to the future of international sporting activities in the spirit of maintaining and implementing the humanistic values of sport.

The Role of Sport in Social, Governmental and Human Interaction

Sport has become a partner of mankind in the twentieth century; even more - it has become an active co-operator in various social conditions and relations as well as in the individual life of millions of people. Like every progressive phenomenon, modern sport, having emerged from humble local, regional and national beginnings, has been able to spread across social, political, religious and other barriers throughout the world within a historically short time. Neither two dreadful world wars nor temporary social or political setbacks have been able to halt its rapid development for long. Today sport is reflected in the social consciousness as a phenomenon of almost universal character. This situation has been considerably influenced by the development of sport over the past 30 years. Crystallising more and more as an autonomous socio-cultural field and increasing its significance, influence and attractiveness on a national and internationl scale, sport at the same time has interlinked more and more with other social fields - politics, economics, science and culture.

Knowledge of these scientifically proven, objective facts also leads to growing recognition of sport's involvement in many important present and future problems of mankind. Directly and indirectly its rate and level of development are influenced with long-lasting effects by the political struggles of our time, by the global problems of our epoch, and above all by the problem of war and peace. The laws and motives inherent in its own genesis as well as the factors facilitating or impeding its development, which sport is objectively or subjectively confronted with as a result of its world-wide publicity and mass attraction, put it into the focus of many social questions.

Across continents governments, social organisations, voluntary associations and outstanding personalities of public life understand better and better the value and important function sport possesses or may possess in the modern world, which role it may and must play in social, governmental and human interrelations. Considering the growing socio-political function and the values and nature of physical culture and sport, we can state that a general consensus has developed internationally through science and practice. The essential aspects of this consensus are:

1. Active participation in sport and games has become an irreplaceable field of physical and psychic development and completion of the human being.
2. There is no doubting the contribution of sport to education and the formation of character, knowing well that sport and education cannot be understood separately from the different aims and intentions of the social orders concerned.

3. There is also general accord on the importance of sport for health and social and psychic well-being.
4. But the decisive fact of the accord, which also corresponds to the humanistic idea of sport, is, without any doubt, that sport is a factor of understanding, of co-operation, of the consolidation of relations at international level, that it above all may promote and maintain peace.

Especially these aspects make sport so important for the individual as well as for the society, so interesting and attractive – today and in the future still more so than in the past because we are now increasingly confronted in our daily lives with the various effects of the scientific-technical revolution.

Development in National and International Activities in the Area of Sport and Physical Culture

If we conduct a historical review for the characterisation of international sporting activities, so we can see that just as economy, technology and culture in the mutual interest and for the benefit of all strived for internationalisation, so modern sport is striving for co-operation. The foundation of the IOC and of other international bodies and associations, especially of International Sports Federations, has created ever better conditions for increasing international and intercontinental sports competitions and contacts, and for establishing all over the world an extensive and effective network of international sporting activities in various fields and at various levels.

If we study the great number of facts known about international sporting activities during recent decades, we can put forward the following thesis: The higher the level of development of sport in a certain country, especially its integration into the process of education and the degree of participation of the population in sport exercises, in training and in competition to top level, the more sport can exert a fertilising effect on international sport. Conversely, the more consolidated international sport is, the more effectively it can inspire and stimulate national sport, transmitting to it knowledge, experience and often practical help too.

Apart from the increasing organisation of international competitions, there has also been greater exchange of experiences in various fields of physical culture and sport and of sport science. It is quite intentional if we understand the term "international sporting activities" in such a broad sense that it comprises both the direct sporting competitions in individual and team sports as well as meetings of sports scientists or consultations of sports representatives at international level.

An analysis of the literature makes it clear that a presentation of all the aspects, levels, institutions and organisationl structures which may be understood under the term "international sporting activities" would go far beyond the time limit of my report. Therefore, I would like to concentrate on only two categories. In the first category I include all sporting competitions – meetings of athletes of various nationalities at international sports meetings, continental and world championships in a variety of sports, and especially the Olympic Games. To the second category belong all other international meetings directly concernig sport and its surrounding fields: co-operation as well as the exchange of knowledge and experience in various fields in the form of congresses, symposia, colloquia, seminars etc.

I would first like to draw attention to some basic problems which in my opinion are of priority in discussion of past and future development in the international system and field of relations of sport.

If we ignore the specifics of the individual international bodies, then the following thematical complexes determine to a high degree the aims and effectiveness of sport and its international activities:

- Training and education
- Health and physical fitness
- Social and personal communication
- Mutual respect and understanding

This conclusion is based on a critical analysis of scientific literature as well as of the topics and results of congresses held by international scientific, pedagogic and medical organisations of sport.

The above-mentioned themes are reflected at the Olympic Congresses and IOC sessions and in the activities of UNESCO, e.g. the Conference of Ministers of Sport with representatives from 101 countries in 1976, the international and regional seminars, the Charter of Physical Education and Sport (adopted in 1978 at the XXth Plenary Session), the Intergovernmental Committee for Physical Culture and Sport, created by UNESCO in 1979, and the European Sports Conferences (ESK), which have been held every two years since 1973. From the world congress of physical education in 1956 in Melbourne over the eight world congresses of ICSPE/CIEPS and the more than 100 international conferences, congresses, symposia, seminars and annual meetings of its committees, the 34 FIMS congresses, the more than 80 international FIEP events and the manifold activities of other international bodies – the dominance of these themes can be proven. Together with the regulations for the organisation of sporting competitions they essentially form the character of bilateral and multilateral agreements and exchange, and determine – in a concrete sense – the contents of meetings, conferences and discussions of different types at the international level.

Especially during the last two decades there has been a turn towards such fields of physical culture and sport as sport for the young generation and sport for leisure time and recreation (sport for all), and towards such problems as sport for older citizens and the handicapped.

As sport became an objective of the whole society, its potentials and possibilities became important for the whole society, i. e. for the personality in a concrete social environment and for the way of life of a nation in the corresponding social order. Thus the necessary social expenditure on sport has clearly increased, as have the conditions necessary for the rate and level of development of sport. This process has been accelerated by scientific-technical progress – science, medicine and technology having been used within and for sport as well as for spreading sport. This development has been internationally reflected by the proliferation of existing and the foundation of new institutions and bodies to tackle individual aspects of sport. A survey of the present situation underlines this; international bodies are working, for instance, in the following fields:

- Scientific research in sport
- The preparation and completion of sports programmes and curriculae
- Sports medicine and sport-medical care
- The training of coaches, physical education teachers and other sports personnel
- Sports information and documentation
- The design and construction of sports facilities and equipment
- The sporting press

International bodies such as the Fair-Play Committee have turned to the ethical problems of sport, dealing with developmental problems of sport under certain political, social, age and sex specific criteria. We must especially underline that in international sporting relations in the most recent past, developmental problems of sport have arisen more clearly in the states of Africa, Latin America and Asia, and correspondingly more attention has been paid to them. The representatives of these countries have become respected and esteemed partners in international sporting bodies, but this process needs to be still more comprehensive and at the same time requires concrete support.

We may state that there is at present no essential sphere in the field of physical culture and sport which does not facilitate in an overlapping or specific form the direct co-operation, consultation and mutual support between the representatives of sport of all continents. There are, however, surely some essential areas where there is room for further improvement. This concerns statutes and principles, projects and objectives, and the knowledge and effectiveness of some international sporting bodies. It also concerns (a) their work to achieve a democratic solution of new problems in the spirit of equality of rights and mutual respect as well as the full implementation of the principle of political and geographical balance, (b) their attitude towards social and political developmental tendencies, (c) their engagement for progress and détente and against discrimination of any kind, and, above all, (d) their clear and unmistakable dedication to and work for the maintenance and strengthening of peace.

I stress these aspects also because of the consensus for which we are striving here, and which is in my opinion an indispensable condition for the fruitful co-operation of international sporting bodies. An understanding of and increasing accord for the solution of these problems, in which the sporting bodies of the German Democratic Republic will also actively participate, creates better conditions for the main field of international sporting activities - the meeting of athletes in the sports stadia all over the world.

International Sport as an Element of Peace Policy

As a vital expression of internationalism, international sporting competition is a cultural achievement which can effectively contribute to acquaintance between countries, to mutual acceptance and respect, and to the overcoming of prejudices. It can also promote the moulding of a humanistic, moral consciousness and behaviour.

The number of international sporting events has reached a dimension which even statistically cannot be registered in its totality, even though its extension in some regions of the world has only just started. To give to these irrevocable international contacts an orientation and practical help will remain the main field of activity in international sport. As we know, this cannot be done if one ignores the processes of social development and the international relations in the other fields of life. It is a historical experience that the character, the scope and the quality of international sporting activities are substantially determined by the general political international relations between states, especially between social systems.

It is obvious that the better implementation of the policy of peaceful co-existence in the relation between states with different social systems during the first half of the seventies has affected international sporting relations extremely positively and was simultaneously effectively promoted by international sporting activities. This is expressed by, for example:

1. The substantial improvement in sporting relations on a multilateral and a bilateral basis. This improvement has been promoted by the UNESCO activities as well as by the European Sports Conferences, which every second year bring together governmental and non-governmental representatives to exchange their views.
2. Olympic Congresses have again become a firm part of the Olympic movement. We consider it no coincidence that this has occurred at the same time as détente.
3. The influence in international sport of nationally liberated states in Africa, Asia and Latin America has increased enormously. For instance, between 1970 and 1980 26 National Olympic Committees from such countries became recognised members of the Olympic movement.

To my mind these few examples make plain the manifold possibilities for further extension of international sporting relations as part of a policy of peace and social and cultural progress.

Looking at the example of my native country, the GDR, I intend to illustrate this progressive development with the help of only a few facts. In 1973 we received 632 delegations and 7428 athletes and sent 667 delegations and 7766 athletes abroad; the figures for 1981 were 847 delegations and 9800 athletes visiting our republic and 734 delegations and 11,302 GDR athletes being received in countries all over the world. Other proof of the positive tendency during the seventies includes (a) the doubling between 1973/4 and 1977/8 of the exchange of coaches, experts and other specialists in sport with the non-socialist countries which took part in the Conference on Security and Co-operation in Europe and (b) the fact that the GDR in 1975 signed agreements/ annual protocols with 12 national sports organisations and that this figure today has increased to 30 countries from four continents.

Sport Needs and Promotes Peace

Consequently it must be obvious to everybody that sport needs peace and a climate of détente. Apart from this requirement for the future development of sport and international sporting relations, sport is at present confronted with problems which threaten its humanistic content and even its existence, problems involving actions alien to the character of sport and aspirations for its abuse. This mainly refers to international top-class sports, but to some extent it is true of all sport. Thus the commercialisation and professionalisation of world sport are having serious results which at present can hardly be surveyed. The dangers involved include even the disregard of personality and unfair and conscious injury to the competitor, and there are opportunities for manipulation and corruption which can scarcely be controlled. As early as 1920 Pierre de Coubertin warned: "As regards corruption, one must consider not only the monetary enticement of the athlete or master-sportsman in thousands of inventive ways, but also the decline and soon the death of chivalry." (Coubertin 1920).

The actuality of this question claims our attention today: Will sport retain its character in respect of humanistic education and learning, of health and fitness, of the universality of personality, or will it become a "merchandise" that is marketed according to principles of profit?

Reflecting current social conflicts, sport is confronted with further challenges: People hostile to sport continually try to undermine the exclusion of racism and apartheid from sports. Each aspiration or attempt by reactionary forces to sanction anti-communist doctrine by means of sport must consequently be unmasked and categorically fought on an international basis. There are indications that world-wide aspirations for democratisation in international sports and realistic ideas for the further extension of international sporting activities are being insufficiently backed by all responsible people. Consequently all international sporting bodies have an increased responsibility to counteract all abuse of sport and all operations hostile to sport, and furthermore to give the future extension of sport purpose and direction by way of balanced and constructive measures.

During world, continental and regional championships and the Olympic Games, athletes from many countries and often from every continent are united. Only this proves the wish of peoples to live in an atmosphere of mutual respect, understanding and mutually beneficial co-operation. It is here that the most important mission of modern sport is expressed - its internationalism, which entails contributing to the peaceful co-existence of peoples. Sport is devoted to peace, it needs peace and promotes it. This was emphatically and unanimously expressed in the final document of the Fifth European Sports Conference in 1981 in Warsaw. The document says that "...the further consolidation of European and international co-operation in sports in the spirit of friendship, understanding und peace is the main task." (European Sports Conference, 1981).

More than ever before the value of international sporting relations is measured by their contribution to the main question of our time - peace or war - in the interest of life and a peaceful future for the peoples of the world.

References

Breshnev LI (1981) XXVIth Congress of the Communist Party of the USSR report of the Central Committee of CP and the future tasks of the party in home and foreign policy. Dietz, Berlin, p 8

Coubertin P (1920) Opening speech of the 18th IOC session, 1920, in Antwerp. Special edition of IOC-Publ., without year, ("Discourse de Monsieur Baron de Coubertin, tenu à l'hôtel de ville à Anverp 17.08.1920")

European Sports Conference (1981) Final Document of the Fifth European Sports Conference, Warsaw.

Final Act of the Helsinki Conference (1975) Final document of conference on security and co-operation in Europe. Neues Deutschland, Berlin, p 5

The Role of International Sporting Ties in Strengthening Peace and Understanding Between Nations

V. Stolyarov and L. Sanadze

The World Situation: Thunderclouds on the Horizon

The main topic of discussion in this session of the congress is: "Do international sporting ties promote the strengthening of peace and understanding between nations?" Why is the question brought up in this form? First of all, of course, we believe that it is because of the present situation in the world. Lately, owing to the activity of the imperialist circles headed by Reagan's administration, the international situation has sharpened greatly. As many political and public personalities believe, the 1980s may be of principal significance for the result of the world-historical battle to prevent nuclear conflict. The situation is very difficult, intense and heated. Of course, there are no reasons to affirm that the world is now in a prewar period. But thunderclouds on our horizon are bringing a potentially growing danger for the future of all mankind.

International Sporting Ties

A further reason for the posing of the aforementioned question concerns the further development of international sporting ties in the modern world. During the last 20 years the many-sided and fruitful system of varied international contacts was formed, incorporating most countries of the world. Now, for example, the USSR maintains sporting contacts with more than 90 countries (in 54 kinds of sport), the GDR with 80, and so on (see Pavlov 1977; Prokhorov 1978). These international sporting ties are becoming broader because of (a) an increase in the social significance of sport in the world and (connected with this) in the interest in sport, (b) sporting ties on the part of national and international organisations, and (c) the participation of young independent states in international sporting ties.

Sporting contacts have become more multifaceted, regularly becoming traditional bilateral short-term or long-term agreements on co-operation between various countries. Thus at present the Soviet Union maintains contacts with 26 countries on the basis of long-term agreements.

During recent years an increasing number of new sporting competitions have been established on a regular basis. For example, no week goes past in Europe without an international sports meeting being held. A large number of tournaments, cups, children's and junior competitions, memorial tournaments, cycle races and matches in a variety of sports are held, not counting championships in nearly 50 events.

However, this burgeoning of international sporting contacts has not been confined to the usual tournaments and matches; rather sporting ties have become more varied.

They are components of cultural and scientific ties between nations, and in this respect one can mention such forms of sporting contact as sports film festivals, the organisation of exhibitions, scientific symposia on problems in sport and participation of the representatives of sports organisations in interstate exchanges of experience in environmental protection etc. (see Prokhorov 1978). In the Soviet Union, sporting ties occupy an important place in the structure of cultural contacts with other countries. Nowadays the USSR has cultural ties with more than 120 countries around the world, and the cultural exchange of our country with foreign states constitutes one-third of all the cultural exchange of our country.

Broad and varied international sporting ties with the various countries of the world are thus the reality of our time. Analysis of the dynamics of their development shows that they have a tendency to broaden and diversify and to assume a greater role in the general system of international contacts. As was mentioned above, this is the second reason for putting the question to the congress: "Do international sporting ties promote strengthening of peace and understanding between nations?"

The Problem of the Humanistic Significance of International Sporting Contacts

There is at least one more reason for the above question which deserves special attention; this concerns the evaluation of the humanistic significance of international sporting contacts in strengthening peace and international understanding.

On the one hand it is not difficult to cite many examples of how the contacts between various nations and countries came into being and became broader and stronger as the result of sporting ties, even when the countries concerned had had very tense relations before this. A striking example is the history of the relations of the D.D.R. with a number of countries, the F.R.G. included, and the positive role of sporting contacts in these international relations. The history of the formation of international relations by the People's Republic of Cuba with capitalist states contains analogies with this example. Based on these facts, a positive answer can be made to the question under discussion. However, other instances are known when sporting contacts have strained the relations between nations, leading to international conflicts. The most striking example of this is the famous "football war" between Honduras and El Salvador, so named because it broke out after two qualifying matches in the World Football Championship between the teams of these countries. Facing these facts and the acts of violence, hooliganism and vandalism connected with sport, some journalists, public men and even scientists from the West began to speak about the negative influence of sport and international sporting contacts on understanding and interrelations between peoples and nations, about the inevitability of aggressiveness in connection with sport, about "estrangement" of men in sport, and hence about antihuman content in sport and sporting contacts (see Rösch 1972; Gerth and Wright Mills 1954; Lorenz 1966).

The Real Effects of International Sporting Contacts

In these conditions it is right and necessary to pose and discuss the question: "What is the real meaning of international sporting contacts – do they promote the strengthening of peace and understanding between nations or prevent it?"

It should be noted that this question is a component part of a broad question about the humanistic value of sport, about its role and significance for individuals and mankind. The question has been discussed repeatedly of late, many reports and speeches being dedicated to it, along with various international symposia, conferences and congresses, including the congresses in Munich (1972) and Quebec (1976), and the World Scientific Congresses "Sport in Modern Society" (Moscow 1974 and Tbilisi 1980) (see Abstracts 1976; Grupe et al. 1972a,b; World Scientific Congress 1978, 1980). The subject is also touched on in many publications (see e.g. Saraf 1975; Vidyin 1980; Jen 1972; Lüschen and Sage 1981; Kulturowe wartosci sportu 1981; Krawczyk 1976, 1978, 1981; Lüschen and Weis 1976; Loy et al. 1978; Wohl 1981; Zeigler 1977).

Analysis of the opinions expressed shows that often certain facts concerning the role and significance of sport in social life, including international relations, are quoted at random and overstressed, giving only one side of the argument. In some cases the facts cited concern the positive influence of sport and sporting contacts on the personality, on the strengthening of friendship among nations etc., while in other cases the violence, aggressiveness and international conflicts connected with sport and sporting contacts are overemphasised. By contrast, the report of the President of the International Sport Sociology Committee, G. Lüschen, at the IInd World Scientific Congress "Sport in Modern Society" (World Scientific Congress 1980) called upon us to adopt a rather cautious position on this question, because in his opinion sport and international sporting contacts may play both a positive and a negative role in the causation and settlement of conflicts between various countries, nations, social groups etc. There was, however, no clear explanation of what this role depends on. There is a danger in this approach of either an eclectic understanding of the humanistic role of sport and international sporting ties or of avoiding a clear-cut and accurate answer to the question. In fact, it is important not only to state that sporting contacts may have a contradictory influence on international relations, but to elucidate why they have a particular influence and, on this basis, to answer the question of whether it is possible to preclude any negative consequences.

The Methodological Approach

From the point of view of methodological principles, there are in our opinion two exactly contrary approaches to the solution of this problem. The first (sometimes clearly formulated, but more often vaguely assumed) originated from the recognition of some abstract, invariable essence, an eternal "nature" of sport, the claim being that the functions, role and significance of sport and sporting contacts in society are predetermined by this eternal nature. Such assertions, as was shown in some of our publications (see, e.g., Stolyarov 1977a,b) are groundless. The opposite approach is the only right one, we feel. It is based on the Marxist methodology of study of social phenomenon, including sport. According to this methodology, in discussing any social phenomenon one must not *abstractly* (proceeding from the concept of an eternal "nature") consider its humanistic value or antihuman direction. This should not be done because the content, character, direction and value of a social phenomenon greatly depend on concrete historical conditions, on the structure of society as the framework in which it functions and develops, and on the conscious activity of the people who use it for definite aims.

This position of Marxist sociology found its full confirmation in the analysis of such social phenomena as science and technology, the humanistic value of which has been and is still being questioned. It is similarly correct in respect of sport and sporting contacts.

The Contradictory Potential of Sport

If we consider them by themselves (from the point of view of their "nature"), then there are possibilities in sport and sporting contacts not only for various, but even for directly contrary influences on people and their interrelations. In fact, on the one hand there is the idea that participation in an honest, just fight and respect of rivals for each other (irrespective of race, colour of skin, religion, ideological views and so on) is the basis of sport. Sporting contacts are supposed to consist of direct contact between sportsmen, experts in the field of sport, fans etc., in the course of which they can get to know each other better and become acquainted with other customs and cultural traditions. But on the other hand, the rivalry of people is at the basis of sport, and this reaches its uppermost limit in so-called top-level sport. This rivalry ends with the victory of one and the defeat of others. And who likes to fail? All the more so, when such values as glory and prestige and material considerations are connected with victory in modern sport. There is consequently some potential for conflict between victors and vanquished. The process of competition may promote it, especially in such events as boxing, ice-hockey, football and rugby, where there is direct contact between sportsmen. Victory cannot be gained without a feeling of "sports anger" natural for a sportman. It is supposed that he is angry with his rival not because of any personal antipathy but because of his eagerness to win. But this anger can develop into hostility to the personality of his rival (see Podolskyi and Starshinov 1975). In modern sport, victors and vanquished as a rule have their own "fans", and victory or failure touches the prestige not only of one person but of definite groups of people, and often of the whole country. Large groups of people can thus be drawn into conflict.

From the above it can be seen that sport and sporting contacts, if theory are not considered in isolation, involve contradictory possibilities. It is no mere chance the founder of the modern Olympic movement, P. de Coubertin, warned: "Athletics can arouse both the most noble and the most mean passions, it can be... human or savage. It can be used both in the aims of strengthening of peace and in the preparation of war" (Vidyin 1980). Which of these possibilities of sport and sporting contacts will be realised? And what does it depend on?

The Influence of Conditions on the Significance of Sport

All possibilities, including those under consideration here, are known to be realised under *certain conditions.* It is thus precisely the concrete conditions of the sporting contacts that determine the character of the latter's influence on people and the interrelations between them. Negative effects are likely when there is no just, objective judging; when sportsmen have the possibility to insult each other with impunity; when there is discrimination between sportsmen (on the basis of race, nationality or some other factor); and when the press, radio and TV use all possible means to arouse interest in a sports meeting, stirring towards the rival etc.

Much depends on what aims are set and achieved during sporting competitions and contacts. Aiming merely at a good sporting result, at gaining victory over the rival by any means, at the subordination of sport to commercial interests in oder to achieve profit maximisation (cf. professional commercial sport in capitalism), at the use of sport for mercenary political motives (e. g. the boycott of the Olympic Games in Moscow by Carter's administration) - all this, naturally, leads to the humanistic direction of sport and sporting contacts being obscured and retarded.

The Social Responsibility of Those Involved in Sport

It is not difficult to observe that the above-mentioned factors above all depend on the social-economic system of society and the system of ideological views and the values built on it. However, this does not answer the question about the *social responsibility,* in terms of propagating humanistic values, of all those who are involved in sport and sporting contacts. This depends on the honesty, uprightness and decency of the organisers and hosts of sporting competitions, coaches, doctors, representatives of the mass media, scientific workers in the field of sport and leaders of national and international sports organisations. How they handle their social responsibility for the humanistic values and direction of sport and sporting contacts will influence the effect of these contacts on peace, friendship and understanding between nations. This side of the question was, of course, stressed especially at the IIIrd European Meeting of Ministers on Sport held in Copenhagen in 1977.

The Results of International Sporting Contacts

If we look from this point of view at the history of international sporting contacts and their modern state, then it can be said with confidence that much is done in organising and broadening sporting exchanges firstly to avoid giving sprout in the souls of sportsmen, spectators etc. to the poisonous seeds of racism, ambition, envy and cruelty and secondly to make a maximum effort to bring up young men in the spirit of understanding and friendship between the peoples of various countries, promoting in this way the preservation and strengthening of peace in the world.

A positive trend in this respect is the special dedication, over the past few years, of manly popular international competitions to the strengthening of peace and friendship between nations. For example, the Peace Cycling Races over the territory of the G.D.R., Czechoslovakia and Poland became traditional. The races gathered more and participants from various European countries and aroused great interest in many thousand of cycling fans all the way from Berlin to Warsaw. The international yachting competitions called the "Druzhba", the "Druzhba" Cup in figure skating and other competitions have become more popular. And quite unique among these similar competitions is the Cup of International Friendship for sailors of the ships of the Pacific and the Indian Oceans. The motto of the Cup is "Oceans and seas unite the people".

Various sporting competitions are included in the programme of international meetings held with the aim of strengthening co-operation and friendship between nations, e. g. at the World Youth and Students' Festivals and the Festival of people from the Arctic regions of Norway, Sweden, Finland and the USSR.

Sports organisations in many countries have responded to the calls of the World Peace Council concerning the conduct of a broad campaign of peace-loving forces for unisversal disarmament and detente by devoting many competitions to this aim. The World Peace Council valued highly the active participation of sportsmen in the movement of peace supporters and awarded many of them diplomas.

Lately we have noticed an important phenomenon, namely sportsmen uniting in a struggle for peace in a number of countries. An example is the movement "Sportsmen Against Nuclear Missiles", which is widely supported in the F.R.G.

The sports organisations of the USSR and other socialist countries believe international sporting ties must serve the cause of bringing up youth in the spirit of understanding and friendship. That is why they have always paid serious attention to this side of sport. Competitions of young sportsmen under the motto *Druzhba* (friendship) are held regularly in the socialist countries. It is traditional in the Soviet Union that our youth organisations devote much attention to foreign sportsmen, e. g. improving their knowledge of the life of Soviet youth and organising cultural programmes for them.

Our people are proud not only of the sporting achievements of our athletes but also of their high moral qualities at the Olympiad: honesty and courage in competition, sincerity, kind feelings for the sportsmen from other countries. It is no mere chance that as the result of a mass questionnaire held by West German TV during the XXth Olympiad in Munich, our young men and women were recognised as being the most sociable and of great erudition among the Olympic family of sportsmen.

The Role of the Olympic Movement

As for the Olympic Games and the Olympic movement in general, they play a special role in strengthening peace, friendship and understanding between nations. Analysis of the history of the Olympic movement shows that the Olympic games have always been directed towards the realisation of humanistic ideals. The founder of the modern Olympic movement, P. de Coubertin, in searching for the rationale of the Olympic movement launched by him in 1912, introduced the term "the Olympics" and explained it by the following: "The Olympics unites as in one brush stroke of sunny rays all those principles which promote the perfection of a man". Following the example of the ancient Greeks, he saw the ideal of human personality in a harmonic unity of high spirituality and perfect physical culture of the body. The sense of the Olympic movement for him was the realisation of this ideal on the basis of sport and sporting competitions. At the same time he considered the Olympics to be a "movement rising with the age-old striving of a man for peace and fraternity„.

Nowadays this direction of the Olympic movement still prevails. It is written in the working Olympic Charter that the aims of the Olympic movement are "assistance to the development of physical and moral qualities, which are the base of sport; the upbringing of youth with the aid of sport in the spirit of understanding and friendship, which will promote the creation of a better and more tranquil world; the spreading throughout the whole world of the Olympic principles for the creation of goodwill amongst nations". However, the modern Olympic movement, in contrast to the movement in the past (for example, in Coubertin's day), has a broader social basis for realising its aim. First of all, it is not only a movement of persons or small groups. At present, it is one of the greatest mass social movements. Second, it not only propagates pacifist principles and makes declarative calls for humanity and peace; rather it is supported by the organised global antiwar movement, based on the real strength of socialist countries, the politics of which is directed towards the elimination of wars from humanity.

The successful organisation of the XXIIth Olympic Games in Moscow (1980) despite the attempt of reaction to organise a boycott demonstrated the strength and fighting ability of the modern Olympic movement. As was noted at the Olympic Congress at Baden-Baden, the holding of the Olympic Games in Moscow represented a victory of the Olympic movement over the forces of reaction, which aimed not only at destroying our Olympic family but in essence at depriving mankind of the Olympic Games.

Although, as was noted, much has been done and is being done to use international sporting ties to strengthen peace, understanding and friendly co-operation, new possibilities and means of achieving these ends must still be sought.

The Relisation of Humanistic Values in Sport: Proposals for the Future

The Chairman of the USSR Sports Committee, S. Pavlov, has repeatedly proposed broadening international sporting ties beyond the level of the "sporting elite". This would greatly promote the active participation of previously "non-active" people in sporting competitions and would combat excessive ambition and other attitudes contrary to the spirit of understanding and friendship.

The Soviet Union and other socialist countries have, with success, combated in sporting competition any manifestation of racism, national discrimination, the penetration of commerce and the use of anabolic steroids because all of these are extremely negative for the realisation of humanistic values by means of sport. On anabolic steroids one cannot help but agree with the opinion of the NOC member for Finland, Kaarlo Hartiala, who declared at the Congress in Baden-Baden that "not one world record should be registered officially if anti-doping control conditions are not executed".

Not everything has been done to impel coaches, organisers of competitions, journalists and others involved in the sporting sphere to recognise fully their social responsibility for the realisation of humanistic values by means of sport and to base all their actions on this recognition. It would be advisable, for example, to try to work out and put into practice a moral code for sportsmen and sports specialists. Nowadays such work has begun in some countries, and attempts are being made to work out a moral code for sports journalists. This is really very important, because much depends on the nature of representation through the sports press, radio and TV. These media influence the humanistic effect of sporting ties - whether they will promote a feeling of friendship between youth, and understanding and respect for the representatives from other countries and nations, or whether they will arouse unhealthy passion, a feeling of hatred for other nations, aggressiveness etc. It is no mere chance that the International ICSPE Committee "Sport, Mass Media and International Understanding", the Chairman of which is the famous English scientist Peter McIntosh, appealed in various countries of the world to all sports journalists and radio and TV commentators to make a greater contribution to the strengthening of peace. Analogously, an "Appeal to the sports journalists of the world" was adopted in May 1982 at the Plenary Session of the USSR Federation of Sports Journalists.

It is important not only to work out such codes of practice but also to consider how effective encouragement can be given to those who follow them and strict punishment meted out to those who neglect them. For example, there was the well-known incident during the last World Chess Championship in Merano when the challenger verbally abused - it was heard by everybody - the world champion; but he received only a warning.

As is known, the participants in the IInd World Congress on Sport in Modern Society, held in Tbilisi in 1980 under the aegis of the International Council of Sport and Physical Education (ICSPE-UNESCO), appealed to scientists, teachers of physical education, coaches, sports doctors and specialists in the field of physical culture and sport to strengthen the friendship and to establish understanding and co-operation between nations.

And now we, the participants in the Congress on Sport and International Understanding, have come together in this historical "Finlandia" Hall, where 7 years ago the heads of the 33 countries of Europe, USA and Canada signed the famous agreement on security and principles of peaceful co-operation and coexistence in Europe and all over the world. In the present difficult situation we propose that all the participants at the Congress make an appeal for sportsmen, coaches, scientists, journalists and all others involved in sport all over the world to unite their efforts for a broad use of sport and international sporting ties in the fight to preserve peace and prevent nuclear catastrophe.

References

Abstracts (1976) The international congress of physical activity sciences. Quebec City, Canada

Gert H, Wright Mills C (1954) Character and social structure. Routledge and Kegan Paul, London

Grupe O, Kurz D, Teipel JM (eds) (1972a) Sport im Blickpunkt der Wissenschaft. Perspektive, Aspekte, Ergebnisse. Springer, Berlin Heidelberg New York

Grupe O, Kurz D, Teipel JM (eds) (1972b) Sport in the modern world - Chances and problems. Papers, results, materials. Scientific Congress, Munich, 21-22 Aug. Springer, Berlin Heidelberg New York

Jen B (1972) Le sport, la most, la violence. Editions Universitaires, Paris

Krawczyk Z (1976) Pod red. Kultura fizyczna i spoleczenstwo. (Physical training and society.) Warsaw

Krawczyk Z (1978) Studia z filozofii i socjologii kultury fizycznej. (Research on philosophy and the sociology of physical training.) Warsaw

Krawczyk Z (1981) Pod. red. Sport i kultura. (Sport and culture.) Warsaw

Kulturowe wartosci sportu (1981) Materialy VI miedzynarodowego sympozjum socjologii sportu. [The cultural merits of sport (1981) Proceedings of the VIth international symposium of sport sociology.] Jablonna, 20-24, 1979. Warsaw

Lorenz H (1966) On aggression. Methuen, London

Loy JW, McPherson D, Kenyon G (1978) Sport and social systems. University of Waterloo. Addison-Wesley, London

Lüschen GK, Sage GH (eds) (1981) Handbook of social science of sport. Champaigne, Ill.
Lüschen G, Weis K (eds) (1976) Die Soziologie des Sports. Soziologische Texte. Luchterhand, Darmstadt
Pavlov SP (1977) At the finishing line. FIS, Moscow
Podolskyi TV, Starshinov VI (1975) About moral debt and responsibility of a sportsman. Theory and Practice of Physical Culture 3:9–11
Prokhorov DI (1978) Integration in sport. FIS, Moscow
Rösch HE (1972) Ist das noch Sport? Kritische Anmerkungen zum Sport und zu den Olympischen Spielen. Herder Freiburg, Basel
Saraf M (ed) Sport and personality. FIS, Moscow
Stolyarov VI (1977a) Humanistic value of sport as the element of people's way of life. Theory and Practice of Physical Culture 5–8
Stolyarov VI (1977b) On a humanistic value of sport. Int Rev Sport Sociology 3:75–84
Vidyin VM, (ed) (1980) Sport in modern society. FIS, Moscow, p 73
Wohl A (1981) Soziologie des Sports. Pahl-Rugenstein, Cologne
World Scientific Congress (1978) Sport in modern society (Moscow, 1974). Collected scientific materials. Moscow
World Scientific Congress (1980) Sport in modern society (Tbilisi, 1980). Philosophy, history, sociology. Moscow
Zeigler EF (1977) Physical education and sport philosophy. Prentice-Hall, Englewood Cliffs, NJ

Sport, International Conflict and Conflict Resolution[1]

G. Lüschen

Introduction

When assessing the contribution of sport to international understanding, one encounters a large variety of claims, many of which assert that sport makes a positive or negative contribution while lacking definitional and methodological clarity. Often such claims are statements of belief, being based on limited experience or express normative demands. Everybody will probably agree that behind this question are very complex issues, particularly when dealing with the political level of international relations and peace; rarely is this complexity sufficiently considered. Moreover, to the already difficult question of how to secure international peace is added the expectation that sport has a function in this regard.

One of the most respected authorities on matters of peace in West Germany, the physicist and philosopher F. von Weizsäcker, flatly stated in a recent interview (Weizsäcker 1982) that he had no scientific solution, no theory for peace between nations, while at the same time indicating that he had probably thought out the problems of peace and international understanding as much as anybody else. In discussing the role of sport in conflict and conflict resolution, Max Gluckman in 1972 summed up his experiences both as an observer of sport and as an eminent social scientist by saying that the "balance (between conflict instigation and resolution through sport) is often delicate" and that he does not "on present evidence agree… that the discharge of aggression in games might lead to games replacing war… indeed, the game may breed as much excitement including aggression as it releases among players and spectators" Gluckman 1972). The present paper will briefly review prominent events and major theoretical approaches, and then, after giving an account of substantive and methodological problems, discuss praxeological suggestions for sport policy dealing with sport and conflict.

Factual Accounts and Theoretical Explanations

A review of individual cases concerning sport, conflict and conflict resolution easily generates examples for or against a function of sport in conflict resolution. A number of accounts to which I referred in an address to the Tblisi Olympic Congress in 1980 and in a recent article (Lüschen 1982), as well as some more recent cases, support the conclusion that the effect of sport is contradictory and thus provide no clear insight.

---

1 Originally published in Goldstein (1983) Sport and violence. New York 1983.

Here are two recent examples: In the World Soccer Championship in 1982 the game between Austria and West Germany resulted in a score that deprived Algeria from advancing to the next round. German citizens, because of the conduct of their team, were so embarrassed that they apologised to the Algerian Embassy. Comments in the media stated that international relations and the general reputation of West Germany would need years of repair. This sporting event certainly was not in line with most previous arguments and obviously had a number of consequences. Perhaps after the team rehabilitated itself through a victory over Spain little impact was left from this event, while in the special reality of the mass media it was a major problem for days. The second example, demonstrating the limits of sporting events, stems from the 1982 French Open Tennis Tournament. British TV barred broadcasting of the final because the Argentinian Vilar was playing. Sport was deprived of any chance of easing relations between Argentinia and Great Britain during the war over the Falkland Islands. But one may also ask whether it would really have done so. Were not the officials of British TV assigning an importance to sport that it does not really have? Obviously, the officials thought that it would - and thus one may as a sportsman find something positive in this incident after all.

The case of the Argentinian Vilas and British TV provides another point for discussion: problems of interpersonal relations between individuals, mainly a matter for psychological explanation, are often hopelessly mixed up with intersystemic, international relations, which are mainly a matter for sociological and political scientific explanation. Vilas, after all, is very much an individual, privately and in the international tennis world, representing Argentina to only a limited degree. The famous love relationships, that occur every now and then at international sporting events between members of nations seemingly unfriendly to one another are other cases that often are given credit for having consequences in terms of intersystematic relations. To be sure, there may be some slight impact owing to some symbolic meaning assigned to such events. In general, however, argumentations citing any impact of interpersonal incidents between individuals definitely lack an understanding of the difficult and entrenched nature of the relations between nation-states, which are the result of long traditions, alliances, and economic and other interests.

In addition to the present unsystematic approchaes and general inconclusiveness of results in terms of intersystematic relations, observations very often focus on the incident accompanying sporting events, such as the conduct of fans and riotous outbreaks in and around sports arenas. What one might call the *individualistic fallacy* abounds here again, insofar as explanations are mainly offered in psychological terms referring to aggression and aggression release. To be sure, the psychological approach may be more appropriate for this type of event. Spectators and fans roaming around the sporting arena or prior to and after the actual sporting event are not greatly structured in social terms. Indeed, Le Bon in his *Psychology of the Masses* assumed an absence of social structure and thus unpredictability. More recent analyses have, however, discovered even here the Rules of Disorder (Marsh et al. 1978) and given sociological analyses much more credence than was previously admitted (McPhail and Wohlstein 1983). While in the treatment of "fandom" and external riots a nation of the consequences of sport is present, these analyses and descriptive accounts place rather too little emphasis on the very core event, the sporting contest itself. To a considerable degree psychological explanations, if only implicitly, are the basis of two major groups of theoretical approach to the consequences of sporting events. Konrad Lorenz is the major representative of a school of thought expecting catharsis as a consequence of sporting contests. His expressed belief that through sport international relations will be helped (Lorenz 1963) is probably more an outcome of his generally positive evaluation of aggression than it is a differentiated account of the peculiar structure of international relations. The Sherifs may be cited as representing a school of thought that expect as a consequence of competition increased aggressiveness and a breakdown of intersystemic realtions. Again, their studies (Sherif and Sherif 1961) and subsequent discussions (C. Sherif 1972) as well as the observations of others, articularly with regard to crowd behaviour (Goldstein 1979), lack an understanding of, let alone a systematic account of, intergroup and intersystematic structures. One of the few who shows an awarness of such structures is Arno Plack (1973), when he criticises Lorenz and others for neglecting the *moral* level in their dealings with sporting events that are only "seemingly harmless".

The two approaches, implying catharsis or aggression, are to be found in many variations in the bulk of discussions and research. They were put to an empirical test on a cross-national level by Richard Sipes (1973), who, however did not in only detail spell out and control for a number of variables. Nevertheless, his comparative, global treatment represents a major empirical insight with regard to the theories of Lorenz and Sherif and also with regard to the question of whether sport in general supports good intersystematic relations or not. He used 20 cases of mainly tribal societies from the *Ethnographic Atlas* that could be classified as being either warlike or not and as having combative sport or not. The seemingly low number is due to the fact that he needed sufficient information for both of his categories and thus was forced to eliminate quite a few societies from his sample.

Table 1. Correlation of warlike character and presence of combative sports in 20 selected societies from the *Ethnographic Atlas* (Sipes 1973, p. 71)

		Combative sport Yes	No	Total
Warlike	Yes	9	1	10
	No	2	8	10
Total		11	9	20

The results in Table 1 apparently indicate that combative sports will reinforce warlike systems. The correlation is even stronger when one considers that one of the two societies that were not warlike at the time of the analysis had a history of heavy involvement in warfare. The deviant case, being warlike without combative sport, had, according to Sipes, such a fragile infrastructure that it had to avoid any type of internal strife for fear of destroying its internal social fabric. While not provoding any information on actual processes, in terms of the two cited approaches this study supports Sherif and rejects the functionality of sport for conflict resolution. Sipes also points out that his results suggest a role for cultural learning and sociocultural selection in aggression rather than an innate propensity for aggression, as suggested by the ethologists. Some 16 years ago Heinilä had already provided us with a careful analysis showing that inter-group conflict and hostility could be expected as a result of sport, rather than conflict solution (Heinilä 1966). To this one might add a few disastrous outcomes of sporting events, the most prominent among them being the 318 deaths at an international soccer match in Lima, Peru in 1964. However, single incidents do not lead to final conclusions, and the fact that they are reported in the mass media is certainly not a valid indication of their importance in terms of scientific insight. But to overlook them is equally unscientific. And the results of Sipes are, of course, seemingly overwhelming evidence for the destructive potential of sport; at least, his results indicate a structural interdependence of sport with war, a fact that Lorenz might still be able to interpret positively. In any care, this finding certainly runs counter to our expectations that sport will foster international understanding.

One should, however, be reminded again that this result does not indicate anything about the actual process within these societies, only a guess that sport reinforces a warlike structure. Moreover, one may note that Sipes, results are based on a selection of mainly tribal societies with a lesser level of cultural development outside such institutions as their kinship system and religion.

Norbert Elias (1971, 1976) has argued, particularly with regard to the control of violence, that throughout the history of modern societies one can observe a "civilising process". He points to the fact that we have by and large an incorrect perception of violence in the sport of Antiquity: The at times brutal outcome of sporting contests would not be tolerated today. Karl Weinhold (1856, p. 297) also mentions that sporting contests in Iceland were so serious in their consequences that they were legally outlawed in 1013. The history of American football provides another example. President Theodore Roosevelt making the football association develop better rules for violence control. Modern sport in its organisational set-up and control can thus well be understood as having, in a civilising process, provided better control of the destructive outcomes of sporting contests. At this level, however, we are no longer dealing with some material commodity called sport; we are dealing with a matter of social organisation and control. In a way, modern sport, through its differentiated system of rules, controls and new, emerging forms of contest may have provided a major cultural accomplishment in the evolution of modern society. Most previous discussions and analyses cannot account for this; their simple form of causal thought is not appropriate for our problem, and our expectations in general that sport as such materially provides accommodation and conflict resolution are wrong. Rather it provides only an opportunity or challenge for accommodation.

In line with this interpretation the modern Olympic Games are probably considered a form of accommodation of conflicting parties through sport. The most recent analysis seems to indicate otherwise, however. According to Keefer, Goldstein and Kasiarz, the number of athletes participating in the Olympics correlates positively with months at war of a country (Keefer et al. 1983). They state "our research suggests that at the present time Olympic Game participation does not reduce international conflict". However, they also add, taking up our previous argument about the neglect of the level of social structure, "the study examines a number of personal variables... and relates them to suprapersonal variables". Specifically, a causal relationship can thus not be implied – at best it is a contextual one. But the evolution of a civilising role for sport cannot be so easily taken for granted as Elias̀ theory implies; also, sport in Ancient Greece was not as violent as his theory suggests (cf. McIntosh 1981).

A Structural Interpretation of the Sporting Contest

Before we address the problem of the external consequences of a sporting contest, it is necessary to take a new look at the structure of the contest itself. In many theoretical attempts to explain conflict and sport, a much too simplified model of sport and the sporting contest prevails. Neither is the great variety of sporting disciplines accounted for, nor is there a deeper understanding of the structure of the sporting contest as it is, for example, represented in the encounters between two parties or teams. Many statements on the positive consequences of sporting events for social relations and those of higher intersystematic levels probably depend on a surprising and yet correct observation – that as a rule sporting contests go on properly despite the fact that the opponents engage in some severe form of physical violence or aggression that would not be tolerated elsewhere.

Bernard Jeu (1973) has referred to this quality of modern sport as providing a counter-society, while Sutton-Smith (1978) in respect of children's games and myself in respect of sport in general and top athletics in particular (Lüschen 1970, 1981) have described this quality of sport as dialectical. In a different way Georg Simmel (1908) has described the sporting contest (Kampfspiel) as providing "Einheit im Kampf" (unity in struggle). There are many other interpretations accounting for association (Lüschen 1970) or communication (Schelling 1960) in sporting contests and other social encounters. Even in war, as Kant acknowledged in his essay on eternal peace, there is some form of accommodation. The mutual understanding between competing parties in a sporting contest is a systemic condition under which the contest can proceed. The rules and organisational set-up, but also the mutual agreements between apponents, provide for such an association. In the end it is a matter of conditional structure, not necessarily individual feeling and motivation.

The dialectical structure of a sporting contest also has one other consequence. Statistical relations between variables, such as those of Sipes and Keefer et al. above, may show no causal explanation at all – they may to a high degree be spurious. Who is to say that those countries and tribes engaging in destructive warfare with others would not do so to an even higher degree, were it not for the fact that they can also involve themselves in bloodless sporting contests? That the dualities of competition in sport and war belong structurally to the same form of systemtic interaction goes without question; that they have the same consequence and reinforce one another is not so certain. Indeed, they may with due organisational caution and preparation replace warfare; but this would no longer provide a causal explanation of the relationship of sport to peace or war.

Under the circumstances, one may well suggest that direct consequences for systems at large should not be expected. Indeed, hostile state of affairs may well be a condition under which a sporting contest cannot even be allowed. And there may be conditions external to sport, such as systems being reference groups for one another (Heinilä 1966) or having developed severe strains in other areas, e. g. the feuds between Protestants and Catholics in Glasgow, which can overburden the system of the sporting contest and/or lead to violent incidents.

Only two consequences of sporting contest for internsystemic relations external to sport may be expected with some likelihood: (1) A contest between two parties otherwise at odds with one another in international relations may take on a symbolic meaning and thus indirectly have an impact. At the same time, there is a danger that a sporting event may even cause a violent clash or war, as in the Soccer War between El Salvador and Honduras in 1969. (2) A sporting contest may provide a model of accommodation and structural insights that can be helpful in intersystematic relations. The wide acceptance of the principle of fairness as a normative guideline, in ordinary life is a slight indication of such an impact. But one should take note that this again refers mainly to the level of interpersonal relations. Countries are not *fair* to one another, rather they *accommodate* or *associate.*

Some Methodological Observations and Structural Theory

As should have become obvious by now, providing a comprehensive theory for the whole set of questions posed with regard to sport and conflict resolution on an intersystemic level is exceedingly difficult. In formal terms such a theory would predict an outcome of a situation involving two competing parties. Moreover, such an outcome is supposed to have an impact on the situation at large, of which these parties are a part. In addition, these parties interact in a rather unimportant, symbolically fairly charged subculture - namely that of sport. The expected outcome, however, happens in a rather complex sphere - namely the system of politics or the relations between societies overall.

If one follows the so-called *statement approach* to theory, then a theory consists of a whole number of verified law-like statemants derived from hypotheses. The topic under question would not only have to account for a great number of variables and consequently for quite a few statements of a partial theory; these statements would also have to be leveled within different spheres, from intergroup relations over competing national teams to competing nations. In addition, considering the multiplicities of sport, all types of qualifier to such theoretical statemants would have to be introduced. From this argument an all-encompassing theory based on the "statement approach" is difficult and probably impossible. To meet the requirements of testability and observability, one would with a great many observations probably produce some rather low-level generalisation. In a strict sense it would not be the type of theory that was stated at the beginning of this discussion. In particular, the extension to a general statemant of international relations on the basis of sport appears difficult. Moreover, as was argued previously, systemic and social structural variables or indicators have hardly been introduced, even in explaining the interaction of competing systems in sport. Most of the previous common-sense claims have not seriously attempted this, for they have used psychological concepts (amongst others) where systemic ones are needed. Under the circumstances one has to ask whether the previous unsatisfactory type of research and theorising will have to suffice, with the expectation that more detailed study and more careful design will enlarge our knowledge at the systemic level within the contest itself. I am not so sure about the feasibility of extending and testing sport's function for intersystemic conflict .

With regard to sport and the civilising process, Dunning has put forward the concept of *bonding*, pointing to a lower level of structural interdependence of a social nature between persons and groups (Dunning 1983). For nations the question is whether they will, over a sporting contest that mainly has a bonding or associational quality, put aside their divergent interests in terms of power, economic resources, ideology and longstanding historical identities. Putting the question this way begs the answer and anticipates minor impacts at best.

Owing to recent advances in epistemology a new type of theorising is now being advocated, which Stegmüller orginally labelled the non-statement approach and more recently renamed *structural theory* (Stegmüller 1976, 1979). This should not be mixed up with what is commonly referred to as structuralism in the social sciences. What Stegmüller has in mind is a theory based on a type of insight that one intuitively feels to be true after examining sufficient information. Advanced previously in mathematics and physics, such a notion sounds almost like an invitation for renewed vagueness in sociology and other social sciences. Yet arguments like those of Simmel and Jeu concerning the structure or form of the sporting contest in terms of its unity in conflict appear to be just such theoretical insights, based on a high level of informational input and yet difficult to break down into propositional statements and rigid testing. It may well be that through such theoretical problems like the unity in conflict of the sporting contest, further light can also be thrown on such new methodology in social science theory. In the end it may also provide an opportunity of overcoming the rigid formality and irrationality of the dialectical method, which at first glance and after referring to the structure of the sporting contest as substantively dialectical is quickly advanced as a solution to our methodological problems.

Conclusion: Some Praxeological Suggestions for Sports Policy (in Place of a Comprehensive Theory)

In summary our results may look meagre in terms of our general expectations with regard to sport and international understanding. They may also look meagre in terms of a neat social science theory. Too much seems to be missing, there is not enough information and not enough research, and on top of that are the almost insurmountable methodological problems, with structural theory perhaps offering a way of explaining the unity of the sporting contest itself. Actually, however, I do not think that the result is meagre. The review of previous research and discussion will hopefully instigate further research and thought. The simmelesque concept of unity in conflict, of structural dialectic, can easily be extended to a notion of a basic structural disposition, at least in ethnic societies with so-called dual organisation (Lévi-Straus 1967, 1969). Moreover, while the result is inconclusive and any statements concerning sport's function for intersystemic and surely international relations must be rather cautious, there is sufficient information, insight and theoretical reasoning to advance some praxeological suggestions as a basis for futute policy in sport. Some of these suggestions may not be so new, but our discussion will hopefully have provided a more informed, and in the end more rational, approach. In this regard, it is also important to know what we cannot be sure about.

For the policy suggestions which follow, it is assumed that we are dealing with conflict in the system of the sporting contest only – at this time neither conflicts of an interpersonal nature nor conflicts between sports organisations are of interest to us. The former, as has been discussed, are actually very much in the centre of analysis, whereas the latter have been almost totally overlooked (Matejko 1975). For the sporting contest as a form of conflict and possible outcomes for relations between systems at large represented in such a contest, the following points may be suggested as a basis for sports policies:

1. Sporting contests are not uniform and involve a variety of structures that need to be handled differently, i. e. a gymnastics contest has a different form and potential from a rugby match.
2. Even the most vigorous encounters need a consensus or, better, an association between parties in order for the contest to go ahead. It is essential to understand such structural disposition of association and to support it through rules, values like fair play and organisational contexts as much as possible. However, it would mean impeding the associative challenges of the sporting contest were it strictly and rigidly ruled and policed by sanctions and quasi-legal personnel.
3. The symbolic meaning of a contest between rival parties may take on added significance, i. e. when those systems are reference groups for one another or when they are engaged in other forms of conflicting interest in economic matters or international power. It is essential for an appropriate policy to consider these contextual factors; a consequence may be either (1) not to allow a contest to go ahead at all if there is a danger of overburdening the sporting contest in its structural disposition, or (2) to provide carefully for controlling arrangements and thus to make use of the contest for general if only symbolic accommodation. It is even possible, through special arrangements such as the use of the mass media, to increase the general significance of a sporting event. But even then one should not expect much beyond some symbolic significance. On the level of international relations the final arrangement will have to come from political moves.
4. There may be certain conditions under which an impact (positive or negative) of sport on international relations is possible. This can go beyond the symbolic sphere under very special conditions. In purely formal terms, however, the association in the sporting contest between competing parties may provide a structural model that could be useful in intersystemic relations. Because of the complex nature of the latter, even such formal and theoretical use will be limited.
5. Despite the general claims concerning sport's impact on system relations, it is not unusual for sports organisations to abandon their responsibility for such impacts in the wider range of the institution of sport. In particular this holds for crowd behaviour and its control at sporting events. Sports organisations have to recognise this.
6. With regard to the latter and for its general handling in policies, it is paramount to understand that the sporting contest is a system of conflict itself, that some sporting events clearly value violence and concflict. Under the cricumstances a belief in sport's peaceful mission as a matter of course is dangerous. In its consequence it would be destructive for the system of sport itself.
7. Even if the impact of sport on intersystemic conflict and relations is limited, as has been argued in reference to many exaggerated statements, some impact is a matter

of reality and needs to be incorporated in to appropriate organisational effort and a policy in sport that involves two major lines of action: strengthening the internal and external controls to bar as much negative impact as possible, and advancing any potential positive impact to the greatest possible extent. The last point implies the recommendation that sport should be given as much appropriate organisational support as is possible, ranging from the regular forms of control of contestants and crowds to the public discussion of sport's potential for accommodation and even conflict resolution when parties are otherwise at odds with one another. Thus, what so far has been regarded as a matter of reality and proven scientific insight may well be understood as a function of necessary controls to channel conflict potential and even turn it into an opportunity for accommodation. Actually, the statements of officials and many publicly expressed beliefs concerning the peaceful mission of sport are in functional terms no more than normative demands and honest beliefs which fulfil important social controls even if they are wrong in scientific terms or as a matter of reality. Who carries out the suggested organisational control is an open question. Public and political agencies will often have to be called on or take on their share of responsibility. But there is no question that many such controls can be provided within and by the system of sport itself.

References

Dunning E (1973) The structural-functional properties of folk-games and modern sport. Sportwissenschaft 3: 215-232
Dunning E (1979) The figurational dynamics of modern sport. Sportwissenschaft 4:341-359
Dunning E (1983) Social bonding and violence in sport: a theoretical-empirical analysis. In: Goldstein J (ed) Sports violence. Springer, New York, Heidelberg, Berlin pp 129-146
Elias N (1971) The genesis of sport as a sociological problem. In: Dunning E (ed). The sociology of sport. Cass, London, pp 88-115
Elias N (1947) Sport and violence. Actes Recherche Sci Sociales 6: 2-20
Firth R (1930) A dart-match in Tikopia. The sociology of primitive sport. Oceania 1:64-96
Gluckman M (1972) Sport and conflict. In: Grupe O et al. (eds) Sport in the modern world. Springer, Berlin, Heidelberg, New York, pp 48-54
Goldstein (ed) (1979) Sports, games, and play. Erlenbaum, Hillsdale, N.J.
Heinilä K (1966) Notes on the intergroup conflicts in international sports. Int Rev Sport Sociology 1:30-40
Jeu B (1973) La contre-société sportive et ses contradictions. Esprit 10:319-416
Keefer R, Goldstein J, Kasiarz D (1983) Olympic games participation. In: Goldstein J (ed) Sports violence. Springer, New York, Heidelberg, Berlin, pp 183-93
Kiviaho P (1974) The regional distribution of sport organizations as a function of political cleavages. Sportwissenschaft 4:72-81
Kotarbinski T (1963) Praxeology. Oxford University Press, London
Lang G (1976) Der Ausbruch von Tumulten bei Sportveranstaltungen. In: Lüschen G, Weis K (eds) Die Soziologie des Sports. Luchterhand, Darmstadt, pp 273-295
Lévi-Strauss C (1967) Structural anthropology. Doubleday, Garden City, N.J., pp 128-160
Lévi-Strauss C (1969) The elementary structures of kinship. Beacon Press, Boston, 1969 (orig. 1949).
Lorenz K (1963) Das sogenannte Böse. Borotha-Schöler, Wien
Lüschen G (1970) Cooperation, association, and contest. Conflict Resolution 14:21-34
Lüschen G (1981) At the edge of human existence: the regularities and contradictions in top athletics. In: Simri U (ed) Proceedings of ICHER-Europe Congress. Wingate-Institute, Natanya, pp 131-147
Lüschen G (1982) Sport, conflict and conflict resolution. Int Soc Sci J 34,2:185-96
Lüschen G, Sage G (eds) (1981) Handbook of social science of sport. Stipes, Champaign, Ill.
Marsh PE, Rosser E, Harre R (1978) The rules of disorders. Routledge and K. Paul London, Boston
Matejko A (1975) The diagnosis of conflict in sport. Revue Int Sociologie (Madrid) 33:63-87

McIntosh PC (1981) The sociology of sport in the Ancient World. In: Lüschen G, Sage G (eds) Handbook of social science of sport. Stipes, Champaign, Ill., pp 25–48
McPhail C, Wohlstein R (1983) Individual and collective behaviors within gatherings, demonstrations, and riots. Ann Rev Sociol 9:579–600
Plack A (1973) Der Mythos vom Aggressionstrieb. Piper, München
Sartre JP (1976) Critique of dialectical reason. NLB, London
Schelling T (1960) The strategy of conflict. Harvard, Cambridge
Sherif C (1972) Intergroup conflict and competition. In: Grupe O et al. (eds). Sport in the modern world. Springer, Berlin, Heidelberg, New York, pp 60–69
Sherif M, Sherif C (1961) The Robbers' Cave experiment. Oklahoma University Press, Norman
Simmel G (1908) Soziologie. Duncker und Humblot, Berlin
Sipes R (1973) War, sports, and aggression. American Antropologist 75: 64–86
Smith M (1975) Sport and collective violence. In: Ball D, Loy J (eds) Sport and social order. Addison-Wesley, Reading, Mass.
Sprenger J (1974) Zum Problem der Aggressionen im Sport. Sportwissenschaft 4:231–257
Stegmüller W (1976) The structures and dynamics of theories. Springer, New York, Heidelberg, Berlin
Stegmüller W (1979) The structuralist view of theories. Springer, New York, Heidelberg, Berlin
Sutton-Smith B (1978) Die Dialektik des Spiels. Hofmann, Schorndorf
Weinhold K (1856) Altnordisches Leben. Berlin
Weiszäcker F (1982) Interview on peace. WDR 3. 30 June 1982. WDR, Cologne

The Idealistic and Factual Role of Sport in International Understanding

P. Seppänen

Introductory Notes on the Role of Sport

In his notes on education, Baron Pierre de Coubertin (1901), Father of the Modern Olympics, tells us that sport is a factor which engenders a form of "pacific nationalism". The same type of conviction about the role of sport is also expressed in the Charter of the International Olympic Committee (IOC), which suggests that better mutual understanding can arise through sport and that sport thereby helps to create a more peaceful world. The Olympic Rules and Regulations allow no discrimination against any person on grounds of race, religion or politics (International Olympic Committee 1979). The only other qualification for participation is that a National Olympic Committee (NOC) must exist in the country concerned.

Similar suggestions as to the role of sport have also been made by some scholars. Milshtein and Molchanov of the Soviet Union state that "sport due to its nature is a factor promoting peace, friendship and mutual understanding" (Milshtein and Molchanov 1976). For his part, Günther Vonneberger (1978) is convinced that the GDR's top-level sport has promoted peace and understanding with peoples and states that have different social systems because "There is no place for chauvinism in sport in the GDR."

On the other hand, the critics for sport seem to regard sporting contests as an activity which causes and strengthens conflicts rather than relives and solves them. Sporting events are seen as polarising participating groups and audiences and as leading to disorders and violence. Descriptions of sports-connected rioting by polarised teams or crowds are not infrequent. At the Olympics of Melbourne in 1956, just after the Hungarian uprising, newspapers reported fist fights and bloodshed between players in a waterpolo match in which Hungary defeated the Soviet Union. When a Hungarian player was injured, the pro-Hungarian crowd, including many Hungarian emigrés, rushed to the pool and had to be dispersed by the police (Morton 1963). References have also been made to the broken sporting relations between Finland and Sweden in the 1930s, to interracial conflicts in American football in the 1960s, to the "post-hockey victory riots" in Czechoslovakia in 1969 and to several soccer conflicts of which the "football" or "soccer war" between El Salvador and Honduras in 1969 is the best known (see, e.g. Lang 1981).

Ambiguous and Deficient Knowledge of the Role of Sport

Actually, the statements which strongly take a stand are not convincing, because they are not analytic and because their factual evidence is often insufficient. Characteristic of them is the *exaggeration of the role of sport.* On the one hand, this means idealisation, on the other, distortion in the opposite direction.

Even though it is possible that sport promotes both mutual understanding and conflicts between nations, acceptance or rejection of this kind of position needs to be based on evidence. In fact, the very first difficulty concerning the suggestions as to the role of sport in mutual understanding is apparently that they *mix up the normative and factual* order of things. Even if values play a role in scientific work, the first requirement of scientific analysis is to emphasise the factual order of things or what is evident and what is not. The factual order of things, or what actually happens in sport, regardless of what is considered ideal, is the main target of the present analysis, too.

The factual role of sport in international understanding is not, however, easily explained, because serious research work in the field is almost non-existent. The available research findings are more or less indirect and their evidence for making firm conclusions is not very convincing. In fact, the first conclusion I want to make is that there is *very little* that we really know about the effect of sport upon mutual understanding between people.

We know only that sporting exchange between nations is quite extensive and a continuously growing phenomenon. We also know that a great part of this exchange is limited to top-level sport and its concomitants like spectator sport, and the increasing coverage of sport in the mass media. Additionally, we know that sports teams visit and sometimes also have a special privilege to visit places which are not visited by ordinary tourists. Cross-national marriages and mutual ties of friendship between individual sportsmen are occasionally reviewed in newspapers and magazines[1]. But of the social functions of sport in international relations, our knowledge is very limited.

The Role of Interaction in Increasing Understanding

In analysing the problem it seems necessary to separate *interaction in general* from *interaction akin to sport.* As sport is a type of human activity, it might be that some of those features which are characteristic of interaction in general are also characteristic of sport. And yet on the other hand, sport cannot be understood without reference to its special nature. George C. Homans 1950, one of the most eloquent spokesman for the exchange perspective in human behaviour, said in one of his basic statements on the regularities in interaction between individuals that: "If the frequency of interaction between two or more persons increases, the degree of liking for one another will increase and vice versa (see also Mulkay 1971). In other words, Homans' hypothesis - which is based on a wider selection of studies - supports the proposal that interaction as such increases individuals' liking for each another. This appears even more clearly in

1 For example: the marriage of the gold medal winner in track and field events Harold Connolly of the USA and Olga Fikotová of Czechoslovakia, and the close friendship between the gold medalists Heikki Hasu of Finland and Simon Slåttvik of Norway in the 1950s.

Homans' further statement (1950) which is worded: "The more frequently persons interact with one another, the more alike their activities and their sentiments tend to become, and vice versa". If interaction as such is a precondition for decreasing prejudice and increasing goodwill, the rule should hold for sport too.

This kind of argumentation is, however, questionable. First the suggestion does not give any evidence of the behaviour of groups and nations. Second, further qualification concerning the type of interaction is also needed. If the relationships between interacting groups or nations we are previously hostile, increasing contact between them will hardly diminish prejudice and hostile attitudes. On the contrary, it is obvious that negative stereotypes concerning each other will only be reinforced. In orther words, the possibility of increasing goodwill through interaction is conditional, and this is also true in sports.

Sport as a Reducer of Tension and Aggression

As a special type of activity sport is most often analysed by starting with an individual. It is regarded as an activity which has some functions - often unintended - from the point of view of an individual. Or more precisely, participation in sporting activities as well as watching sport has been explained by scientists as a compensatory reaction against the requirements and impacts of industrial society and life in it. The compensatory function of sport is identified in several ways, of which an *instinct-releasing* function or relief of aggression, as Hans Lenk (1981) puts it, is interesting from the standpoint of interpersonal co-operation and understanding.

One of the most prominent defenders of the aggression-relieving theory is Konrad Lorenz (1965). According to him sport is an activity with a function of reducing the aggressive potential of human beings. Eibl-Eibesfeldt (1970) also talks about an aggressive drive of man being displayed in sport. Nevertheless, the role of sport as an associative or unifying factor receives very little attention in his thinking, although he does refer to single combats and duels as potential forms of controlling aggression.

The suggestions made by Desmond Morris (1978) are also of great interest. He sees sporting activities as essentially modified forms of hunting behaviour based on man's permanent hunting instinct. The triumph of a hunter is, however, transformed from the original goal of killing the prey to a symbolic one - winning. By distinguishing between the warlike blood sports of past centuries and the bloodless sport of modern man, Morris comes to strongly emphasise the great importance of modern sport as an activity reducing the chances of war breaking out. Or, as he literally puts it, "The ancient sport or war-hunting exploded into the uncontrolled savagery of modern total war", but, as he furthermore states, "In planning future work-styles, attempts to involve workers in a pseudo-hunting sequence of some kind would seem to be essential, if we are to avoid the damaging alternatives of riots, violence, and total war".

The argument that everyone needs to release tensions and that sport is one of the most important vehicles for this is actually quite widely accepted. This kind of release of tensions is considered especially characteristic of modern industrial society (Elias and Dunning 1970). Similarly, it has often been stated that vicarious or secondary involvement in sport, as in spectator sports, also acts as an important institution by providing for the release of man's aggressive, combative and chasing instincts (Spinrad

1981; Brill 1929; Loy et al. 1978). Gerth, Mills and Wright (1954) for example report in their study on character and social structure that many mass audience situations, with their "vicarious components", serve psychologically the unintended function of channelling and releasing emotions. Thus great amounts of aggression are, at least theoretically, released by crowds of spectators cheering their favourite stars and jeering at the referee/umpire (see also Loy et al. 1978).

The Sherif's Experiment

On the other hand, some studies suggest that observers may be more aggressive after reviewing battle than before (e.g. Berkowitz 1929; Bogardus 1931; Heinilä 1966; Goldstein and Arms 1971), and some outbursts may spread beyond the sports arena to become fanatical public riots, city-wide riots and destructive behaviour (Lang 1976). Similarly, the Sherifs' account for an increase in conflict and aggression in a contest situation. Sherif et al.'s (1961) famous experiment on young American boys at a summercamp illustrates how the boys who were randomly divided into two main groups soon began to develop strong loyalties towards their own group, or in-group, and negative attitudes towards the others, or out-group, when pitted in various sporting and other competitive activities. Furthermore, Sherif created some emergency situations which could not be solved without co-operation as a single team. Only in these particular situations did both groups began to interact co-operatively, forgetting their old hostilities. Co-operation did not, however, become permanent, lasting for a while only. As a whole Sherif et al.'s experiment clearly shows how feelings of in-group loyalty tend to be preferred and how antagonism between the groups lessened only when the members of both groups were obliged to unite in the pursuit of common goals (Sherif et al. 19161; Sherif 1973).

In other words, the research findings in the field are not unequivocal but rather a challenge for further research and qualification. One greater difficulty with them is the fact that they mainly concern individuals and small groups without any attention to larger social unities like societies and nations. As everybody knows, it is one thing to talk about experiences of an individual or face-to-face groups and quite another to show the effects of sport upon societal behaviour and cultural patterns.

The Presence of Both Associational and Conflict Elements

By analysing sport from a socio-cultural point of view Günther Lüschen (1981) states that one of the most essential characteristics of sporting contests is a kind of duality. A sporting contest includes *both associational (unifying) and conflict elements* depending on the type of sport, situation and other similar qualifications. Or, as he puts it: "Seemingly we have here structural contradictions which fit the label *dialectic.*" He additionally concludes that the effects of the sporting contest upon society are less negative than one would expect after reading the Sherif's work and less positive than one would believe after reading Lorenz.

Although sport obviously includes elements of both conflict and co-operation, peaceful rather than militant characteristics of it are primarily emphasised. The sporting contest always takes place under socially approved rules. Or, as Georg Simmel (1923) expressed it about 60 years ago: "One unites in order to fight, and one fights under the mutually recognized governance of norms and rules". The observance of rule and the consideration of an opponent (or fairness), which are the most important ideals of sport, also refer to the unifying rather than the destructive role of sport.

According to some critics of sport, the pacifying role of sport goes so far that it suppresses aggressive and other potentials which otherwise could develop "socially explosive power" and become dangerous for the existing system (e.g.Marcuse 1955; Habermas 1958; Vinnai 1970; Böhme et al. 1971). Hoch (1972) goes even further than these representatives of the so-called "critical school of sociology" by suggesting that sport in capitalist countries is an opiate or tranquilizer, distracting the underprivileged and keeping them from confronting the source of their alienation.

Even though suggestions of this type greatly exaggerate the role of sport as a neutraliser of explosive potentials of people (Lenk 1981), there seems to be something in the very essence of sport and even in the essence of sporting contest which entitles us to speak not only about the "safety valve" function of sport on the individual level but also about its function as a moderator of tensions within a society. To have evidence of the role of sport as a reducer of internal tensions in society does not, however, mean that sport automatically decreases tensions in international relations too. When this role of sport is hypothesised, it is thought that sport can act in the world as a kind of humanistic and civil religion which has a considerable impact on modern thinking and the modern way of life. This was one of the basic ideas that de Coubertin had in mind and one of the important sources of the Olympic movement (see, e.g. MacAllon 1976).

Obscurity in the Role of Sport

It is also possible to argue that there exists a special ideology of sport which emphasises such things as fairness, justice and competition on equal terms. Additionally, it can be concluded that the ideology of sport is different from other out-looks on life. But has the sports ideology any essential impact on the modern way of life and the relations between nations? There are at least two resons to doubt this. Firstly, sport with its goals and values is not a sufficiently coherent phenomenon to unify people, but a widely varying institution with different functions in different societies and cultures (e. g. Loy et al. 1978; McIntosh 1981; Sutton-Smith 1981). Secondly, it is not independent enough to carry through the values and ideals that it represents. In fact, sport lacks power. Even though it may look independent like the Catholic Church or any other supranational and non-governmental organisation, it greatly depends on other institutions and especially on those in power. Actually, *the social and cultural role of sport in international relations is obscure rather than clear,* and the capacity of sport to carry through a universal ideology of its own seems to exist more in theory than in practice.

The instrumental role of sport in international relations is clearer and also more thoroughly discussed. The focus of discussion has primarily been high-performance or top-level sport. One characteristic of international top-level sport is that it usually takes place as a contest between national teams. The athletes of different nations fight for superiority not only amongst themselves and one against the other but also as representatives of their countries. As the international success of individual athletes and teams is highly valued and widely visible, it seems to be in the interest of nations to make use of this visibility and to manipulate it with their national sports policy. The results of sports policy are seen not only in international success (Seppänen 1972, 1981) but also in the growing dependence of sport on those in power. Or more precisely, the role of sport is becoming increasingly subordinate to national political interests. A good example of this kind of tendency is given by Dieter Voigt (1975) when he states that the function of sport in the GDR is "to enhance the prestige of the GDR and document the superiority of the socialist system in comparison with the capitalist one". If this type of sports policy is generally characteristic of modern sport, it can be concluded that the *internal integration of society rather than international solidarity is the main function of international sport.*

The most mordant critics of modern high-performance or top-level sport go considerably further in their suggestions. Kalevi Heinilä (this volume, Chap II.1.) talks about totalisation as being the main characteristic of present top-level sport and argues that not only the intervention of politicians but also the basic ideology of sport itself is changing with the overvaluation of top-level sport. Top-level sport with its "victory ideology" has become a frightening weapon of cold total war.

Even though there exists evidence, like the role of drugs and cheating in modern top-level sport, which supports Heinilä's thesis, there is also evidence which supports a more optimistic view on the role of sport in international relations. Like Desmond Morris I want to argue that institutions such as sport - even international top-level sport - are needed to reduce the chances of war breaking out. It is, however, *uncertain if sport ever can have such a role that international conflicts can be solved or even reduced through it.* On the other hand, it is certain that sport as such neither brings about nor inspires wars or other international riots. The examples of football wars and other instances of unrest connected with sport have never had their origin in sport but in already existing conflicts of national, political or other interests beyond the realm of sport.

Conclusion

Although the utilisation of sport as an instrument of international power struggle and cold war is apparent and a matter of well-founded concern, there also seem to be some elements of sport which can serve as a safety valve in reducing tensions between peoples and nations. In fact, the role of sport in international understanding is at present inadequately clarified and a lot of further research in the field is needed.

References

Berkowitz L (1929) The frustration-aggression hypothesis revisited. In: Berkowitz L (ed) Roots of aggression. Atherton, New York, pp 1-29

Bogardus ES (1931) Golf galleries as social groups. Sociology Social Res 4:27-276

Böhme JO, Gadow J, Güldenpfennig S, Jensen J, Pfister R (1971) Sport im Spätkapitalismus. Limpert, Frankfurt

Brill A (1929) The why of the fan. North Am Rev 228:429-434

de Coubertin P (1901) Notes sur l'Education Publique. Librairie Hachette et Cie, Paris, pp 201

Eibl-Eibesfeldt I (1970) Liebe und Haß. Piper, Munich

Elias M, Dunning E (1970) The quest for exitement in unexiting societies. In: Lüschen G (ed) The cross cultural analysis of sport and games. Stipes, Champaign, pp 31–51
Gerth H, Mills C, Wright L (1954) Character and social structure. Routledge and Kegan Paul, London
Goldstein J, Arms R (1971) Effects of observing athletic contests on hostility. Sociometry 34:83–90
Habermas J (1958) Soziologische Notizen zum Verhältnis von Arbeit und Freizeit. In: Konkrete Vernunft. Bouvier, Bonn
Heinilä K (1966) Notes on the intergroup conflicts in international sport. Int Sport Sociology 1:49–69
Hoch P (1972) Rip off the big game. Anchor, Garden City, New York
Homans GC (1950) Human group. Harcourt Brace Janovich, New York, pp 112
International Olympic Committee (1979) Olympic Charter. Lausanne
Lang G (1976) Der Ausbruch von Tumulten bei Sportveranstaltungen. In: Lüschen G, Weis K (eds) Die Soziologie des Sports. Luchterhand, Darmstadt, pp 273–295
Lang G (1981) Riotous outbursts at sport events. In: Lüschen G, Sage G (eds) Handbook of social science of sport. Stipes, Champaign, pp 415–436
Lenk H (1981) Sport achievement and social criticism. In: Lüschen G, Sage GH (eds) Handbook of social science of Sport. Stipes, Champaign, pp 369–382
Lorenz K (1965) On aggression. Brace and World, Harcourt, New York
Loy J, McPherson BD, Kenyon G (1978) Sport and social systems. Addison Wesley, Reading (Mass.) pp 3–26; 312
Lüschen G (1981) The system of sport – problems of methodology, conflict, and social stratification. In: Lüschen GH, Sage G (eds) Handbook of social science of sport. Stipes, Champaign, pp 197–213
MacAlloon J (1976) Religious themes and structures in the Olympic movement and the Olympic Games. Presented at the International Congress of the Physical Activity Sciences, Quebec City, July 1976
Marcuse H (1955) Eros and civilization. Beacon, Boston
McIntosh P (1981) The sociology of sport in the Ancient World. In: Lüschen G, Sage G (eds) Handbook of social science of sport. Stipes, Champaign
Milshtein OA, Molchanov SV (1976) The shaping of public opinion regarding sport by the mass-media as factor in promoting international understanding. Sociology 3:71–85
Morris D (1978) Manwatching, a field guide to human behaviour. Triad/Panther Books, Frogmore, St Albans, pp 305-310
Morton H (1963) Soviet sport. Collier, New York
Mulkay MJ (1971) Functionalism and exchange and theoretical strategy. Schocken Books, New York, pp 135–141; 243
Seppänen P (1972) Die Rolle des Leistungssports in den Gesellschaften der Welt. Sportwissenschaft 2: 133-155
Seppänen P (1981) Olympic success: A cross national perspective. In: Lüschen G, Sage G (eds) Handbook of social science of sport. Stipes, Champaign, pp 93–116
Sherif C (1973) Intergroup conflict and competition. Sportwissenschaft 3:138–153
Sherif M et al. (1961) Intergroup conflict and co-operation. The Robber's cave experiment. Oklahoma University Press, Norman
Simmel G (1923) Soziologie. Duncker and Humblot, Berlin, pp 200
Spinrad W (1981) The function of spectator sports. In: Lüschen GH, Sage G (eds) Handbook of social science of sport. Stipes, Champaign, pp 354–365
Sutton-Smith B (1981) The social psychology and anthropology of play and games. In: Lüschen G, Sage G (eds) Handbook of social science of sport. Stipes, Champaign, pp 452–478
Vinnai P (1970) Fussballsport als Ideologie. Europäische Verlagsanstalt, Frankfurt
Voigt D (1975) Soziologie in der DDR. Eine exemplarische Untersuchung. Analyse der DDR-Soziologie am Beispiel des Forschungsgegenstandes Sport. Verlag Wissenschaft und Politik, Cologne, pp 41–42
Vonneberger, G (1978) The social functions of high-perfomance sports with particular reference to sports in the GDR. In: Landry F, Orban WAR (eds) Physical activity and human well-being, II. Symposia Specialists, Miami, Flo., pp 114

Nationalism and Internationalism in Sport

R. Väyrynen

Introduction

Sport is a social institution which reflects the realities of the society in which it is exercised. The organisation of sport is different in a segmented or polarised society when compared with a fairly unified and homogeneous society. There are a plethora of examples to show that the fragmentation of sports organisations according to class, ethnic or linquistic divisions is rooted in the underlying social and political polarisation of the society. Sports also have their own ideology which ideally stresses fair competition between amateurs on equal terms, but is in reality modified by underlying political and social interests. In a fragmented society sports become an instrument, wrapped in ideological arguments, by means of which various groups in the society try to promote their own goals and interests. From this point of view sports are a form of collective social competition, as well as competition between individuals and teams. This is a *conflict perspective* of the role of sports in society.

Sports do not, however, only reflect the existing social contradictions of a society; they also have a strong unifying function. Sports provide linguistic symbolism and a kind of social dream by which people can be socialised into the dominant culture. In the words of Richard Lipsky (1979, pp 61–88) "the symbolic resolution of tension in sports drama preserves the group's energy for positive social action, overcoming the danger that social order will collapse in the wrangle of insurrection and pent-up frustration." In his opinion sports provide a symbolic refuge in which potentially dangerous political conflicts can be resolved and the legitimacy of a polity bolstered. In this sense sports have become a *safety valve* in almost any society. In addition to that, team games are often described as a microcosm of a good society; players have to behave according to certain rules and limits in pursuing, either collectively or individually, their goals. An athlete in good physical and mental shape is an ideal citizen because of his or her abilities to convert the sporting achievements into "good citizenship" in everyday life. These comments open an *integrative perspective* to the role of sports in society.

This rough distinction can also be applied to the international implications of the sports culture. The integration model has been reflected in the ideal conception of the Olympic movement in which internationalism prevails. Intense but fair competition between individuals or teams – independently of their national, racial or linguistic origins – has been the main characteristic of this ideology. It is true *transnationalism* which is supposed to integrate the youth of the world under the Olympic banner. This vision has never been realised. Rather the conflict model provides a better description of the nature of the Olympic Games; they are a competition between individuals and teams for "honour and gold" which is aggregated into competition between nations for prestige. The Olympic Games have "evolved into a ritualistic struggle, one national community against the others. Olympic athletes have become soldiers of sport who are indoctrinated with grotesque conceptions of national prestige," wrote Alex Natan in his famous indictment of the role of nationalism, "sport's deadlist enemy." In Natan's (1969) view, national governments are responsible for converting sports into a "propaganda weapon in world affairs" and hence for betraying the ideals of the Olympic movement.

The reality is, however, more complex than that. In fact it can be claimed that the prevalence of national competition in sports - for gold medals in the Olympic Games or for world Championships - is due to the emphasis laid on their integrative role within societies. The demand for national integrity logically leads to the division of athletes and players into national contingents. This is a price which has to be paid for universalism, as transnational contacts between nationally segmented teams - such as the Workers' Olympics in the 1920s and 1930s - would obviously be less nationalistic by their character but would also lack the universal representation embedded in the Olympic ideals. Nationalism is thus a part and parcel of international competitive sport. That is why this contribution aims at penetrating into the role of nationalism in sport and into its implications for international sporting exchange. Nationalism in sport can be hardly analysed without anchoring it in the process of *nation-building* which every society has to undergo. Nationalism has, in turn, to be related to the *sports creed* which is an integral part of the mental map of sportsmen and women: amateurs, professionals and fans alike. From this point of view I also seek to explore some interfaces between individuals as well as national and international sports communities, their norms and their authority structures.

The Social Role of Sports

If a society is fragmented by social and political cleavages it is less probable that a unified sports culture will develop. This is reflected in the evolution of the Finnish ski sports during the twentieth century. There were three separate skiing organisations in the country, one of them represented workers, one the Swedish-speaking minority in the country, while the third, a non-socialist one, pretended to be a nation-wide association. Thus political and linguistic cleavages divided the ski sports in Finland. Yet at the same time they were used as an integrative symbol to which every Finn should subscribe. Skiing was said to be a national sport in which everybody has to participate in order to improve his or her physical and mental health. Even though the basic cleavages remained, some national unification could be discerned in the 1930s behind this ideology of skiing. The foundations of this ideology remained, however, different. The workers' movement stressed the importance of sports as a means of enhancing its political strength through better physical fitness. In the dominant culture motivations were naturally different. Skiing could improve the productive capacity of workers and the military preparedness of the people. The economic motivation is visible in the anxiousness of bigger corporations to foster skiing among their workers. On the military side skiing was regarded as an essential ingredient of the Finnish strategy to defend her long wooded borders: "skis are our protection" was a popular phrase in the 1920s. The military argument was dominant in the replacement of flat-country skiing by cross-country skiing in the 1920s (see Heikkinen 1981).

Sports are not naturally dominated only by private or national economic and military motives. They also absorb individual aspirations and provide a good deal of social drama for the sports fans. These functions of sports have to be conceived, however, in their societal contexts. In earlier phases of economic development sports are more individually oriented; big names in track and field or skiing events are the objects of popular admiration. With the progress of economic development societies tend to become mor collectivist, more bureaucratic and less divided by visible class cleavages. The apolitical politics of integration, such as sports and other forms of popular culture, also becomes more important. In these social circumstances individual sports lose ground, relatively speaking, to such team sports as football, basketball and ice hockey. These team games have their counterpart in the teamwork of the factories (developed by the industrial psychology of the human relations school in the 1930s). *Steering* and *control* processes become more important both in sports and in society at large.

In this process sports lose some of their original character which is captured in the definition of sport in *Webster's Dictionary* as "diversion, amusement, or recreation." Sports develop into a *system* which is maintained by an organisation, external economic support and scientific inputs through which the effectiveness of athletes is enhanced. The success of individual athletes becomes dependent on membership in this system and on compliance with its rules and norms, even though they may be distorted and unhealthy (e.g. doping).

This perspective has been used to describe the evolution of the role of sports in "administrative capitalism", in which new social needs give rise to collective rather than individual performance (Lipsky 1979, pp. 82–85). At a certain level of generality these changes can be discovered in the socialist societies as well. They may be signs of a performance society, a *Leistungsgesellschaft*, which has penetrated into the values of both capitalist and socialist countries. In socialist societies sports are seen as a way to develop a many-sided socialist personality in an individual, who can improve his or her physical and psychic capacity to respond to social challenges. These challenges include the needs created by production and national security. In fact, physical culture and sports are indispensable in contributing to enhanced production potential and national defence capability. By contributing to the reconstruction of socialism as well as to its defence, sports also have a class character (e.g. Tappert and Jodl 1973; Enquist 1972). On the basis of these premises, sports in socialist countries have been closely integrated with the economic and political steering of their societies. In addition to this, sporting successes have been used to show the superiority and legitimacy of the socialist political and economic system. The policy of the German Democratic Republic has been an illustrative example of this tendency. In the Federal Republic of Germany a liberal model has prevailed: the lack of deep political cleavages have prevented the division of her sports movement. Partly for this reason the dominant political forces of the country have not shown any major interest in steering the development of the sports movement. Apart from the economic rationales transforming the character of sports, the Olympic and other successes of the GDR bolstered political interest in the promotion of sports. In this way sports were annexed to the ideological competition between socialism and capitalism, East and West (see Ström 1977).

The molding of sports to new dictates of the production life – according to Per-Olav Enquist, team gymnastics was a perfect functional equivalent of the production process in early capitalism – has naturally created countertendencies. The *privatisation* of social life and the emerging culture of *narcissism* have brought about some changes. On the one hand, they have alienated people, making them passive watchers of team games, providing them with a symbolic refuge, while on the other hand they have given rise to such narcissist phenomena as body building and jogging (Lasch 1978), which have become a kind of ersatz sexuality.

Both team and individual sports are still motivated by *military needs* as they enhance the ability of individual soldiers to operate more effectively and in a more co-ordinated fashion in a troop formation (Tappert and Jodl 1973; Reiter 1976). The military motive behind sports may be diminishing, however. The battlefield is increasingly dominated by military machines rather than by the formations of capable and brave soldiers whose operations are dependent on good physical condition. In earlier times military sports were also more closely connected with the national function of the army. Later on, the army was expected to have a similar national function in new nations.

Sports and Nation-Building

In a new nation sports have a dual function in the building of national identity and national competence. Nation-building is intimately connected with social mobility, which implies people's moving physically but even more mentally. Social mobilisation normally starts from the centre of a society and spreads outwards to the periphery. There is some evidence that the dissemination of sporting activities follows a similar pattern (see e.g. Heikkinen1981, pp 6–11, 23–57). Thus one may presume that sports have a role to play in the mobilisation of peripheries to new awareness and hence in social development. The mobilisation hypothesis is also supported by the rather high positive correlations between the Olympic success and the level of education and intensity of mass communication in the country (Levine 1974, pp 356–358).

Social mobilisation helps in tapping the human resources in a new nation and hence provides human "material" for sporting successes. These successes, mostly achieved by individual persons, become almost symbolic of the nation, which is thus raised to the same level as other nations or "run onto the world map". International sporting achievements are especially important when a nation is either struggling for her independence or consolidating it. As examples one may refer to the national importance of the Olympic medals achieved by the Finnish athletes in Stockholm in 1912 - and even in the Olympics of 1920 and 1924 - or by the Kenyan and Ethiopian runners in the course of the 1960s and the 1970s (see Toohey and Warning 1981; Schumacher 1936). Competitive sports thus provide *national symbols*. It is no accident that the medal ceremonies at the Olympic games include the raising of national flags and the playing of the winner's national anthem. Obviously the use of these symbols is important for new nations and for their representatives - much more important than for the old, established nations. It is symptomatic that criticism of the nationalist character of the Olympic games and proposals to reform or denationalise them have mostly come from the old nations of the industrial world. They have experienced the paradox between nationalism and internationalism to be much more burning than, say, the present Third World countries (see Toohey and Warning 1981; Schumacher 1936).

Nation-building necessarily involves the drawing of boundaries vis-a-vis other political entities in the world. The demarcation of political entities, called nations, from each other not only gives rise to national consciousness, but also leads to the comparison of power differentials. These differentials are mostly based on material resources and on their utilisation. The demarcation of nation-states, however, also emphasises the need to show by various symbols the strength, vitality and significance of these constituent units (see Foltz 1981; Deutsch 1953). Boundaries stress competition in political as well as in sporting terms. Sporting successes are visible and easy to quantify. That is why the counting of the medals and points of each national team is the most natural exercise in, for instance, the Olympic Games. They are a manifestation, by another means, of the political competition between nations. In criticising nationalism in sport it has to be recalled that it is a relatively harmless and peaceful form of political competition, even though it is based on the *discriminating function* of sport between winners and losers, on sporting competition as a test which is resolved in favour of the person with the highest overall performance capacity (see Heinilä 1963).

Differentials in Olympic Success

Olympic success, which can be measured both in absolute terms and in relative terms (taking into account population size), has been explained in a number of ways. All of these explanations start from the notion of resources which are assumed to contribute in the competition between nations to a successful outcome. These resources, i.e. the independent variable, are conceptualised, however, in different ways. Some scholars consider economic and population resources to be most significant because they provide a pool from which talented individuals can be drawn. Others tend to think that the character of the political system is the most crucial one as it defines the capability of a nation to utilise her pool of resources. This approach is closely related to the idea that the levels of social mobility and social equality within a country are, after all, the central determinants of sporting success. Finally, somewhat more individualistic is the assumption that performance motivation, which can be operationalised by the religious attitude, is a major driving force behind sporting success. In fact this view is heavily stressed in Eric Liddell's figure in a recent film, *Chariots of Fire.*

Without trying to resolve all the intricacies that are involved in the measurement of Olympic success and in its explanation, I will try to indicate some broad conclusions which pertain to sports as a manifestation of international competition. Practically all the relevant studies come to the conclusion that bigger nations, in terms of area, population and economic size, win more Olympic medals than smaller countries. Large population and area are positively associated with Olympic achievements, though there are also contrary findings. More important are obviously large economic resources and a high level of development, measured by Gross Domestic Product on an absolute as well as on a per capita basis (*Levine* 1974, pp 364–356; Ball 1972; Kiviaho and Mäkelä 1978). Thus Olympic success is distributed roughly in the same manner as any other rewards in the international system: the top echelon receives most of them, and those towards the bottom are able to capture them only occasionally. This tends to increase the relative value of Olympic medals for smaller and poorer nations and to convert them into signs of competence and vitality.

Mere economic size and level of development are not, however, sufficient in accounting for the distribution of Olympic success. Not all relatively big and rich nations succeed in the Olympic Games. There must therefore be additional factors that regulate the diversion of economic and social resources for sporting achievements. One such factor, which is obviously connected with the level of economic development, is the level of social mobilisation, which generates the attention and the human potential to promote competitive sports. A related factor is social equality, as it tends to remove the differential access to sport and hence to push it forward. There is indeed evidence that urbanisation, mass communication and literacy as well as social equality and homogeneity are positively associated with success in sports (see e.g. Ball 1972, pp 195-196; Colwell 1981 pp. 245-246).

Economic development and social mobilisation are, however, the opposite sides of the same coin, and hence "true" additional explanations must be sought from other directions. It is often claimed that a socialist political system is better able - because of its more centralised, effective and goal-conscious steering system - to divert economic and social resources to sporting achievements. Most of the studies indeed show that socialist countries collect more Olympic medals than countries with other types of political and economic systems. This can be further elaborated by observing that in socialist as well as in Third World countries Olympic success is linked with the high level of education and social mobilisation, while in Western countries the overall pool of population and economic resources is the most important determinant of the success. As far as political systems are concerned, achievements in competitive sports are related to the lack of institutional political competition (Ball 1972, pp 196–197; Colwell 1981, pp 245–246). This means, all in all, that in market economies a kind of liberal model is valid; the overall resource endowment defines the limits of Olympic success, which is only partly dependent on the central societal steering of sports. In socialist countries the promotion of sports is much more goal-conscious, as Olympic and other sporting successes are important evidence, both internally and externally, of the legitimacy and competence of the prevailing social system. Roughly in the same manner sports are more goal-conscious in new nations, where they have a role in promoting nation-building. Thus economic resources are only a necessary but not a sufficient explanation of sporting achievements. Some authors have taken a similar point of departure and argued that the explanation must be complemented by religious motives favouring inner-worldly ascetism which is characteristic in particular of Protestants and Catholics. It can indeed be shown that Protestant and Catholic countries succeed better in the Olympic Games than countries confessing other religions, though the authors have to recognise that socialism is the superior "religion" in this respect (see Seppänen 1970, 1981). The religious explanation resembles the analogy between athlete and monk; both have to learn to sacrifice individual glory for the good of the whole, for this is also an integral ingredient of the sports creed (Lipsky 1979). The religious explanation is, however, fairly weak if compared with the explanation based on economic and other material factors (Kiviaho and Mäkelä 1978). It should not, however, be dismissed but rather qualified. The Protestant ethos, which Max Weber postulated was connected with the rising "spirit of capitalism", was apparently important in earlier times in mobilising human resources for competitive sports. This ethos was, furthermore, combined with the needs of rising nationalism and nation-building, which were more prevalent in Europe of the early twentieth century than they are today. The declining importance of "inner-worldly ascetism" as an explanation for Olympic success testifies to the validity of this conclusion (Seppänen 1970 pp. 11-16).

Olympic success is largely explained by the overall resource endowment of a country and the determination to allocate these resources to competitive sports in order to promote national goals and interests in international fora. Olympic medals are a means of communicating both to the domestic and international audience that the country is in a healthy condition and capable of fulfilling its commitments. They are also a means by which the small can occasionally show to the large that the international authority structure can in certain dimensions be broken down. Success in competitive sports has primarily a symbolic value vis-a-vis other members of the international community. From this perspective *internationalism in sports* is inevitable: without international contacts and exchange, national as well as individual goals could not be promoted. Any description of internationalism without paying attention to the national interests involved is patently false. Only the consideration of the national factors involved enables internationalism to reveal its true face, which may not be so ugly after all.

References

Ball DW (1972) Olympic Games competition: structural correlates of national success. Int J Comparative Sociology 13 (3-4):186-200

Colwell J (1981) Sociocultural determinants of Olympic success. In: Segrave J, Chu D (eds) Olympism. Stipes, Champaign, pp 245-246, 254-256

Deutsch KW (1953) Nationalism and social communication. An inquiry into the foundations of nationalism. M. I. T. Press, Boston

Enquist P-O (1972) Släggan (Hammer). Stockholm

Foltz WJ (1981) Modernization and nation-building: the social mobilization model reconsidered. In: Merritt RL, Russett BM (eds) From national development to global community. Essays in honor of Karl W. Deutsch. Allen and Unwin, Boston, pp 25-45

Heikkinen A (1981) Kansallisurheilun suuri nousu. Suomen hiihtourheilun laajuus, yhteiskunnalliset tavoitteet ja merkitys 1918-1940. (The great rise of the national sport. The extent, social goals and significance of the skiing sports in Finland, 1918-1940.) Liikuntiateellinen Seura, Lappeenranta

Heinilä K (1963) Kilpaurheilun teoria. (Theory of competitive sports.) Helsingin yliopisto. Sosiologian laitos. Tutkimuksia 33

Kiviaho P, Mäkelä P (1978) Olympic success: a sum of non-material and material factors. Int Rev Sport Sociology 13 (2):5-22

Lasch C (1978) The culture of narcism: American life in an age of expectations. Norton, New York

Levine N (1974) Why do countries win Olympic medals? Some structural correlates of Olympic Games success: 1972. Sociology and Social Research 58 (4):356-358

Lipsky R (1979) Political implications of sports teams symbolism. Politics and Society 9 (1):61-88

Natan A (1969) Sport and politics. In: Loy JW Jr, Kenyon GS (eds) Sport, culture and society. Macmillan, New York, pp 203-210

Reiter R (ed) (1976) Sport in der Bundeswehr. Offene Worte, Herford

Schumacher J (1936) Die Finnen, das große Sportvolk. Limpert, Berlin

Seppänen P (1970) The role of competitive sports in different societies. Institute of Sociology. University of Helsinki, Research Reports 151

Seppänen P (1981) Olympic success: a cross-national perspective. In: Lüschen GR, Sage GH (eds) Handbook of social sciences of sport. Stipes, Champaign, Ill., pp 93-118

Ström L-I (1977) Idrott och politik. Idrottsrörelsens politiska roll i Tredje riket, DDR och Förbundsrepubliken. (Sport and politics. The political role of sports movements in the Third Reich, GDR and the Federal Republik of Germany.) Rabén & Sjogren, Uppsala

Tappert J, Jodl H (1973) Körperertüchtigung und Sport für die sozialistische Landesverteidigung. Militärverlag der DDR, Berlin, pp 7-11
Toohey DP, Warning K (1981) Nationalism: inevitable and incurable. In: Segrave J, Chu D (eds) Olympism. Stipes, Champaign, Ill., pp 118-126

Possibilities of Understanding Modern Sport on the Basis of Aristotelian Theory

K. Kirsch and I. Schüssler

Introductory Remarks

Why start from Aristotle when considering the extent and content of international co-operation in modern sport? The answer is that Aristotle (and Plato) must be regarded as the founders of the European way of thinking (and also of the American way of thinking which, as is generally accepted, stems from the European). It is only with knowledge of the basic structure of European philosophy as a whole - which has always remained the same even though the contents have become more complicated (as in the case of Hegel for instance) - that we are really in a position to enter into a fruitful dialogue with the philosophical conceptions of other cultures. But if Aristotle (and Plato) are a key to this very European tradition, which determines our own way of thinking even today and which they were the first to elaborate, then the modern sports movement and the appropriate concept of it is to be found within this intellectual unity of European philosophy, too. Thus the question of international understanding concerning problems of modern sport attains a deeper sense.

When not only discussing sport scientifically but philosophizing about it through a world-wide perspective - which is in line with the objectives of this congress - a true and contemporary understanding of modern sport can be developed only from this origin of the history of philosophy. To proceed otherwise involves a danger of becoming separated from one's own tradition and thus at the same time of losing a way of thinking which determines one's own self. Only on this firm basis, on which we all still stand today (though often without realizing it), can philosophical elaborations on sport be attempted which start from classical philosophical thought - in our case from that of the Greek philosophers, but one could also proceed from German idealism or even from the post-metaphysical thinking of a Martin Heidegger - and which vie with this thought on the same level.

Concepts of Mass Sport and Top-Class Competitive Sport

In modern times there has been growing concern at the dominant role played by top-class competitive sport in the assessment of general sporting performance. This is underlined amongst other things by the discussion surrounding mass sport, a discussion which is aimed at conceptualising mass sport. The problem here, however, is that there is a lack of appropriate terms since mass sport itself is considerably influenced by top-class competitive sport. The notion of top-class competitive sport is also reflected in the terminology associated with mass sport and thus prevents mass sport from developing as an independent concept. Even international athletes feel that there is a further aspect to their sporting activity, one which they find difficult to define. They usually describe it as the elevating nature of sporting activity, but critics of modern, performance-orientated sport - especially of top-class competitive sport - dispute this.

It is here that Aristotle provides us with a conceptual aid. According to his theories we can recognize a possibility of understanding sport which corresponds to man as a physically and organically determined being. This does not mean that this possibility can be realized for its own sake in the modern world. It could, however, serve as a critical corrective with regard to the tendency to orientate sporting activity towards top-class competitive sport, which is characterized to a large extent by the modern concept of performance.

The Force of Life

The possibility of understanding sport through Aristotle becomes apparent when we think more deeply about his concept of 'life' and the force of life as laid down in *De Anima* (Ross 1974), one of his later treatises. In this case, however, the word 'anima' in Latin has nothing to do with the modern psychological concept, but refers to the life of all living things, to their state of being alive.

In an initial attempt Aristotle defines 'life' in general as follows (see the first chapter of the second book of *De Anima):* "What we call life is feeding, growing and atrophying in a self-contained process." Feeding, in other words, is the basic feature of life. It takes place in a dual movement: Outwardly towards a possible source of food and inwardly back to the organ itself. Yet this takes place in a self-contained process. And these processes are the living thing itself. They are its own organs, the organs in which the living thing itself lives. If these organs have the possibility, so to speak, of having life, the force of life itself is the realization of what the organs themselves are capable of and destined for.

But Aristotle defines the force of life not only through the term 'reality' but also and primarily through the term 'entelechy', a word which can only be circumscribed: When something appears in the full splendour of its very essence and, in an open vision, shows what it is and what it is capable of being purely through itself ('eidos'), it enters a state of fulfilment and contentment in which it assumes a concrete form. Maintaining this state is what Aristotle calls 'entelechy'. This means that when an organ manifests itself in the force of life, which through itself it is capable of and is destined for - in other words: generates this force of life -, the force of life is its 'entelechy'. It is the plastic, complete phenomenon of what exists like a seed within the organ itself. Thus according to Aristotle an initial definition of life is that life is the force of life and this is "entelechy of a body of this kind"; in other words: entelechy of an organic body which through itself is capable of and suitable for the force of life.

We must, however, differentiate between the various stages of the presence of the force of life: While sleeping the force of life is only present in a reduced and inconspicuous form (breathing, obtaining nutrients like oxygen, nitrogen etc.). The force of life only achieves its full fulfilment when the living thing awakes and in this awake state stands in an open relation to its environment. But this more intensified force of life when awake is only possible on the basis of and through the prerequisite of the force of life, which also occurs during sleep. The former is thus the First Entelechy, the latter is the Second Entelechy. According to its general, full definition, therefore, 'life' is the "First Entelechy of a natural body, which has the possibility of having life". This, however, shows that the force of life as entelechy is basically capable of intensifying and heightening. The more the open, plastic presence of the force of life intensifies and heightens, the more a living thing attains its fulfilment and contentment. For this reason the Second Entelechy, although it originates later than the first, is superior to it with regard to quality of being.

Now modern sport is also a kind of the organic-physical force of life - namely movement towards something else by the organic human body as a whole. As such it is not the reduced life movement of the First Entelechy but the force of life of the Second Entelechy which especially appears in the open phenomenon. In sport, however, the force of life is intensified once again, something which man alone is capable of. For man is not only open to his life through his senses (like animals) but also through his mind. He is therefore capable of distinguishing the eidos of life as such. And for this reason the human body is also capable of representing the eidos of the force of life in such a way that this not only becomes present (First Entelechy) and openly shows itself in its presence (Second Entelechy) but is especially emphasized in the Second Entelechy. This very thing occurs in sport. The sporting force of life therefore would not only be the open presence of the force of life, i.e. Second Entelechy, but the specially emphasized open presence of the force of life, i.e. an even more intensified Second Entelechy. As such it would be a supreme presence of the force of life of the organic human body. The organic human body portrays the plastic form of life in its greatest evidence in the sporting force of life. From Aristotle's point of view sport would be the specially emphasized phenomenon of the force of life of the organic human body. In sport the organic human body reveals itself as the phenomenon to which as a (natural) body it is especially suitable.

Sport in Aristotle's View

In this way a concept of sport is outlined which can only be seen from Aristotle's perspective. According to this concept sport stems from the 'physis', the nature of the human body itself, i.e. from the way it is of itself. But man cannot detach himself from his own body. The body is the natural thing in man and as such man has always to deal with it and at the same time to bear responsibility for it - even in a highly technological world like ours. For this reason this possibility of understanding sport will always manifest itself and therefore has to be taken into consideration time and again even in modern sport - without being able today to be the determining reality.

But modern sport, too, which is fascinated to a large extent by the quantitative maximisation of performance, can be formulated on the basis of Aristotelian theory and his concept of intensifiable entelechy. Thus Aristotle could be a key to defining not only the natural concept, as described already, but also the modern performance-orientated concept of sport. Taking Aristotle's ideas then, the possibility presents itself that the measure and limit concept can give way to the capability of intensification of the entelechy itself. Because if entelechy according to Aristotle is characterized at all by a capability to intensify, then it is possible that the intensification of the eidos and its limit is overcome and, in the absence of any fixed aim of limit, becomes its own sole aim. The entelechy is released into its own, pure capability of intensifying. Ths sporting force of life then has its aim and therefore its meaning solely in the intensification of itself. Since it is no longer a question of the eidos and its appearance, there is no longer anything in the body that reveals itself through its own nature. This at least is no longer of prime importance. But if there is no longer anything in the body which naturally reveals itself in the being, then the reality of the entelechy which has been released into intensification must be created through extreme exertion out of nothing, so to speak. In other words: the entelechy must be created as a counter to nothingness. This means that it must be achieved. The essence of this entelechy exists in the achievement of being. Consequently it appears that modern sport is subordinate to the "achievement or performance principle".

This change in the entelechy, however, also has an effect on the body itself as far as its suitability character has to be adapted to the character of the entelechy. In Aristotle's view the body was adapted to the eidetically determined entelechy: it was the organ that was prepared and suitable for the presence of the eidos (of life). With regard to the entelechy released into the capacity to intensify, the body, too, is adjusted to its pure intensification: it becomes a "potentia", a "potential" of physical energy, an "energy potential" which is basically capable of intensifying. As such it does not exist in nature. In the same way the entelechy for its part is still only created by achievement, the body as a whole has to be specially taken together with the potentials of physical energy which it embraces: This means not only the potentials which become effective by themselves, but also those which lie within the range of the "physiological reserves connected with free will" and indeed finally within the range of the "autonomously protected reserves", which are only mobilized when life is in danger.

Discussion

On the basis of the above, it is possible to cast light on the modern problem of doping. Doping is "... the unphysiological attempt to intensify the performance capacity of an athlete by applying (taking, injecting or administering) a doping substance..." (see official definition of the West German National Sports Federation and that of the International Olympic Committee; Donike and Kaiser 1980, p 76).

Let us consider the problem of doping on the basis of the dual understanding of modern sport as developed from Aristotelian theory. With regard to the natural-organic possibility of understanding modern sport, the body, seen as an organism, manifests itself of its own accord in the appearance of the eidos, which is contained in it like a seed. An intensification of the suitability character of the body which creates its entelechy in the sporting movement in the full splendour of its very essence can only be of a nature in which it helps the body to show itself purely through itself in an open vision. It is care and cultivation of what the body is capable of through its own nature. This means that all possibilities of intensifying the organic suitability character through "technical" (= externally applied) means are excluded. For they would, according to Aristotle, miss the (natural) organic character of the body. What can only be regarded as a means here has to be of such a nature that finally it always remains up to the body – both definitively and initially – to manifest itself of its own accord. This could be what is also implied today in the notion of the "physiological intensification of achievement". Recently, as is well known, the assembly of delegates of the Swiss National Sports Federation took a fundamental decision against all pharmacological and medical influences in top-class competitive sport. It has even imposed sanctions on these condemned influences and has also called for measures so that it will be possible to "enter again into competition from the sole valid platform – physiologically intensified sporting performance" (Sport-Informationsdienst 1977). This demand, which itself is not substantiated any further, may arise from many and also varied motives (for example from the moral and legal motive of what is known as "clean sport"); it may also reflect, however, the Aristotelian concept of the 'physis' of the human body. On the other hand an "unphysiological" intensification of achievement, in the sense of doping, would have been inconceivable for Aristotle. It lies beyond his intellectual horizon, for it would offend against the essence of the organs as such, which consists in the "physis", in their emerging from themselves.

It is another thing to consider the problem of doping from the modern, so-called performance-orientated understanding of sport, which can be outlined starting from Aristotle, but only in certain initial respects. Here, too, the body is determined through its suitability character: The only thing it is still suitable for is to manifest itself through performance in the intensifiable and quantitatively measurable fulfilment of the movement of life. To achieve this it is necessary for the body itself as a whole to gather itself together towards the energy reserves enclosed in its organs; this, however, is not left solely to the individual will, but has to be guaranteed by the methodical intervention of science and technology. Now since the sole purpose of the achievement of the body is intensification, the body as an energy potential has always to be intensified, too. Indeed, this intensification can be and is also achieved initially and usually through a purely "physiological intensification of achievement", which, of course, is methodically controlled by science and technology, because the body is the energy potential to be secured. Science and technology mobilize the "physiological reserves that can be released by the will" and make them available. But since the body is also primarily the energy potential in the "physiological intensification of achievement", which still has to be methodically guaranteed by science and technology, in the final analysis this approach itself, too, already presents the possibility of guaranteeing the intensification of the energy potentia 'body' "unphysiologically". This, of course, is what happens in doping. Through technical manipulation doping methodically demands from the organs those energies which lie within the range of the "autonomously protected reserves" and which are set free naturally only by affect (for example, a danger to life). But through this doping merely realizes a tendency which is the fundamental element of the modern concept of the body. For the (energy potential) body is released solely into intensification of its 'potentia'. Yet even doping faces a barrier, for on the one hand it is motivated by the intensification of the energies of the body, but it moves at the same time within the danger area of the mobilisation of the last reserves of the body. Doping, therefore, also has always to avoid injuring the organs, not to mention destroying them. It must continually keep them available for further intensification. Since this can only be ascertained by empirical facts, the barriers of the possible application of doping will always be fluid. They depend not least on the standard of modern science and technology. Therefore, doping by its very nature will be a subject of controversy time and again. However, this controversy will occur solely within the intellectual horizon of the modern, perfomance-orientated understanding of sport, without the Aristotelian concept of the 'physis' being brought into consideration.

Our reflections proceeding from Aristotle have tried to show that modern man still remains bound and responsible to his own body as nature in himself. Therefore, the organic and natural understanding of the body will always co-determine his consciousness - no matter how much it is pushed to one side. This is the reason why the Aristotelian concept of the body is capable of being a critical corrective in understanding modern sport, not by simply being taken over but by becoming the basis of a new philosophical appreciation of the reality of what we call modern sport.

My discourse has been an attempt to pave the way for this new approach.

References

Donike M, Kaiser C (1980) Dopingkontrollen. Bundesinstitut für Sportwissenschaft, Köln, pp 76–81

Ross WD (ed) (1974) Aristoteles: De Anima. Recognovit... Oxford University Press

Sport-Informationsdienst (SID) (1977) Radikales Verbot pharmakologisch-medizinischer Beeinflussung in der Schweiz: „Nun müssen wir auch glaubwürdig handeln". In: Frankfurter Allgemeine Zeitung 260, p 21

Theiler W (1979) Über die Seele. Akademie-Verlag, Berlin/Ost 1979

Volkmann-Schluck K-H (1979) Die Metaphysik des Aristoteles. Verlag Vittorio Klostermann, Frankfurt am Main, pp 233–258

The Social Significance of International Sporting Activity

N. Petrova

Introduction

The genesis and the specifities of the historical development of international sporting activity are based above all on the progress within nations in respect of economics, education and culture, and are influenced by definite social, political and cultural necessities. By its nature, sport is a social activity of people and is dependent on the development of human society. Undoubtedly, the initial beginnings of international sport were the national systems of physical education and the English system of sport, which represented the first model of modern sport.

A very important prerequisite for the promotion of international sporting activity is the existence, as a social organisation, of institutionalised sporting activity in many countries. Its appearance and progress have significant consequences for the development of physical education and sport.

The Main Social Functions of International Sporting Activity

We regard international sporting activity as a polyfunctional system, which is interrelated with many other systems, such as the sporting activity in different countries, the international Olympic movement and the work of national federations.

In the literature (Savranski 1979), the following three functions of sport are pointed out as being of greatest importance: informative, communicative and governing. These functions and also the fostering of peace and understanding among peoples, are decisive factors for the existence of international sporting activity.

The Informative Function. The informative function of international sporting activity involves the exchange of knowledge about the development of physical culture and the different kinds of sport in all the countries of the world. Thus this function plays an enormous cognitive role, facilitating insight into a variety of sporting problems through exchange of experience.

The Communicative Function. The communicative function of international sporting activity concerns the links formed between people of different race, religion and political views, and their uniting on the basic of unanimous acceptance of the necessity of the systematic sporting activities and their organisation under competitive conditions. The communication achieved through sporting activity provides people with a great deal of information, with the help of which "time, space, social, national and linguistic barriers are overcome" (Popov 1979). During international events everyone gives something and, in turn, receives something, reaching mutual understanding to a greater or lesser degree. When we speak about the communicative function of international sporting activity, we do not have in mind only competition itself, but also the planning of sport, including the work of national and international governing bodies and the mass media. International sporting activity is one of the main channels that ensure exchange of different countries, experience concerning methods and forms of physical exercise and sport; it thus constitutes a practical pedagogic process. We have good reason to point out the great contribution made by international sporting activity to physical culture as a special branch of the general common culture of mankind.

The Governing Function. The governing function of international sporting activity is closely connected with the informative and the communicative functions. The main purpose of the governing function is to increase the effectiveness of physical education and sport through international sporting activity.

Other Functions. The ideological and educational function of international sporting activity is very important, being based on the ideological character of separate phenomena and their influence on the formation of views on life in accordance with different social groups. One can also speak of an adaptive function of international sporting activity, with a view to its contribution to human adaption to social environment.

It can be accepted that international sporting activity realises its social function in two ways (Popov 1979). The first concerns the interrelation between society as a collective body of activity (offering opportunities for physical exercise and sport in suitable surroundings) and separate individuals. The second concerns the interrelation between individuals in their actions to achieve socially important purposes (such as universal physical perfection and the progressive development of physical qualities) and locomotive habits, which are vitally necessary for the practical life of people.

The interdependence between material and spiritual culture helps the development of international sporting activity. From a sociological point of view, the material culture of society affords an opportunity for devoting much more time to rest, which is a very important condition for the development of spiritual culture and for separation of physical and mental labour. In this way, more people realise the necessity of physical exercise and sport and the great moral and emotional effect of a competitive event. If a harmoniously developed person is a purpose of society, international sporting activity contributes to this purpose.

Conclusions

International sporting activity makes possible a valuable exchange of information concerning health care and the physical perfection of man. It acquaints us with the ideological and moral climate of historical periods of peoples' development, being an activity with the aim of realising the main purposes of physical culture in society.

Consequently, international sporting activity is human activity for which are valid the specific characteristics of culture such as activity, social meaning and reformation character (Bogoljubova 1979). It helps to improve common culture, creating definite spiritual values and thus increasing social awareness.

International sporting activity is a branch of physical culture, which in its turn is a part of common culture. Sport is a specific kind of activity with an influence over man's biosocial nature (Savranski 1979), developing both his physical and psychological condition and ensuring association with other people.

International sporting activity has its practical aspect as a part of physical culture. Thanks to international sporting activity, society is enriched materially: In order to meet the needs of sporting activity, stadia which are very interesting architecturally are built, bearing the features of the historical period. Specific facilities are made available for competitive events, and unique appliances are constructed in order to control and direct training, etc.

A great number of national and international federations and unions organise sporting activity. The activity of the International Olympic Committee and the National Olympic Committees is of particular importance. The progress of physical culture and sport in social life is determined by:

1. The ability to study the inheritance of the past and the experience of the advanced countries with regard to mass physical activities and sport.
2. The enrichment of physical education through new ideas and methods.
3. The contribution made by sport to the realisation of the most human ideals of mankind (including the desire for a stable peace in the world) and to international understanding.
4. The optimal usage of all advantages of physical culture and sport for the puposes of harmonious development of all members of society.

References

Bogoljubova E (1979) Culture and society. Moscow
Goncharenko NV (1980) Spiritual culture. Naukova dumka, Kiev
Markarjan O (1973) The genesis of human activity and culture. AH Erevan
Popov K (1979) Culture. Narodna mladej, Sofia
Savranski I (1979) Communicative and aesthetic functions of culture. Nauka, Moscow

2. The Role of Sport in International Politics

Sport in Europe and the Helsinki Agreements

O.Milshtein

Introduction

It is highly symbolic that the present congress on "Sport and International Understanding" is being held in a place which is so historic for the nations of Europe and the whole world - Finlandia Hall, where 7 years ago, on 1 August 1975, the Final Act of the Helsinki Conference was signed. That document has entered the annals of history as the Charter of Peaceful Coexistence and Co-operation. The ten principles of that document established a programme of development and strengthening of peace in the whole world through a bolstering of détente and international understanding.

The role of the agreements reached in Helsinki, to which were affixed the signature of the heads of 33 European states, the USA and Canada, is particularly timely in our days when the reactionary forces of the world are again seeking to exacerbate the world situation, to push the nations of Europe, the nations of the whole world to the brink of a nuclear catastrophe.

Against this background, it is deeply symbolic and very timely that this international congress is being held here today on the theme "Sport and International Understanding". The organisers of the congress, our colleagues, are workers in the area of physical culture and sport in Finland, representatives of sport science and public figures from international and national sports organisations of Europe and the whole world; all of us who are participating in this congress are, as it were, summing up the experiences of the last 7 years. We are endeavouring to generalise that enormous experience of social dealings and scientific theory which in practise will achieve the goal of strengthening peace through sport in working towards the realisation of the Helsinki agreements. It is no accident that the tasks of our congress are "The Scientific Analysis of the Role of Physical Culture and Sport in Developing International Understanding and also the Contribution of Scientific Studies in the Given Field", and the working out of new paths "Towards Removing Obstacles and Strengthening the Positive Aspects of International Sporting Activity."

On the basis of the experience and activity of national and international sports organisations, an analysis of the measures carried out within the framework of international co-operation during recent years in Europe, an analysis of the social practice and functioning of the system of mass media and mass communications in sport, an analysis of the data of concrete, sociological studies, statistical indexes and the results of our own studies, we have set ourselves an undertaking - to show the social mechanism of international co-operation in sport and its social consequences. Hence, the perspective of the paper: a sociological treatment.

Consequences of the Helsinki Agreement

When speaking of the social consequences for sporting co-operation of the Helsinki agreements, there is reason to recall the fundamental provisions of the Final Act of the Conference on Security and Co-operation in Europe (Izvestia 1975).

The Helsinki agreements established the fundamental principles of peaceful co-operation and coexistence between the states of Europe and indeed the whole world. These are the principles of the sovereign equalitity of states and their sovereign rights, including the right to freely choose and develop their social, political, economic and cultural systems, including, of course, the systems of the physical culture and sports movement. This completely excludes the use of force or coercive threats, the violation of frontiers; and it means the territorial integrity of states, the peaceful settlement of disputes, the non-interference in the affairs of other parties, the respecting of human rights and fundamental freedoms. This includes the freedom and right of every citizen to attain spiritual and physical perfection, to take part in physical culture and sports. Finally, this means the equality and right of peoples to decide their own destiny, co-operation between states and good-neighbourly fulfilment of international legal obligations. In this case, too, sport acts as an important factor in strengthening these principles within the domain of contemporary international relations. We are not inclined to overrate its role in these processes and to raise it to the level of a panacea. It would be naive to assume that sport is a kind of universal lock-pick for the solution of all social problems. On the other hand, however, there is no reason not to see the objective reality of the social consequences of sport which are fulfilled by sport in society. The proof of this assertion is the genesis of sport as a social phenomenon, its universal history and ultimately the entire history of social development.

In its very essence sport is a fundamental factor contributing to peace, friendship and understanding. Its development and functioning are not possible without the peaceful coexistence of states, without their co-operation; on the other hand, sport strengthens, develops and enriches co-operation and mutual understanding between the peoples of different countries and nations, states and societies. Even where it leads to conflicts, to unsolved contradictions, this as a rule is a corruption of its humanistic nature, a breakdown of the manifestation of its social functions, which leads to dysfunctions.

The Olympic Movement and International Understanding

The dual dialectical process of interrelationships and interconnections between the peaceful development of sport and society is determined by the complex of political, economic and socio-cultural factors. this has been reflected in a number of fundamental documents of the international sports movement. Thus, in the section of the Olympic Charter entitled "General Principles" it is stated that amongst the goals of the Olympic movement are:

"- the upbringing of youth with the aid of sport in the spirit of understanding and friendship, which will promote the creation of a better and more tranquil world;
- the spreading throughout the whole world of the Olympic principles for the creation of goodwill amongst nations" (Olympic Charter 1980).

The Tenth Olympic Congress (1973), which in the manner of preceding congresses took place in Europe under the motto "sport in the service of peace", addressed and appealed to all the world's sport enthusiasts. This was an appeal to the youth of all countries to carry high the Olympic ideals, an indissoluble part of which are friendship and peace. This appeal contained a reminder of the fact that "The Olympic Games are intended not only for Olympic athletes: they spread the principles and spirit of friendly games between the youth of the whole world, thus creating in international life an atmosphere of trust and good will which lead to the strengthening of peace throughout the world" (Sovietsky Sport 1975). One of the most important conclusions of the tripartite commision of the congress states: "The Congress has demonstrated the goodwill of all participants in wishing to co-operate under the motto 'Sport in the Service of Peace'".

This spirit inspired all the subsequent actions of the International Olympic Committee (IOC), of the progressive majority of international Olympic sports committees, of the sports leaders of the majority of countries of Europe and the world.

A striking affirmation of this peace-loving tendency was the holding on the highest level of the 22nd Olympic Games in 1980 in Moscow; the total failure of the policy of boycotting the Games, which was launched by reactionary forces; the sharp criticism of the commercialisation and professionalsation of sport, of all manner of discrimination in sport and the interference of reactionary policies in sport; the criticism of the attempts to do away with the Olympic rituals (the raising of the national flag, the playing of the national anthem etc.); the banning of doping, bioloigcal substances and other medical preparations in sports practice; the demand that athletes strengthen their role in the solution of the most important problems of the day facing the Olympic and world sports movement - these and other fundamental problems of international sport were the leitmotif of the 11th Olympic Congress held in Baden-Baden in 1981.

The entire work of the congress, its agenda, the representative spread of its participants [it bears reminding that for the first time the participants included many of the world's leading trainers and athletes, and there was strong representation by UNESCO, ICSPE (International Council of Sport and Physical Education), the UNESCO Inter-governmental Committee on Physical Education and Sport and other organisations] and the wide, democratic discussion and its treatment in the world's press, on radio and on television demonstrated the indisputable excellence of the realistic policy of the IOC and other organizations that are responsible for the destiny of sport and the sporting world, for the future of the Olympic Games and the Olympic movement. Indeed, in addition to the 1000 participants at the congress, 500 representatives of the mass media were in attendance.

In our opinion, it was at the Baden-Baden Olympic Congress that the most concrete and constructive statement was heard of the fundamental problems which are envisaged also by the framework of our session today. It was at this forum that wide discussion was given to the measures and principles of present and future sporting co-operation for promoting or hindering international understanding.

Mr. S. P. Pavlov, the representative of the USSR Sport Committee and the National Olympic Committee of the USSR, who was one of the first speakers and whose paper set the tone, expressed the opinion of the entire multimillion army of Soviet physical culture and sports enthusiasts when he said:

> Sport and the Olympic movment are not enclosed in an ivory tower. They develop along with other areas of life, are subject to their influence and in their own turn they themselves are capable of influencing these areas. Wheter we recognize this logically or intuitively, it is an incontestable fact that the problem "the future of the Olympic Games" has arisen not only among the rank and file of athletes, rather, in the context of many other problems it is an objective reflection of the contemporary stage of human life faced with disquieting perspectives.
> From this fact, which in our opinion is incontestable, it is possible to draw the conclusion that in seeking a solution to the problem of the future of the Games, it is necessary to make use not only of specific, technical, sports-oriented methods but also of those methods which are universal and have been proved reliable in other spheres of life. (Pavlov 1981)

The speaker went on to enumerate a number of important theoretical questions and practical conclusions which derive from the experience of the Soviet physical culture movement and from the practice of the international sporting co-operation of countries with a different socio-political system and with a different ideology. Amongst these are the following:

- Will the Games be transformed into an arena of political struggle or, as was demonstrated by the recent Olympic events, will they make an important contribution to understanding and co-operation between peoples?
- Will the Games remain a bright and colourful pageant which every 4 years magnetises the attention of the whole world or will they, being scattering around the world, be transformed into a series of ordinary championships?
- Will the Games retain their amateur character, that high spirit which mankind has borne down through the millenia, or will they become the same kind of uninspired commercial happening as various kinds of professional sport shows?
- Will the Games be the standard of fairness, nobility and justice and a demonstration of the best physical and moral qualities of the world's youth or will they, falling prey to people having no conception of humanism, morals and ethics, become an arena for anti-human and pseudomedical experiments on people, a bazaar for those who see in sport only a means of making a profit?
- Must we go along the path of the so-called denationalisation of the games or will we, having respect for the national work of athletes, of the many millions of sports amateurs, conserve the rituals of the Games?

The speaker then went on to give an accurate and constructive answer to each of these questions. Concerning the last point, I should like to recall the opinion of the Olympic athletes, expressed on their behalf by Vladislav Tretyak, Sebastian Coe and others. In particular, Sebastian Coe stated: "athletes wish to conserve the traditions of the Olympic ceremony..." (Coe 1981)

Sporting Competitions and Other Acitivities for Peace

These brief excerpts from the wide review of the Olympic Congress and the majority of interventions of the other delegates speak in favour of the progressive tendencies in the field of world co-operation in contemporary sport. This is attested by the existing forms of this co-operation which have been worked out in Europe in recent years.

First, there has evolved a multi-faceted and fruitful system of international sporting connections which embraces the majority of the countries of the world. Let us remember that today the IOC unites 150 national Olympic committees and, for example, the federation of light athletics comprises 168 countries! In Europe alone, in addition to championships, thousands of tournaments, play-offs of different regional, institutional, national and memorial cups, memorial prizes, multilateral and bilateral matches and comradely meetings are held every year in almost 50 kinds of sport. Many of these events take place under special mottos in defence of peace and friendship, e.g. the peace cycle race which is held annually on the roads of the GDR, Poland and Czechoslovakia. With each passing year this race draws an ever larger number of teams from the countries of our continent. No less popular have become the European yachting contests, held under the slogan "friendship", and the Friendship Cup for figure skating. Here, too, belong the competitions held within the framework of all-world festivals of youth and students, the festival of the peoples of the polar regions, Norway, Finland, Sweden and Soviet Union.

Many athletes and sports organisation of a number of European and other countries, acting in response to the urgent problems of the modern world and the appeals of the progressive organisations struggling for peace in the whole world, have dedicated numerous competitions to this cause. It is no coincidence that the World Peace Council, valuing these facts highly, has awarded Honorary Degrees to many sportsmen. We certainly must recall that the recent Relay for Peace, the baton of which was carried across the countries of Europe and which reached New York on 7 June, the day of the opening of the second special session of the UN Special Assembly on Disarmament, was lit with the holy fire of Olympia. The torch-bearers of this event were European athletes and physical culture enthusiasts, some outstanding and some rank and file. Quite a number of sportsmen took part in the recently held peace march which was directed against the decision of NATO to deploy nuclear missiles in Europe etc.

Secondly, international sporting contacts are not limited to purely sporting events but assume the most varied forms and organically constitute the cultural and scientific connections between countries. Here can be mentioned the organisation of festivals of sport films, various exhibitions, and scientific conferences and symposia on the problems of physical culture. It suffices to recall the pre-olympic scientific congresses of ICSPE in Munich in 1972, in Quebec in 1976 and in Tbilisi in 1980, the Moscow World Congress "Sport in Modern Society" in 1974 and a number of congresses in other countries.

Special mention should be made of the great contribution made to the solution of the problems we are examining by the European Sport Conference, which set the following goals:

- to make its own effective contribution to the cause of understanding, co-operation and friendship between peoples, irrespective of their race, religion or political convictions;
- to promote close contacts between national sports organizations and state sports institutions;
- to maintain exchanges of information in all fields of sports;
- to treat questions of general interest and work out proposals for the solution of questions of this nature;
- to promote the development of constructive co-operation and strengthening of sports contacts;

- to sum up relevant experiences and search for new paths leading to strengthening and developing co-operation. (Third European Sports Conference 1977).

The upshot of this work as well as the documents accepted at the last five conferences of leaders of sports organisations of the European countries (Vienna 1973, Dresden 1975, Copenhagen 1977, Berchtesgaden 1979, Warsaw 1981) points to the following:

The European sports conferences established the aims and paths for reaching constructive co-operation between sports organisations; they discussed current problems concerning the social responsibility of sport in the modern world, the connections between sport and environment, sport as a factor in upbringing and mutual understanding, sport as a factor in contacts between states and cultures etc.

The work of these conferences is invaluable also in the sense that they served as a basis for the convening in 1976 of the first international UNESCO Conference of Ministers and Senior Officials Responsible for Physical Education and Sport, a conference which drew participants from more than 100 countries of the world (First International Conference of Ministers and Senior Officials Responsible for Physical Education and Sport in the Education of Youth 1976). The results of the work of this conference were such major actions as the creation of a UNESCO intergovernmental committee for physical education and sport and the Charter of Physical Education and Sport.

Thirdly, a great contribution to European sporting co-operation is made by ENOC (the Union of European National Olympic Committees), ICSPE with its research committees and other subsections, and a number of other European associations and organisations.

The Soviet Union and its organisations, which are responsible for a number of the above-mentioned initiatives, in every way expands the practice of bilateral short-term and long-term agreements concerning co-operation between various countries of Europe and the world. Thus, at the present time the USSR pursues sporting contacts on the basis of long-term agreements with 26 countries of Europe and with three countries on the basis of protocols which are extended after 1 to 2 years. All in all, our country carries out sporting co-operation with 110 countries. Worthy of attention and study is the experience of sporting co-operation of the fraternal countries of socialism (Prokhorov 1978) and of countries in America, Africa, Asia and Australia, where a rich experience of international sporting co-operation is available. An analysis of this is to be found in the works of Lowe et al. (1980), McIntosh (1979), Mlodzikowski (1979) and other authors.

Fourthly, the mass media and the means of mass communication play a special role and bear a social responsibility for strengthening the principles of trust and good will in the sporting community of nation and states. It is no accident that this problem was discussed at all four of the most recent universal congresses on sports sciences as well as at a number of special conferences and seminars. Within the framework of ICSPE a special committee on "Sport, Mass Media and International Understanding" has been created; this committee has drafted a document bearing the same name. It is a moral and professional code for the world's sports journalists.

With the help of the mass media, sports become a means of enabling people to learn not only about results and achievements, about the victors and the vanquished, but also about the rules of competitions and the norms of sporting life, sporting ethics, the values of sport and man's potential. They also learn about social and political systems, about the way of life, ideology and culture of peoples, and about their customs and traditions. Herein lies the essence of international understanding through sport. Here is the central point of many social functions of contemporary sport. How objectively, justly, unbiasedly and competently those working in the mass media shed light on these events - on this depend public opinion, social attitude and social creation that are formed with the help of sport.

All readers will know well what an enormous flood of sports information cascades down on us daily through television, radio, cinema and the press. In our own country, the annual printing of the paper "Soviet Sport" amounts to 1200 million issues. In addition, sports papers are published at the republic level in the Ukrainian, Uzbek, Kazakhstani, Georgian, Azerbaijan, Litthuanian, Latvian, Estonian and Armenian languages, with a total print-run of 1,338,000 issues. In the USSR there are a total of 15 sports papers. Their printrun per issue amounts to more than 6 million copies. The result of sociological investigations show that more than 20 million persons read "Soviet Sport." Each issue is read through by 4 to 5 readers and this includes only the adult population (Vinogradov 1981).

Eighteen sports magazines with a print run of approximately 5 million copies are published in our country. Amongst them are *Physical Culture and Sport* (592,000), *Sport in the USSR, The Theory and Practice of Physical Culture* (16,000), *Football - Hockey* (1,050,000), *Light Athletics* (76,000), *Sporting Games* (160,000), *Chess in the USSR* (68,000), *Olympic Panorama* and others.

During the years of Soviet power, more than 30,000 books and brochures on questions of physical culture and sport have been published in the USSR. Their total print run amounts to 400,000,000 copies. Theres has been particular growth in the number of publications in connection with the preparation and hosting of the 22nd Olympic Games in Moscow - almost 20 million copies of more than 500 separate titles. In addition there is a considerable volume of materials in central, republic, district, town, regional and periodical publications. Today in the USSR there are more than 8000 papers, 5000 magazines and other publications having a total print run of 373 million copies.

Year after year there is an increase in the volume of broadcasts dedicated to physical culture and sport on the radio and television. This is what the growth in television programmes on our central television looks like: 1966 - 357 hours; 1971 - 565 hours; 1974 - 640 hours; 1978 - 857 hours; 1981 - more than 1000 hours.

The Mass Media and International Sporting Co-operation: A Content Analysis

What, then, is the effectiveness of this widely disseminated and ever-increasing flood of information? What is its contribution to the strengthening of international sporting co-operation? We posed these and other questions in our study of the central press of our country. The study was carried out by us in 1974 and included a content analysis of such papers as *Izvestia, Komsomolskaja, Pravda, Soviet Russia, Agrarian Life, Pioneer Pravda* and *Soviet Sport,* and the magazines *Ogonjok, The Working Women, Agrarian Youth, Sport in the USSR, Physical Culture and Sports,* and *Sports Abroad.* The analysis was conducted within the following chronological limits: one calendar year - 1972 as an Olympic year – and one non-calendar year in accordance with the sporting calendar for 1973–1974. All in all, 516 newspapers and 260 issues of magazines were subjected to the content analysis. The various elements of the content were taken as units for analyses. Each element included the indices of categories chosen by us. A total of 15 elements of content were determined: international competitions, the national championships of foreign countries, the results of athletes in international competitions, materials dealing with foreign athletes, materials on foreign trainers, the principles and ideals of the olympic movement, problems of the international Olympic movement, the international contents of Soviet sport organisations, the state and development of physical culture and sports in various foreign countries, criticism of anti-humanitarian phenomena in sport and the international sports movement, materials on the candidature of Moscow as the venue for the 22nd Olympic Games in 1980, materials on separate types of sport, a typology of authors, the representatives of information agencies and organs of the press of various countries, and types and genres of materials. As can be seen from this list, all the elements of the content embrace the object of the study in its entirety and derive from its content.

The number of empirical indicators in each element ranged from 3 (materials on foreign sportsmen: of socialist, capitalist and developing countries) to 35 (materials on separate kinds of sport). Thus, for example, for the second element of content – the national championships of foreign countries – the categorial indicators selected were: socialist, capital- and developing countries, and the countries of Europe, Asia, Africa, Latin America, North America, Australia and Oceania, i. e. nine indicators. The sixth element – the principles and ideals of the Olympic movement – contained three indicators: ideational, pedagogic and organisational as well as methodological. Each of these was broken down into more concrete indicators. For example, the indicators of the first type were:

- The principle on internationalism, understanding and co-operation of peoples and states through sport
- The principle of democracy and equality as a fully justified part of the Olympic movement in general and of the Olympic Games in particular and also the absence of any discrimination
- The principle of the many-sided development of the personality of the sportsman as a citizen and a patriot of his country and people
- The principle of viewing sport as a component part of society or the unity of sport with the economy, politics, ideology, culture and art

Element 10 – criticism of anti-humanitarian phenomena in sport and the international sports movement – also contained three indicators:

- Criticism of political discrimination in sport
- Criticism of religious, national, racial and other discrimination in sport
- Criticism of the essence of professional sport, and of the professionalisation and commercialisation in bourgeois sport in general.

The unit of calculation for the indicators selected was the frequencly of mention of one or another indicator and the number of lines. The conceptual unit was the paragraph. On the basis of this a coding instruction was worked out and a model of a coded form was established.

The quantity of materials was determined by the generally accepted method - a line counter - and it was measured in printed lines. Ultimately it was reduced to a single indicator of the amount of space per element selected.

We shall not go into the results of this study in detail, as they have been widely treated both in our own scientific literature (Milshtein 1974) and in foreign scholarly sources (Milshtein and Molchanov 1976; Mass Media, Sport and International Understanding 1980). We shall only say that we carried out according to the very same methodology comparative studies of the same sources in 1980-1981 and received results that not only confirm the conclusions of the first study but indicate also that there is a growing tendency in the Soviet central press towards such an international orientation with regard to sporting information. Of course, this is largely explained by the hosting of the Moscow Olympics. This was an enormous social factor which increased the interest of the public in sport. It also considerably influenced the strengthening of international sporting contacts and their role in strengthening friendship between peoples.

At the same time a comparative analysis of the content, structure and volume of materials on the international aspects of physical culture and sport in the Soviet indicated that these materials are highly varied in terms of the themes they treat. They cover, in fact, all aspects of international sporting life. By objectively treating the variety of current and urgent problems of international sporting life and by revealing the essence and humanism of sport, the Soviet sports press fulfils not only an information function - it simultaneously contains considerable cognitive educational and ideological values and constitues an important organisational link in the Soviet physical culture and sports movement. In summary, the Soviet press provides a many-sided, fully objective and unbiased treatment of international sporting life, strives for the democratisation and progress of the international sports movement, including the Olympic movement, and in every way reveals the humanistic and international essence of sport.

The Need for International Research

The present study must be viewed only as an attempt, as a concrete experiment in the sense of a sociological study of one side of the problem. For a detailed study it is necessary to carry out an analogous study of both of the mentioned sides of the process, formed by other means of mass information: television, radio, cinema and literature. Establishing the relative impact of these means, the size and structure of their audience, readership of the press will allow us to approach the question of these stereotypes formed through sport and the real behaviour of the reader (or listener spectator).

Finally, when comparing similar data obtained in different countries by different authors using the same methodology, it is necessary to elucidate the reasons for the negative influence on public opinion (and this means on social and individual consciousness) of the mass media in sports public relations: the case which instead of friendship and international understanding, sport is used by certain representatives of the mass media for anti-humanitarian aims, as a factor of schism between peoples, creating nationalistic enmity between peoples and spreading chauvinism and misanthropy, the base passions of the mob. The practical experience of the reactionary, gutter press, the commercial bourgeois press, radio, cinema and television furnishes a good number of such examples.

Only through an integrated, many-sided study of all the above enumerated aspects and facets of the problem, through the concerted, collective efforts of sociologists, progressive sports figures and the mass media can we reach positive results in solving this difficult problem. On this level it seems to us that several of the premises which are advanced in our study (above all the structure of the elements of content, revealed with the aid of contact analysis and others) may be quite utilisable in realising an international research project.

In conclusion, we should like to point out that the basic provisions of measures carried out within the framework of European international co-operation are based on general political principles and the decision of the European Conference on Peace and Security in Europe. Reflecting the universal tendencies of peaceful coexistence and co-operation, the struggle for preace, and actions directed against a nuclear catastrophe in order to preserve life, civilisation and mankind, sporting co-operation plays an ever greater role in the modern social life of Europe and the whole world. It enables us to bring into effect the principles of the Helsinki Final Act, to realise the ideas of peace and peaceful co-operation.

References

Coe S (1981) Future of the Olympic Games. XI Olympic Congress. Journal Diary, Baden-Baden, p 4

First International Conference of Ministers and Senior Officials responsible for Physical Education and Sport in the Education of Youth (1976), Final Report. UNESCO, Paris

Izvestya (1975) Final Act of the Conference on Security and Co-operation in Europe, August 2

Lowe B, Kanin D, Strenk A (1980) Sport and international relations. Stipes, Champaign

Mass Media, Sport and International Understanding (1980) A Summary of a review of literature and research. UNESCO, Paris

McIntosh P (1979) Fair play. Heinemann, London

Milshtein OA (1974) Sport, mass media and international understanding. Theory and Practice of Physical Culture 5:75–76

Milshtein OA, Molchanov SV (1976) The shaping of public opinion regarding sport by the mass media as a factor promoting international understanding. Int Rev Sport Sociology 3 (II):71–84

Mlodzikowski G (1979) Politika i sport. (Politics and sport.) Sport i turystka, Warszawa

Olympic Charter (1980) FiS, Moscow, p 6

Pavlov SP (1981) Future of the Olympic Games. XI Olympic Congress. Journal Diary, Baden-Baden, p 4

Prokhorov DI (1978) Socialist integration in sport. FiS, Moscow

Sovietsky Sport (1975) October 5

Third European Sports Conference (1977), May 11–15, 1977, Records, p 19

Vinogradov P (1981) Portrait of our reader. Sovietsky Sport, May 5, p 2

Sport, Political Autonomy and International Understanding

B. F. Booth

My presentation is based on the assumption that societies, like human beings, are engaged in a constant battle for autonomy. Since societies are composed of human beings, human beings are constantly being exposed to tension as their individual needs compete with societal needs for expression and fulfilment. It is in the management of tension that the process of autonomy may be observed.

The struggle for autonomy is a struggle for power and for control over others. Play is basic to the well-being of mankind, and since it often requires leisure time and physical resources, it becomes a scarce resource to be competed for. However, the stage of development reached by a society will govern the kinds of controls exercised over its play forms. For example, a simple society like the Inuit will require its members to learn to be self-sufficient yet co-operative. Inuit games will not stress strategy since this society requires more sharing of its resources than competition for them. Inuit games' forms, therefore, are a great deal less complex than the team sports of nineteenth century urban England. Social behaviour among the Inuit is more equal than among the social classes of nineteenth century England.

By examining the games of the Inuit or the sports of the Victorian English, for example, we can learn a great deal about the way these respective societies are structured, and about these respective social constraints. Simple societies reflect a greater belief in magic and witchcraft as they seek to control supernatural forces through supernatural means. But as society progresses to a more rationalised system of technology, religious beliefs give way to a consensus achieved through ideology. Table 1 illustrates the cybernetic system described above.

Table 1. Cybernetic system

↓	Cultural system	↑
↓	Social system	↑
↓	Personality	↑
↓	Physical-organic world	↑

If we apply this model to the simple society we can see that since it is dominated by concerns of the physical-organic world, a great deal of its energy is spent on translating superstitious beliefs (culture) into social practices (games) which train the young to adapt to the constraints of the physical-organic world. The same model tells us that in a complex industrial society certain segments of the population (the upper classes) manage to achieve enough power to fashion a set of beliefs which sustain their power and help to suitably mould the behaviour of the respective social systems, and their personalities. Obviously, this model is quite useful for providing us with a comparative framework for examining the role of sport in the evolving society. The corollary, of course, is that if we, as sport planners, realise the extent of this tension-management process then we may be more justifiably optimistic about planning for greater international understanding.

Games of the Inuit and the Motu

Games are an expression of cultural values. Much less structured than sport, they reflect the socialisation patterns of a society and may be an index of cultural evolution (Roberts et al. 1959).

Games may be defined as play activity, with rules, specific goals, contest, boundaries of time and space, and a sequence of repeatable actions. They have been classified by Sutton-Smith and others as games of physical skill, of chance, of strategy and of memory (Roberts et al. 1959). Traditional Inuit society subsists on hunting and fishing. Its values therefore emphasise behaviour associated with the skills of hunting and fishing, and of individual and group interdependency. Individuals must be able to rely in themselves to cope with emergencies. They live in a uniform environment where small details may extremely important for survival. Yet, the individual is also extremely dependent upon the goodwill of the group, and the traditional Inuit value system puts a gremium on behaviour that encourages goodwill. Hence, while it is important for the hunter/fisherman to develop individual skills, they must not be cultivated at the expense of other group members. It is, therefore, not surprising that Inuit games stress self-testing like tag, strength contests, wrestling, juggling and physical and memory skills like string weaving.

But one will not find games of strategy in traditional Inuit culture, because strategy implies seeking superiority over an adversary. While competition exists in Inuit culture, it is non-malicious. Games are characterised by physical skill and quick recall, and are somewhat competitive, but their competitive nature dies not extend to acquiring the possessions of other persons or of humiliating them. Where groups of spectators witness a contest, there is a striking informality between contestants and spectators.

Inuit society does not practise the formal hierarchical relationships of Western society: equality is predominant. This lack of social rigidity may explain the preferences of children for informal play. However, Roberts et al. (1959) have documented that as society assumes greater social structuration and as hierarchical lines of authority appear, the games children play assume new combinations. The relationship between games of strategy and cultural complexity is increasingly accepted. Roberts et al. (1959) argue that acceptance of strategic games is consistent with new values regarding the ability to cope with the stresses and strains of modern life. Studies of Inuit who have been exposed to southern Canadian culture over long periods illustrate that games of skill and strategy are becoming more common, with a resultant loss of the non-competitive, non-malicious goodwill of the traditional society.

When the cybernetic model is applied to traditional Inuit culture, it appears that the integrative function of the social system is predominant. Individual hunting and fishing skills and collective survival are the predominant values. Material possessions are shared; hence there is no point in teaching children to seek ownership. The game is valuable, but so is the goodwill to be retained. Hence games and contests occur within an environment of humour. Such situations are ideal for socialising the young into informal relationships by teaching them not to take themselves too seriously.

The Motu are a Papuan–Melanesian people who inhabit a group of 18 villages scattered over the south-eastern coastal area of New Guinea. The physical environment is threatening. The soil is shallow and infertile and because of the tropical climate, agricultural products cannot be stored. The Motu subsistence culture revolves around gardening, hunting and trading, and is supported by a network of social and religious practices. Once a year the Motu make a journey to the Gulf of Papua to exchange pots which they have made from saga and wood. Motu beliefs emphasise a strong, wicked spirit world, which preys upon unfortunates. The environment of the Motu, therefore, is harsh and unpredictable.

Motu mainly practise games of physical skill. Their games perform an integrative function within a relatively static society. The Motu is exposed, from birth, to a continuous form of social interaction. Swinging from a tree or fastened to its mother's back, the child is free to watch the activities of older siblings and of parents. There is no need for a division of labour and hence no social distinction between the sexes. Girls and boys play group games together.

The sea is their physical environment. Motu children learn to swim very early, to build and sail and hold miniature races on small crafts; such skills will be very important in later life. Sea games also become social games in which competition is evident, when, for example, one group tries to penetrate another group's space. However, when entry has been achieved the groups simply reverse roles; attackers reverting to defenders and vice versa.

As with the Inuit, the games are non-competitive and lacking in materials significance. What is important is learning to maintain status from victory or defeat while trying to develop the essential skills that will be useful in adulthood. As amongst the Inuit, stringing threads together is considered an important preparation for net-making. Boys and girls practise hurling grass spears at each other and may become quite proficient at it even before they are 8 years of age.

The game of the Motu exist to reinforce the status quo. Group games reflect social dependency as roles are reversed or changes individually during the game. One example is a child balancing on a plank held aloft by its friends. The child who completes the act is caught by the group and replaced by another child. Games and social role-playing serve the function of teaching the Motu child certain contraints of his society.

Games and Social Organisation

The study of play and games has thrown light on several relationships: cultural customs and differentiation, social class, economic or adaptive strategies, family structure, sex roles, child-rearing practices and integrative functions. Games teach adaptive strategies in a harsh environment, help to educate children in the kinds of motor skill they will use in later life and, as a by-product, provide a social occassion for value reinforcement, as in the case of the Inuit when losers are expected to laugh at themselves.

Salter (1967), in his survey of North American tribes, found that games are associated with rituals. Despite certain differences between tribes, he concluded that it was the manner in which the game was played, rather than the outcome, which had the greatest spiritual effect. Salter also found that games of physical skill and strategy occurred more often in these contexts than games of chance, leading to the conclusion that man, in his search for autonomy; invents games that allow him to control his environment. The concept of control is central to our understanding of the function of games and sports in development. Salter further concluded, in his study of Australian Aboriginals, that economic or survival reasons accounted for the largest number of games, followed by social interaction games. Political activity and cultural identification games were much less common.

Frederickson's (1960) studies of wrestling in various cultures showed that this sport was used in settling boundary disputes, expressing puberty, selecting a mate, demonstrating power and controlling the uncontrollable, i. e. the weather. Roberts and Sutton-Smith (1962) have studied game complexity and sulture and have concluded that physical skill is usually present in games. However, as in traditional Inuit society, games of physical skill are often practised without strategy. Societies that lack competitive games exhibit low social complexity and are usually characterised by subsistence economies. Where games of strategy are played, this is usually an indication of increased complexity of social organisation and possibly of severe child-rearing methods. Where games of chance predominate, this us usually an indication of economic uncertainty and a feeling of inability to control the environment.

However, Ball (1974), who studied the control factor in games, concluded that games are capable of modelling a cultural control scale, where players exercising more control over risk emerge at the top of the scale, the reverse being true for players feeling helpless and controlled. Ball argues that the attitude of rationality and control associated with sport and games, rather than the organisational structure the games appear to reflect, should be studied. This concept of control, or autonomy, is central to the study of sport and societal development. The premise argued, so far, has been that societies, through their socialisation practices via games and sport structures, are attempting to control their destiny. The relative complexity of the games, as they reflect cultural values, are an indication of the status of that society on the development scale.

Sport in Complex Societies

A brief historical review of the social factors that have contributed to the rationalisation of sport will illustrate the nature of the struggle between different social groups for the control of sport. This will enable us to see sport as a mirror of society while illustrating the social function of sport in the process of striving for autonomy.

Joseph Strutt divided "rural exercises" into those practised by "persons of rank" and those practised by the "common masses". It was during the nineteenth century that many of the spontaneous, ritualistic and local sports began to die out as a rural preindustrial society changed into an urban industrial society (Cone 1981). In the emerging industrial society, sport began to take on national characteristics. Rules were formalised and administered by private governing bodies of sportsmen whose authority extended throughout the nation. The high degree of rationalisation of sport, which is so evident in the modern world, had its antecedents in the first half of the nineteenth century.

Until then, only the leisured gentry had the time to engage in sport. There was no social conflict and consequently no social incentive to develop rules. Rules became important when different social classes began to meet in competition and the rather sedentary gentry were tested by the physically stronger labouring class. The notion of professionalism was introduced to keep a barrier between the gentry who were enjoying sport socially, and the emerging working class which engaged in sport for a living. By traditon, sport was to be enjoyed more for the opportunity it provided to engage in social interaction than to discover winners.

In socialist societies sport has served an integrative and adaptive function. Because of its visibility, and because it is capable of functioning within social units as diverse as the factory, the sports club, the school, the family and the army, sport has a potentially integrative nature and carries social messages across different groups and regions.

The German Democratic Republic provides an example illustrating the ideological rationalisation of sport. A sport governing body, the Deutsche Sport Ausschuss (DSA), was created by the state and communal sport was integrated within the production system under the direction of this body. The primary purpose of the DSA was to ensure adherence to the ideological principles of the new state, and to co-ordinate sport and youth activities (FDJ) with the German Gymnastics Association (FDGB). Later, the FDJ and the FDGB were incorporated within the DSA to plan and develop sport along community lines. All sectors of the economy came to be represented in the sports clubs. Hence sport was established as a co-ordinating mechanism to help the development of the emerging state's autonomy. A few years later the DSA was replaced by the Deutscher Turn- und Sportbund (DTSB). This body was given the task of developing the rationalisation of sport. It should be noted that the German Democratic Republic's excellence in sport helped it to gain international recognition.

Cuba provides an illustration of the way sport may be used to rationalise the popular effort towards national development. A suitable index of Cuban development tensions is found in President Castro's speeches. They are published regularly in *Granma Weekly Review*, and are of historical value for studying Cuban development. The role of sport in the developing Cuba state has gradually changed. In his first speeches, in the early 1960s, President Castro suggested that Cuba's poor record in international sport was a product of laissez-faire capitalism. The 1960s were the period of moral incentives, whereas in the 1970s greater attention was given to a more centralised economy, the urbanisation process and a centralised sports system patterned along the Soviet model (Ritter 1978, Both 1981). The 1970–79 speeches reveal a greater concern with the microsystem of the economy and attention to particular segments of the population. The tension between the state and the people was initially mediated symbolically through a system of moral incentives. But with progress in sporting accomplishments, the system of moral rewards gave way to more tangible rewards, thereby creating a new tension to be dealt with. International success in sport (Olympic Games in Munich 1971, Montreal in 1976 and Moscow in 1980) brings a certain amount of pride in its wake but not permanently. There is plenty of evidence, however, that Cuba has put its people first, and sport is no exception to this (Booth 1981).

These brief illustrations of sport show it may be playing a tension-management role in the autonomy process. What remains to be examined are some of the theoretical questions that ought to be asked to better understand the function of sport in the tension-management process between state and individual.

Theoretical Discussion

Metcalfe, McIntosh and other scholars have documented how certain dominant groups have controlled sport, historically, by establishing rules and procedures with respect to the inclusion and exclusion of particular social classes. I have tried to show that it is this social cut and thrust that is the basis of societal autonomy, but more importantly I have tried to illustrate how autonomy is a process of man, the player, trying to assert himself and establish himself against the forces of nature. As he wins the battle against nature his battle then turns inward against himself and he is forced to re-create some of the controls that nature imposed naturally. These controls are found within his social make-up and take the form of ideology, social class relationships and so forth.

It is very ease to see the play process in the simple society; less easy in the complex post-industrial society. In the latter, the state is forced to take on a personage and create social meanings for itself. Sport, at this stage of societal development, takes on a wider set of meanings as state may pit itself against state. Consider the effects of the South African tour of New Zealand and the resultant threat of the African nations to boycott the Commonwealth Games in Australia if New Zealand should be allowed to take part. Sport has clearly moved from man the player to state the player with a much vaster set of collective meanings than occurred in the simple society. Finally, what does it all mean? How should we use this knowledge to promote peace and understanding?

In conclusion, may I suggest that we recognise that society needs to play in the same way that man needs to play, that collective meanings and collective identities must continue to balance with individual meanings and satisfaction in sport in much the same way as it does in the Inuit society. The threat is much greater now in that society has collectivised and polarised its loyalties but the converse is equally true; the social rewards will be much greater. Let us, therefore, try to teach to our young the tenets of peace and fairness, implicit in sport, and show that we are capable of learning that sport does mirror the social cut and thrust of competing interest groups. Our capacity today for autonomy is greater than in the simple society because we have the knowledge and the means to make it work; primitive man was less fortunate.

References

Ball D (1974) Control versus complexity – continuities in the scaling of gaming. Pacific Sociological Rev 17:1

Both BF (1981) Communist sport and urbanization in Cuba. Paper presented at the 12th International Congress in International Development. Ottawa, 30 October 1981

Cone CB (1981) Hounds in the morning. University Press of Kentucky

Frederickson FS (1960) Sports and the cultures of man. In: Johnson W (ed) Science and medicine of exercise and sport. Harper, New York

Ritter A (1978) The Cuban Revolution: A new orientation. Current History. February
Roberts JM, Sutton-Smith B (1962) Child training and game involvement. Ethnology 2:166–185
Roberts JM et al. (1959) Games in culture. American Anthropologist 61:597–605
Salter M (1967) Games and pastimes of the Australian Aboriginals. Unpublished M.A. Thesis. University of Alberta, Edmonton

The Integrational Functions of Competitive Sport and Its Role in Shaping International Competition, Co-operation and Mutual Understanding

A. Wohl

Improvement of Motoric Skills and Civilisational Needs

Man, as the producer, is an indispensable component of the production process beause without him, without his skill and his motoric abilities, no production process could take place; consequently, at each stage of the development of our civilisation the need existed for the proper adjustment of the human motor apparatus and of peoples' motoric skills to the needs and tasks connected with the development of the productive forces that had been achieved.

This simple truth about the connection between production needs and the drive for motoric improvement of human beings, as well as the importance of this connection, was not fully understood. This was in part due to the fact that during historical development the course of motoric improvement developed features of far-reaching independence and became separated from the production process. This entire process was also connected with many shperes of human life and human civilisational needs, sometimes having little in common with the production process.

The more all these undertakings departed from the production process itself, the more people forgot about the connection between these undertakings and the production needs objectively motivating them. As a result, the true reasons for human aspirations to achieve motoric improvement turned into mystifications in human consciousness, and pride of place was instead given to subjective motivations and manifestations connected with human likings, ambitions and beliefs. The conviction took root that precisely individual motivations were the basic stimuli of existing aspirations of people to achieve better results in motoric activities. But such a way of shaping these aspirations was nevertheless a natural one, since the mechanisms of social co-operation are always bound to be connected with individual motivations. After all, they are the most all-round instrument of human activity, which must always be initiated by the head, must "pass through the human brain." The essence of the humanisation of nature, its adjustment to human needs, consists in the fact that we transform it in accordance with our own human, subjective needs, that we create a stimulus of a cultural type in order with its help to put into motion our own energy resources, the resources of our mind and body. Such motivations turn into a factor automatically arousing human energy, bringing to the fore human talents and skills and supporting the human ability to develop activity. That is why human co-operation is always based on elements of competition, mutually interwined in a dialectical way.

It should, however, be added that irrespective of their course and motivations, all such aspirations directed towards improvement of motoric skills were always to some extent connected with the existing needs of the historical stage of development of the given society. This is also true of our present-day aspirations to achieve development of human motoric skills and of the aspirations of contemporary systems for motoric improvement in the form of various types of physical culture, but above all in the form of sport.

The Civilisational Role of Competitive Sport

The development of present-day technology requires increasing rationalisation of physical culture. After all, we have created a world in which the rate of technology is increasing as never before, and there is some doubt as to whether the motoric skills of man's organism are sufficient to keep up with this progress. The ever more urgent task that faces humanity is no longer merely the protection of health and preservation on a certain level of motoric efficiency; it is becoming increasingly obvious that the present goal is adjustment of the human organism to the world we have created.

Competitive sport, with its mechanism of rivalry, is in its very essence a school for the improvement of motoric skills. The necessity to compare the results achieved with those of others compels competitors constantly to control their body, forcing them to wrest from their body as much as possible and to employ means of doing this which are not open to average people. Their entire mode of life is subordinated to this goal, as is true of people in other fields who want to rise above the average. Thus, this is an authentic humanising process, a process forcing the competitor to check a hundred times what has already been checked, to reject hackneyed truths and prejudice (in this case, prejudices connected with our body).

Competitive sport, basing itself on mass sport and physical education in schools, is in its very essence a modern school of motoric improvement for large strata of the population - an instrument for the introduction of new forms of motoric activity for the masses. It is a means of maintaining the equilibrium between constant improvement of our intellectual abilities and the improvement of our motoric system. That is why one may assume that the motoric improvement of man and the broadening of the limits of his motoric possibilities are the most fundamental functions of competitive sport. One should oppose the thesis occasionally voiced that the drive for the best possible results in sport is something negative. One should rather support the idea that each means of improving our motoric system provides opportunities to improve our knowledge of the properties of our body, which so far continue to remain a secret.

But, side by side with this basic social function, competitive sport performs one other very essential social function which is most significant today and which is based on its integrational values. Below I wish to analyse this particular function of sport.

The Integrational Functions of Sport

Recent decades have been marked by exceptionally dynamic social integrational processes and a growing participation in these processes of factors related to culture, customs, education and ideology. Sport is also one of these factors.

Sport is a form of motoric game that is connected with competition and is subordinated to certain rules and requirements connected with such competition. It consists in a drive constantly to break one's own records and to compare them with the achievements of others. This forces those participating in sport to go beyond the boundaries of the local community, their own courtyard and playgrounds. That is why, in contradistinction to games and entertainment involving movement, which are of a local and sporadic nature, sport is a continuous game. The accidental, loose circle of participants out of necessity has to be replaced by a regular team, with a strictly defined, formalized structure; personal ties in this case are subordinated to larger impersonal structures. In the eagerness to obtain the best possible results, sport breaks through local barriers, links and unites competitors across towns and settlements, provinces and countries, and reveals tendencies towards institutionalisation of the very nature of the game. This brings in its wake the establishment of a network of organisations: clubs, associations and federations with an entire staff of instructors, activists, referees and sports doctors. Sport develops on the state and international level, bringing people from various countries and continents closer to one another.

Thus, side by side with the structure of formalised sport there arises on the periphery an exceptionally widespread informal structure made up of large numbers of sports fans and readers of the sporting press. The number of competitors in various sports sections, clubs, associations and national federations already amounts to tens of millions, while it is difficult even to assess the number of sports fans in the stadiums. In this way the wide range of the integrational values of sport is revealed.

In these reflections one should not, of course, forget to mention the fact that sport as a factor of social integration is not a primary factor. This funtion takes place only under certain definite conditions of social life, when the barriers dividing local, territorial and ethnic societies have already been markedly undermined by the rapid processes of industrialisation and after the natural aspirations of a wide strata of the population to satisfy their motoric needs have been stimulated by this development and sufficiently sanctioned to be transformed into a universally accepted value.

The National Integrational Role

Factors indicating the national integrational role of sport can be found in many contemporary national movements. Along with motives for sport such as entertainment, and motoric features and social gatherings, there are also patriotic motives. Each victory of a national team in an international match turns into a national holiday, is treated as a symbol fo national vitality, is enjoyed not only by spectators present at the game and the fans but also by people not directly connected with sport. It is used as an argument to change the minds of those who are not yet interested in the national aspect of competition in sport. Proof of the fact that sport undoubtedly plays such a role can be found in the history of the German "Turner" (gymnastic) movement, the Czech Sokól (Falcon) movement and Polish sport during the period of Poland's loss of statehood and in the years of Nazi occupation (into which there has been much research).

Analogous integrational functions of sport can be found on the class level, too. During the period between the two world wars, especially in the years of the Great Depression in 1929-1934 and the intensified class struggle, workers' sports organisations played an undeniably important role in integrating the working class and provided a significant reserve from which many activists of the workers' parties could be recruited in many European countries and elsewhere. Many workers keep to this day as cherished souvenirs evidence of their membership in these sports organisations, which not only served as an outlet for their need to improve their motoric skills but also helped them to find many loyal friends. In these organisations they received their first lesson in class consciousness ans their first experiences of class struggle. In their memoirs members of workers' sport organisations in many countries provide documentary evidence of the role of sport as a factor of class integration.

The International Integrational Role

Exceptionally characteristic however, is the integrational role of sport in the international sphere. Like on other field of cultural activity sport requires international contacts. Having said this, clearly all spheres of culture and sciences require some such contacts. The interaction of various national and regional cultures and of various fields of science and technology enriches their content and speeds up their development. This is, at any rate, inevitable in the circumstances of the present-day international division of labour and the international marketplace. This is why, irrespective of the deep differences and lines of division that still exist and are always difficult to overcome, mankind is becoming more and more consolidated, turning into an entity. Many forms of limited international contact virtually always cause damage or lead to stagnation. However, any attempt to limit contacts in sport would mean betrayal of the very essence of sport and would lead quickly to its decline. This is exactly what turns sport into an irreplaceable instrument of integration on an international level. One simply cannot imagine contemporary sport without the Olympic Games and international championships, without international co-operation. Such co-operation began when many fields of culture were still limited to the national environment. It survived hot and cold wars. Almost the first day after the end of the First and the Second World War, as soon as the two sides declared an end to hostilities, athletes from both sides fixed dates for meetings. And to this day these are the most systematic and most regular of all the international meetings.

As far as integrational functions are concerned, a distinct difference exists between mass sport and competitive sport. The role of sport for the masses does not surpass the framework of local integration and thus plays rather a secondary role. But competitive sport participates exceptionally actively both in integrating national communities and on the international level.

Integration and the Social Systems

When dealing with features of the integrational function of sport on various levels we should also bear in mind that the definition "integration" does not at all mean that processes of shaping new ties and imbuing them with lasting features do not take place without conflicts and resistance, without the need to overcome opposing forces. And the result of such processes is not always unequivocal. After all, the creation of new ties does not only mean the establishment of additional ties, but very often consists in replacing former ties by new ones. In such cases integration is the reverse side of disintegration, or the alternative of disintegration.

But the integrational functions of sport are not performed independently of the structure of relations and tendencies in the macrostructure. Because of its specific values sport can therefore play a certain integrational role, but only to the extent to which this is possible in the existing system of social relations.

The interdependence between the consolidation of peaceful relations in the world and the development of international co-operation in sport and international sporting competition was well understood by Coubertin. That is what made him combine the Olympic movement with aspirations for peace. It is true that the develeopment of competitive sport is inseparably connected not only with international understanding and co-operation but also with the fight for peace. Competitors are deeply and personally committed to the fight for peace. Democratic forces within the sports movement should deepen and develop these interests, turning them into the basic slogan of the sports movement throughout the world. No democratic sports movement has a right to renounce this role if it does not want to become disloyal to the needs of sport itself as well as to the foundations of democracy. That is why one reaches the conclusion that the next indispensable condition for the development of competitive sport is democracy in social relations and, what follows, democracy within the sport movement. Any lack of democracy and democratic relations hampers the possibilities for the development of competitive sport and its ability to exert an influence on youth; it holds back from sport the most active and far-sighted people, and prevents feedback between sport and social life as a whole.

Therefore, the more progressive the system of economic and social relations the greater the possibilities for sport to carry out its integrational functions and the more favourable the conditions for its development. Thus, if we would want most concisely to express the sense of our reflections, we could say that it consists in the statement that there exists a concurrence of two tendencies, namely: developmental tendencies of competitive sport and the general tendency of present-day social development. Sport needs international co-operation, peace and democracy and for its part it supports these tendencies in the contemporary world.

The New International Sports Order: An Appraisal

A. Hietanen

Introduction

One of the magic phrases of the 1970s was without doubt "new international order". All kinds of orders were brought into discussion: economic, military, communication – and the sports order. Discussion of a new economic order dates back to the Sixth and Seventh Special Sessions of the General Assembly of the United Nations in 1974 and 1975. The Sixth Session adopted the Declaration and the Programme of Action on the Establishment of a New International Economic Order (United Nations General Assembly 1974), and later two Conferences on International Economic Co-operation were held as a continuation of the North–South dialogue. The communication order was discussed at the Fifth Conference of Heads of State or Government of the Non-Aligned Countries in 1976, and the declaration of the conference regarded a new information order to be as vital as the economic order. Two years later, at the 20th UNESCO General Conference, a resolution on establishing a new information and communication order was adopted (UNESCO General Conference 1982; Pavlic and Hamelink 1982). As to the new international sports order, it was not perhaps a mere coincidence that the 1976 Conference of the Non-Aligned Countries included sports in the action programme and that a refenrence was made to "the democratization of international sports organizations and the abolition of apartheid in sport" (Fifth Conference 1976). After the 1976 Conference the interest of the non-aligned countries in international sporting relations grew visibly.

The Contents of the Sports Order

In 1978 the non-aligned countries made a decisive step towards clarifiying their sports policy. In Algeria a "Manifesto and Plan of Action for Co-operation in and Development of Physical Education and Sports among the Non-aligned Countries" was signed, including the following objectives:

- To encourage countries to give priority, within their respective means, to the development of national physical education and sports plans that are closely related to existing education, health and recreation plans;
- To stimulate exchanges and various forms of bilateral and multilateral co-operation and assistance among the non-aligned countries in the field of sports;
- To participate actively in the events of the international sports calneder and the activities of specialized governmental and non-governmental organizations, intensifying the struggle to democratize the decision-making structure and eliminate all forms of racial, political and religious discrimination, especially *apartheid* and zionism;

- To give priority to the training, advanced training and retraining of cadres through seminars, courses and short- and long-term scholarships;
- To organize the exchange of experts and forms of co-operation among countries of different geographical areas by taking advantage of the resources of those areas and the opportunities offered by international organizations;
- To hold international meetings for the purpose of evaluating on a yearly basis the degree of implementation of the Plan of Action in this field and the status of the ongoing struggle for democratization and against apartsheid;
- To promote the broadest possible sports exchange among the non-aligned countries by organizing special competitions and/or extending invitations to national and international events sponsored by members of the Movement;
- To continue to strengthen the work of the non-aligned countries in the UNESCO Intergovernmental Committee for Physical Education and Sports by ensuring that they are adequately represented and their positions co-ordinated in that forum.

However, the movement of the non-aligned countries has not been the only forum in which this issue has been discussed. The Charter of Physical Education and Sports, which was approved at the 20th UNESCO General Conference in 1978, includes some principles relevant to the new international sports order. This international charter refers, for example, to national sporting traditions, whereas the non-aligned countries have preferred discussing in broader terms self-reliance, "a firm determination in the part of developing nations to secure their legitimate rights in international dealings through the use of their collective bargaining strength" (see Fifth Conference 1976; Väyrynen 1978).

This issue of the sports order has its roots in the decolonisation process of the 1950s and 1960s, but at the level of principles it dates back to the beginning of the modern Olympic movement and to adaptation of the structure of international sporting co-operation. During this century, the international sports system has been relatively successful in its adaptation to the changes in the external environment, although quite the opposite has sometimes been argued. Anyhow, there have been few challenges or alternatives posed vis-à-vis the present system of international sports. The two major challenges were the Red Sportintern in the 1920s and the Games of the New Emerging Forces in the 1960s. The Workers' Sport Internationals of the 1920s constituted an alternative in the sense that sportsmen from the countries defeated in the First World War (Austria, Bulgaria and Germany) and from the Soviet Union could participate (Steinberg 1978). The Games of the New Emerging Forces (GANEFO) had their origins in the 1955 Afro-Asian conference in Bandung. The Indonesian refusal to invite Israel and Taiwan to the Asian Games gave birth to a conflict between the IOC and Indonesia (i. e. Sukarno). As a result, Indonesia decided to organise new Games outside the Olympic framework. Thus the Games of the New Emerging Forces were held in 1963 and 1966. As to the sports included in the Games, no cultural alternative based on the national sporting traditions of the developing countries was presented; rather the programme consisted of the traditional European sports with European rules (SIE 1978). Nevertheless, the GANEFO can be defined as an effort to produce an alternative to the Olympic system, since there were participants from countries which were not members of international federations (e. g. North Vietnam, North Korea and Palestine) and the developing countries played the main role in the organising of the Games. In 1969 the story of GANEFO was ended, mainly because of the cultural revolution in China (von der Laage 1977).

The objectives of the plans for a new international sports order (NISO) have not been defined very accurately. Up till now the principle has been the main thing and the term NISO has appeared as an embodiment of the developing countries' growing awareness of their largely disadvantaged position in the sphere of sports - as well as of economy and communication. The practical measures have not yet been thoroughly analysed, but something can be said about the changes to be expected. The demands for the democratisation of international sports are focused on the International Olympic Committee and the international federations. In the case of the IOC, the traditional argument has been that the IOC has representatives only in some 70 countries although there are 150 countries with National Olympic Committees. Another issue has been the low number if representatives in developing countries, since only some 40% of the members of the IOC come from developing countries. As to the international federations, the developing countries have often referred to the weighted voting system in some major federations, including the amateur athletics federation (in which there are over 110 member associations outside the industrialised world) and the tennis federation. In some federations there are other kinds of organisational imbalances, e. g. in the international association football federation (FIFA): in the executive committee of the federation the British associations and the USSR have their own vice-president quotas and in addition Europe has as many vice-presidents and members as for example, Asia and South America together.

The New International Sports Order in Practice

Besides the organisational issues mentioned above, there has not been any comprehensive analysis of the future practive of the NISO. As is known, the new international reforms in the spheres of economy and communication have met with significant difficulties and thus the prospects for the sports order are not encouraging. In addition, the structure of international sports as such causes problems: thus far there are few international governmental organisations in the field of sports. This non-governmentalism means that the organisations involved - i. e. the IOC and the international federations - are exceptionally independent in their activities. Furthermore, within the United Nations framework no agency exists which would not face major problems in carrying out such reforms. Much depends on the activity of the non-aligned countries in the United Nations and in UNESCO. Anyway, some progress has already been made in eliminating racial discrimination in sports: A convention on the prohibition of apartheid in sports is being prepared in the United Nations.

Finally, the actual meaning of NISO deserves some comment. It is quite possible that such reforms could improve international understanding in the North-South dimension. As far as the future prospects are concerned, it seems to be wiser to try to improve the present order instead of leaving the reforms to the NISO of the next decade or of the 21st century. Organisational reforms combined with increased and specified development co-operation in sports could be carried out in a relatively short time - if only the essential political consensus were to be found.

References

Fifth Conference of Heads of State of Government of Non-aligned Countries (1976) Political Declaration. In: Review of International Affairs 634:September 5
Pavlic B, Hamelink CJ (1982) Interrelationship between the new international economic order and a new international/world information-communication order. Ljubljana
Sie S (1978) Sports and politics: the case of the Asian Games and GANEFO. In: Lowe B, Kanin D, Strenk A (eds) Sport and international relations. Stipes, Champaign, pp 279–296
Steinberg A (1978) The workers' sport internationals 1920–1928. J Contemp Hist 13 (2):233–251
UNESCO General Conference (1982) Resolution 20 C-DR 311
United Nations General Assembly (1974) Resolution 3201 (S-VI), 1 May 1974
Väyrynen R (1978) Interdependence vs. self-reliance. Two approaches to international economic relations. Tampere Peace Research Institute, Research Reports No. 16, Tampere
von der Laage R (1977) Sport in China – Eine Entwicklungsskizze und Bestandsaufnahme. Bartels & Wernitz KG, Berlin

The Objectives of Sport and International Understanding

D. Happel and R. Kramer

When discussions emerge around, for instance, a boycott of the Olympic Games or some other spectacular sporting event one often hears the axiom, or "natural truth", that sport contributes to international understanding, or even to a more peaceful world. Notably, the charter of the Olympic Movement, being the mother of contemporary international sporting activities, refers to: "helping to build a better and more peaceful world". If one looks at how often this objective is invoked, it is obviously of great value. This value can be traced to the psychological need of every group or society to set a goal or to develop an ideology. Another more practical reason could be that this objective serves as a justification for organising sporting activities.

So much for the background of this objective. Now, our question, as advisors to a Minister responsible for sport, is: "To what extent do international sporting activities contribute to such a faraway as the one we are talking about?". "How can sports organisations realise this objective?". Before attempting to answer these questions one has to define the subject. What is sport? What is international understanding? What is a better and more peaceful world? What, indeed, is better and for whom and by what standards? And more peaceful? In what sense? From our point of view, we will try to shed some light on these questions before we draw some conclusions.

First, one can observe a difference between top-level sport and everyday competitive and recreational sport. From a politician's point of view this difference is mainly based on the level of publicity surrounding an activity, which is decided upon after journalists and reporters have deemed a sporting activity to contain news or amusement or not. It would go too far here to explore the motives of newspaper editors and the like on this subject. But clearly it is possible to discern a difference between top-level competitions and tournaments and everyday international sporting exchanges between, for instance, two or more youth teams in some kind of sport. In the same way this difference in publicity can also create differences in ranking as to the sport which is reported on (or not). It is easy to see that the world championships in football attract more publicity and, with it, spectators, than, for instance, a tug of war championship. It is these differences in publicity that largely determine the public interest and, together with that, the political interest shown in an event.

This brings us to the second distinction which is of importance here. This is based on the question: what is international understanding? Roughly, two levels can be observed in this respect: First, there is international understanding as the state of peaceful co-existence and relations between nations. Second, there are friendly relations between individual citizens from different countries or nations. International understanding, however, can be seen as: peaceful *political* co-existence and peaceful *political* relations between nations. Friendly relations among private individuals, however important these may be, can be described as merely friendly relations between people who are in a privileged position to travel around and meet other people. The first and foremost aim in sport, however, is to compete and if possible to beat your opponent on the track. This in no way means that human contacts are subordinate to this aim; rather they accompany it. Sport therefore provides a means of bringing people together, across borders and independently from political systems. Herein lies the immense value of international sporting activity: it creates conditions for people from all over the world to meet each other and to talk to each other.

Being brief means that you have to generalise and simplify to an extent which could have a negative influence on the absolute truth of your conclusions. Brevity is the main reason I cannot be specific as to all the occasions when sport has had an impact on international understanding, either positively or negatively. The so-called US ping-pong diplomacy was one example of a positive effect, while the boycott of the Moscow Olympics demonstrated the possible negative effect. Given the dangers caused by brevity, however, I could be justified in drawing the following conclusions.

In today's world sport and politics are becoming more and more involved in each other's affairs and domains. National governmental and sports policy even coincide in some countries of the world. In most of the so-called Wester countries, however, sport has always had a more or less independent position in society. This does not preclude colissions every now and then. On the other hand, admittedly, sport and politicians often have the same objectives as regards, for instance, the human and social development of the individual through active or passive participation in sport. At the international level interests diverge more often. The organisers of large tounaments and championships have as their main objective that the event is well organised. Then, together with the mass media two potential actors appear: commerce and politics. We are not dealing with commercial influence an sport here, so we shall concentrate on the interest of political groups or politicians in these events. This is where we come to the objectives of sport in relation to international understanding. Let's take the IOC's "helping to build a better and more peaceful world". This goal or objective is a political one, *by nature.* Let us explain why. "Better" in this context means that one has chosen between two or more situations and called one of these "worse" and the other(s) "better". This choice is a political one, as all choices in principle are. The same holds for the word "peaceful". If peaceful means "the absence of conflicts or war" it is quite clear that sport has never directly had any influence on the realisation of a "more peaceful world". Perhaps even to the contrary.

Finally, we would like to state that we are not labelling the present situation as good or bad. Our only aim is to make clear that by having objectives of a political nature, sport is offering itself as an instrument for policy-makers and politicians in *their* search for the attainment of *their* goals, which may well be the same as that of the IOC. The distinction between top-level sport and the average competitive and recreational sport becomes significant in this respect. Top-level competitions and spectacular tournaments are, mainly because of the publicity that surrounds them, often a far better instrument for political persons or groups in their search to attain their goals. Less spectacular events are the ones in which the phenomenon of vast personal, human contacts is not overriden by the effect of publicity. This is the domain where international understanding means meetings between "people" from different countries and political systems. This is the area in which values are upheld or even strengthened *through sport,* and the way in which sport is an instrument of individual mutual understanding. But this is not the only level on which international sport takes place. There is this other, often mentioned level of the Olympic Games, World Football Championships etc. We think it is on this level, as well as through publicity, that politicians legitimately make use of the fact that sport offers itself as a political instrument. The results of the relationship caused by this "togetherness" at the level of objectives are known only too well to all of us.

To conclude, what we have tried to do is to analyse, rather roughly how "things work". This description is meant to contribute to mutual understanding between sport and politicians, which is a different mutual understanding from the one we are talking about generally. Our hope is that in the future a sincere dialogue between these two emerges, on the basis of knowledge of each other's premises and objectives.

Fairness, Democracy and Justice

F. de Wachter

Fairness: A Model for Social Institutions?

There is a persisting tendency to consider the ethics of sport as a model of democracy and justice in the life of society. One may be reminded of the famous poem written by de Coubertin (1967) for the 5th Olympic Games in 1912: "Oh Sports, you are Justice. The perfect equity men are looking for in vain in their social institutions, is established spontaneously by you." One may be reminded also of the words of the former President of the International Olympic Committee, Avery Brundage (1964): "In the Olympic Games victory is based on merit. Everyone is entitled to equal rights and to equal opportunities, and if so, the race will be won by the fastest man regardless of colour, creed or political affiliations. This is the kind of world we all seek." The purpose of this paper is to analyse this claim. Is this the kind of world we all seek? In what sense and to what extent can the ethics of fairness, as embodied in sport, be represented as a model for democratic and just human institutions? We do not want to repeat the excellent work done by Küchler (1969), McIntosh (1979) and others in the *ethical* relevance of fair play. We shall only try to establish *the socio-political connotations of the concept of fairness,* using the vocabulary of political philosophy.

Substantial and Procedural Democracy

The societal and ideological background of the concept of fairness is the concept of "procedural democracy". As we all know, the original meaning of democracy has led to two different definitions in Western political philosophy. The first, content-oriented or *substantial* democracy, claims that the results of legislation must offer a maximum of welfare, freedom and human development to everyone. Here the criterion of democracy is related to the content of a set of values (freedeom, equality, brotherhood). The second, formal or *procedural* democracy, relates the criterion to a set of procedures mutually agreed upon. What does this second definition mean, why is it so important and what has it to do with sports and fairness?

The importance of the procedural definition arises from the problem of how the obligatory character of a political decision can be legitimatised. When one proceeds from content legitimation (I respect the decision because its content is good, because it promotes specific values), two difficulties are encountered. First, the achievement of consensus over these values is utopian in modern society, which is very highly stratified and which embraces enormous conflicts of interest and an extensive pluralism of values. Second, content legitimation is potentially bellicose. Presenting a decision as the correct or the best one makes everyone who does not agree wrong. No one can protest against truth, and everyone must be brought into the consensus, if necessary by coercion. To avoid these difficulties, one can legitimate a decision procedurally, not on the basis of the values that are promoted by it, but because it is itself the result of a reasonable procedure, the rules of which are established beforehand by a reasonable contract, a contract with which everyone involved in the results of the procedure can concur. This would imply, for instance, that everyone is directly or indirectly involved in the discussion, that the rights of minorities are guaranteed, and that concrete agreements are made in advance about how valid decisions are made (competent authorities, majority rule etc.). Only then would a reasonable person agree with the results of the procedure, whatever the content might be.

This procedural interpretation of democracy has always been present in Western political thinking (for a survey of the discussion, see Stankiewicz 1980 or Nelson 1980). It is not by chance that our modern Western sports originated in the same Anglo-Saxon context that is also the cradle of Western liberal-democratic thought: the notion of fairness in sports fits in closely with the procedural aspects of this thought. How?

The Social Value of Fairness: Procedural Respect

First of all, fairness is respect for game-constitutive *rules,* just as the democratic attitude in its procedural definition can be formally described as respect for the "rules of the game" that themselves constitute democracy. Second, it involves respect for *decisions,* not on the basis of their truth, but on the basis of the legitimacy of the authority to which decision-making competence is assigned by contract, in this case the referee. Third, fairness in sports teaches the acceptance of *opposition* and rivalry, as democracy accepts opposing parties and various conceptions of social values and does not force everyone into a Procrustean bed of content consensus.

Sports do show that peaceful co-operation with others is not a conflict-free paradise of a consensus society where the interests of each coincide with the interests of all. Such a utopian ideal would cause the very opposite. Suppression of contradictions would lead to pressure for conformity, to criminations of those who do not identify with the universal (Lübbe 1978). The Olympics have been wrongly accused of being a utopian ideal. For de Coubertin, they were not a utopian feast of brotherhood and love: "To ask people to love each other is a sort of childeshness. To ask them to respect each other is not utopian" (de Coubertin 1967). Democratic society is not a society of the one, but of the many (Lefort 1981). What is celebrated in the Olympics is not man's homogeneity or brotherhood, but the capacity of man to live their heterogeneity and to enter self-confidently into confrontations that, however sharp, are lived out within the rules of the game, the procedural nature of which is a guarantee of peace. Thus sports could indeed, on the international level, be a model for a *pacific coexistence,* where we do not share each other's doctrines and interests, but where we do share common conflict-resolving procedures.

The Limits of Fairness

The procedural model does not exhaust, however, the claims of justice and democracy in real life, unless one considers life a super-game, where the only ethical claim would be that the competition is fair and open to all. In sports, equality of chances and procedural respect or fairness are required to measure more accurately *inequalities of game capacities*. The original symmetry (equal opportunities and identical rules for both sides) has a disjunctive effect: its end is the establishment of a difference between players or teams where originally there was no indication of inequality. As Lévi-Strauss (1974) points out, ritual games in primitive societies are the exact inverse: starting from an original asymmetry (for example, between the dead and the living), they establish a union, a symmetry, an equlibrium, as is exemplified by the Gahuku-Gama's or the Fox Indians, who arrange their ritual ball games in such a way that there are no losers; by contrast in modern games the whole purpose is to differentiate between winners and losers.

When we try, as de Coubertin and Brundage suggest, to transfer sportive fairness to the whole of social life, we reach an extremely competitive view of society, where equality of opportunities must enable everyone to compete for success, that is to become unequal to others. In this view, all justice is reduced to fairness, i. e. to commutative justice in competitive interaction. This is defended theoretically by the famous economist Hayek (1976), who bluntly denies the possibility of such a thing as social or distributive justice. He says that the distribution of wealth, even if extremely unequal, is just when it is the outcome of fair market game procedures where, as in games, original equality of opportunities and fair behaviour guarantee that only skill, strenght and chance determine success.

But here, the limitations of the games model become quite obvious. In a moral perspective, each human being has an equal right to all primary goods necessary for a human existence (health, education etc.). If we transfer the idea of fair competition to the whole of social life, even those primary goods would be determined by factors so arbitrary as talents and chance in some market game of an economic nature (Rawls 1980). We cannot play games, not even fair games, where primary goods are at stake. Equally, international justice should mean more than that nations with poor initial assets or poor economic game capacities should enter a fair competitive race with highly developed countries in which, being good sports, they would be predictable losers. Is it always just, as Brundage suggests, that the race is won by the fastest man? Not always: sometimes there should be no race at all.

Conclusion

Fairness exemplifies an attitude of procedural respect, i. e. the readiness of any party not to force the opponent into its own truth (which is violence), but to confront him according to contractual procedures mutually agreed upon (which is pacific coexistence). In this sense the ethics of sport do embody important aspects of democracy, the respect of democratic procedures of formal equality in competitive interactions. In real life, however, some values are too fundamental to be legitimated only as the outcome of a fair competitive game. Here procedural concepts of democracy and justice, as exemplified in sports and as glorified by de Coubertin and Brundage, are too limited a model because they are designed for interactions of a competitive nature. The ethics of sport do not embody democracy in its broader and more substantial meaning of a set of social conditions that guarantee also substantive effects for all individuals and all peoples of the world.

References

Brundage A (1964) Speech by the President of the International Olympic Committee. Bull Comité Int Olympique, pp 63–65
de Coubertin P (1967) L'idée Olympique. Discours et essais. Hofmann, Schorndorf, pp 38, 133
Hayek FA (1976) Law, legislation and liberty, vol 2: The mirage of social justice. Routledge and Kegan Paul, London, pp 107–132
Küchler W (1969) Sportethos. Barth, Munich, pp 141–165
Lefort C (1981) L'invention démocratique. Fayard, Paris, pp 102–172
Levi-Strauss C (1974) The savage mind. Weidenfeld and Nicolson, London, pp 30–33
Lübbbe H (1978) Praxis der Philosophie - Praktische Philosophie - Geschichtstheorie. Reclam, Stuttgart, pp 73–77
McIntosh P (1979) Fair play. Ethics in sport and education. Heinemann, London, pp 79–163
Nelson WN (1980) On justifying democracy. Routledge and Kegan Paul, London
Rawls J (1980) A theory of justice. Oxford University Press, Oxford, pp 83–90
Stankiewicz WJ (1980) Approaches to democracy. Philosophy of government at the close of the twentieth century. Arnold, London

3. The Role of the Olympic Games

The Notions of Peace of Selected Leaders of the Olympic Movement and Their Realisation in the Olympic Games

A. Krüger

Introduction

Ever since the ancient Olympic Games with their truce for participants, coaches and spectators, the Olympic Games have been considered a symbol of peace. The longing for peace is written into the Olympic charter. On the other hand, physical education and sport in classical Greece were performed to prepare able soldiers; in more recent times, the victory of the British over Napoleon was supposed to have been prepared on the playing fields of Eton and de Coubertin recognised "war" as the root of German gymnastics, an Olympic sport from the very beginning (de Coubertin 1894).

This dichotomy of war and peace has been predominant in modern Olympic history. Both the countries in which the Olympic Games have been staged and the countries which have participated have been involved in wars and war-like activities between 1896 and 1980 (Krüger 1982 a, b, c). The purpose of the present study is to show the attitude of the three presidents of the International Olympic Committee (IOC) with the longest terms of office towards war and peace, as expressed in their writings as well as in noteworthy decisions.

Pierre de Coubertin (1863-1937)

The question of war and peace is of great importance in the writing of de Coubertin as a historian, educator and philosopher. From an early essay on *L'èducation de la paix* (1889) until his late work in the Union Pédagogique Universelle (1927) and the Bureau International de Pédagogie Sportive (1933a), the question of education for peace was one of his main concerns (Krüger 1980). His notion of peace does remain fairly constant, however. Peace for him was armed (1904); he was against pacifism (1903), as he saw wars as breaking out "like a tempest". He was therefore in favour of physical education that included education for courage and a notion of one's own strength. He claimed that this could best be achieved through sports, as a strong self-confident athlete could best defend his rights and produce a balance of fear (1923) which would hinder the outbreak of wars (1933b). This internationalism was based on a firm patriotism, resenting cosmopolitanism that would lead to shortcomings in moral principles without a firm root in a homeland (1898).

As a logical consequence, de Coubertin volunteered for military service at the beginning of World War I, although he was above the normal age limit. The war taught him a lesson, however. He moved his home outside the sphere of blind nationalism to Lausanne, where he started to educate foreigners in internment, and wrote a 100-page monograph on mutual respect as his answer to the atrocities of modern warfare (1915).

Avery Brundage (1887-1975)

The second longest presidency of the IOC was that of Avery Brundage. Although all of his papers are readily accessible (Brichford 1977), very little can be deduced. Neither his speeches (1968) nor his autobiography (1972) are very helpful. Twenty-four years younger than de Coubertin, World War II came almost exactly at the same point in his lifespan as World War I in de Coubertin's. Their reactions were completely different. Brundage was in the forefront of the "Keep the U.S. out of the war" movement. He was an ardent supporter of Willkie against Roosevelt (Brundage 1940). While de Coubertin was asked to run for a seat in parlament and refused three times (Boulogne 1975), Brundage ran for governor of Illinois - and lost, although he used his prestige and prominence as a sporting personality. His campaign theme was isolationism. Brundage tried to ignore wars as much as he could. During World War I he built up his construction business and was athletically successful. With his theory that sport and politics should not mix, that the world of sport should stay aloof from the political world, he avoided educational, moral and political questions, if they were not directly related to sports. More general questions which he dealt with in the first draft of his autobiography he crossed out before publication (Brundage Collection Box 330, 331). As Brundage looked at the world through the eyes of a self-made businessman and not as an educator like de Coubertin, peace education had nothing to do with sport for him. Mutual respect on the basis of knowing and understanding are also of no concern for a businessman from the Midwest, quite naturally assuming that the American way of life is right anyway (Guttman 1979).

Henri de Baillet-Latour (1876-1942)

The third longest term of office is that of de Baillet-Latour, 1925-1942. Although little is known of his attitude towards war and peace, he was very pragmatic in these matters. As the organiser of the 1920 Olympics in Antwerp he succeeded in using the military machinery for the success of the Games. In his term of office World War II began. Interestingly enough he did not take any personal decisions but let the committee as a whole decide how to deal with the aggressor. Already when he took office in 1925 he had announced that he would execute the wishes of the executive committee while de Coubertin and Brundage tried manipulate the committee to agree to their wishes (IOC 1925).

Political theory differentiates between "just" and "unjust" wars. The latter include invasions of other countries. The relationship of the IOC to such actions can best be studied using the example of the German invasion of Czechoslovakia in 1939. After the Munich Treaty of 1938 had given an outer ring of Czechoslovakia to Germany, Germany had itself invaded the rest and occupied it - not honouring a treaty just signed which was supposed to have guaranteed "peace in our time".

After St. Moritz had turned down the Olympic Games for the winter of 1940, the IOC met in full session on 6 June 1939 in London. The IOC had the choice of either giving in to Swiss demands to have non-amateur ski-instructors competing as amateurs and have the Olympic Games in St. Moritz, or dropping the winter games for 1940, or giving them to the organisers of the last games, as they were the only ones who had the necessary installations ready in time. By a vote of 2:27 the games were not postponed to 1944. In spite of the German invasion less than 3 months before, the Olympic Games were given to Germany unanimously (Krüger 1982a). The Olympic rule that the games must be held every fourth year was considered more important than the moral question of whether the Olympic Games could be held in a country considered an aggressor.

Two weeks after the outbreak of World War II de Baillet-Latour asked the members of the executive committee what should be done now that Europe was at war. The answer have been the guiding principles of the IOC ever since. He asked his fellow members: Can the Olympic Games take place in a country fighting a war? "Yes", by 4:3 votes. Should countries fighting a war be excluded from the Olympic Games? "No", by 7:0 votes. Are the Olympic Games technically organisable during a war? The question was handed over to the international federations and answered positively by the majority of them. Is it conceivable that athletes of countries which are at war with one another can compete peacefully with each other at the Olympic Games? "Yes", by 7:0 votes. Should the executive committee alone decide the question of cancelleation in the event of ermergency or should the whole IOC be asked? The whole committee should be asked (4:3). Therefore the IOC did not cancel the 1940 Olympic Games; instead they were cancelled by Germany on 25 November 1939 and Finland on 6 May 1940.

Discussion

The Olympic movement bases itself on the thoughts of de Coubertin. Brundage and de Baillet-Latour held the second and third longest terms of office and can therefore also be considered very important for the development of Olympism. Although the national importance of other personalities for the Olympic thought of their respective countries may be considered large, examples being Carl Diem in Germany (Krüger 1980, 1982a, b), Ferenc Kemény in Hungary (Kereszténvi 1982), Messerli in Switzerland and Ketseas in Greece *et al.*, one may safely assume that the influence of the three aforementioned president on the whole Olympic movement has been the strongest.

German Nazism, a creed that can be considered incompatible with the Olympic rule of non-discrimination on political or racial grounds, can be considered the test of the thoughts of these three personalities, as Nazi rule occurred during their lifetime and all three were required to take a stand. This test serves least well for de Coubertin, who died in 1937, at which time the atrocities were not as obvious and the war had not started. However, in a recent paper de Coubertin has been linked with Nazi thought as he had permitted himself to be exploited for the benefit of Nazi propaganda (Teichler 1982). Although this fact cannot be denied, one should not overlook that de Coubertin was the only major Olympic leader who publicly rejected the burning of books, the leaving of the League of Nations and the reduction of civil liberties in Germany (Krüger 1982c). How can you respect one another if you do not learn the opinion of the other? de Coubertin also used a radio lecture one year prior to the Olympic Games to explain to the German people that internationalism, democracy and mutual respect are of historical importance (de Coubertin 1935).

Brundage worked actively in favour of the Nazi movement both prior to and after the 1936 Olympic Games (Krüger 1972). His pro-Nazi stand was acknowledged by the German government by helping him to obtain the contract for the construction of the German Embassy in Washington (Brundage Collection Box 127). While Brundage's straightforward anti-semitism has been described elsewhere (Krüger 1978), de Coubertin's racialism is far more complicated. Whereas de Coubertin readily accepted the cultural superiority of whites over blacks (de Coubertin 1903b), Jews were among his oldest friends and collaborators. In his analysis of the Dreyfus affair, the touchstone of French anti-semitism, he came up with a political rather than a racial analysis (de Coubertin 1899). The 1904 Olympics Games were the only ones which de Coubertin did not attend while he was in office. They took place in St. Louis, where racial segregation among spectators and participants obviously took place. de Coubertin had fought for Chicago as the site of the Olympic Games, but lost (Krüger 1980). de Coubertin's life credo *mens fervida in corpore lacertoso* can accommodate the Nazi views on strength, but his notion of mutual respect runs counter to all Nazi philosophies (Krüger 1979).

de Baillet-Latour did not take any stand in matters concerning Nazism. Prior to World War II he did not use the moral authority of his office to defend the aims of the Olympic chàrter against the German usurpation. Acting on behalf of the executive committee of the IOC, this cannot surprise, as from 1937 onwards this had a pro-Nazi majority. Later on it was obvious that he could move freely from occupied Belgium to Lausanne and back as he did not cause any trouble for the Nazi aims (Diem 1942).

Brundage's "The Games must go on" has been criticised as perverted reduction of the Olympic ideal to athletic actionism. de Coubertin wanted this last stand of Olympism, as he saw sport as a basis for better understanding and mutual respect. As can be seen from the Nazi era, the Olympic Games cannot be considered a symbol for peace or love of peace, not are they a symbol for pacifism - but one of a longing for peace which is represented by common respect for the rules of the game, by staging the games and by taking part in them.

From these writings and the action taken concerning the Olympic Games, one can see that it is not easy to consider the Olympic movement a peace movement. Therefore one need not be surprised that initiatives to confer the Nobel Peace Prize on the IOC have failed. The Olympic movement has, however, as its core a belief in history. By taking over the tradition of the ancient Olympic Games, a historic role within Western civilisation is taken over. Sporting leaders who consider the Olympic Games nothing but super world championships where therefore like "leprosy" to de Coubertin (1903), and men without a conscience in history, "monsters" (1915). In this respect even the mere fact that the Olympic Games do go on can be considered a sign of hope; they constitute a sign of the unity of man.

In his last major interview in late 1936 de Coubertin pointed out that he wanted the Olympic Games the way they had become. But he also explained that they were but a small part of his educational plans. Since education starts with children and not with top international athletes, in the last 12 years of his life de Coubertin worked for these aims outside the Olympic movement, as this did not achieve all he had hoped for. Brundage realised this deficit very late in his life and created a scholarship fund in his will to help the athlete and scholar. Baillet-Latour died in office during the war.

Considering the limited concern regarding the use of the Olympic movement as a peace movement (over and above the mere fact that talking to and being in contact with each other is better than fighting each other), it can be concluded that de Coubertin was right in placing more emphasis on his educational rather than on his Olympic initiatives in the latter part of his life.

References

Boulogne Y-P (1975) La vie et l'oeuvre pédagogique de Pierre de Coubertin. Editions Leméac, Ottawa
Brichford M (1977) Avery Brundage Collection, 1908–1975. Hofmann, Schorndorf
Brundage A (1940) Address of Brundage and Lindbergh at Chicago mass meeting of the "Citizens Keep America out of War Committee". Chicago
Brundage A (1968) The speeches of Avery Brundage. IOC, Lausanne
Brundage A (1972) Die Herausforderung. ProSport, München
Brundage A (1977) Avery Brundage Collection. Alumni Association of the University of Illinois. Microfilm edition. Champaign, Ill.
de Coubertin P (1889) L'education de la paix. Réf Soc 7:361-363
de Coubertin P (1894) Le rétablissement des jeux olympiques. Rev Paris 1:170–184
de Coubertin P (1898) Does cosmopolitan life lead to international friendliness. Rev of Rev, NY 17: 429–434
de Coubertin P (1899) France since 1814. Fortnightly Rev N.F. 66/67:186–211; 572–585; 817–834; 1026–1037; 240–255; 843–855; 977–990
de Coubertin P (1903a) L'oeuvre de la paix. Figaro, 23.12.1903a
de Coubertin P (1903b) La question négre. Figaro, 26.9.1903b
de Coubertin P (1904) Les bases de la pédagogie prochaine. (2) La paix armée. Figaro, 26.1.1904
de Coubertin P (1915) Le respect mutuel. Lib Félix Alcan, Paris
de Coubertin P (1923) Discours prononcé par le président. IOC session 1923. Rome
de Coubertin P (1927) L'histoire pourvoyeuse de guerre ou de la paix. Union Péd. Universelle 2:5-12
de Coubertin P (1933a) Anthologie. B.I.P.S., Lausanne
de Coubertin P (1933b) Lettre à S.E. le Président du Conseil de la Société des Nations. B.I.P.S., Lausanne
de Coubertin P (1935) Les assises philosophiques de l'olympisme moderne. Le Sport Suisse, 4.8.1935
Diem C (1942) Der olympische Gedanke im neuen Europa. Terramare, Berlin
Guttmann A (1979) The Games must go on. Stadion 5:253-262
IOC (1925) Minutes. (Microfilm)
Keresztenyi J (1982) Ferenc Kémeny. Olympic Rev 174:212-213
Krüger A (1972) Die Olympischen Spiele 1936 und die Weltmeinung. Bartels und Wernitz, Berlin
Krüger A (1978) Fair play for American athletes. A study in anti-semitism. Can J Hist Sp PE 9:42–57
Krüger A (1979) Mens fervida in corpore lacertoso oder de Coubertins Ablehnung der schwedischen Gymnastik. 8. HISPA Kongress, Uppsala, pp 145-153
Krüger A (1980) Neo-Olympismus zwischen Nationalismus und Internationalismus. In: Ueberhorst H (ed) Geschichte der Leibesübungen, vol 3/1. Bartels und Wernitz, Berlin, pp 522–568
Krüger A (1982a) Deutschland und die olympische Bewegung (1918-1945). In: Ueberhorst H (ed) Geschichte der Leibesübungen, vol 3/2. Bartels und Wernitz, Berlin, pp 1026–1047
Krüger A (1982b) Deutschland und die olympische Bewegung (1945-1980). In: Ueberhorst H (ed) Geschichte der Leibesübungen, vol 3/2. Bartels und Wernitz, Berlin, pp 1048–1081
Krüger A (1982c) de Coubertin und die Olympischen Spiele als Symbol des Friedens. (to be published) 3. ASSAS Seminar, Fribourg, 9 pp (in print)
Teichler H-J (1982) de Coubertin und das 3. Reich. Sportwissenschaft 12:18–55

Pierre de Coubertin and World Peace

R. Petrov

The life-work and deeds of Pierre de Coubertin have been the object of numerous analyses and evaluations by scientists, journalists, workers in the field of sport and writers from different countries. One can find in these analyses all shades of opinion from adoration to nihilistic nagation. The reasons for such discrepancy are not only the contradictions and inconsistency of de Coubertin's ideas but also the different ideological and political points of view of the research workers. Very often a subject of discussion has been the attitude of this great humanist towards the opportunities for transforming sport into a factor for improving understanding among people and stabilising world peace.

Pierre de Coubertin entered world history with his work in connection with the resumption of the Olympic Games (Diem 1967). Basing this work on giants of the past, he had probably far more grounds than Newton for saying that he looked into the future better than his contemporaries. The great philosophers of the Renaissance had rediscovered man and rehabilitated the ideal of a harmonious human body. Furthermore some prominent scientists and pedagogues had created national systems of physical education; the archaeologists Chadler, Fovel and Curcious had revealed the secrets of the ancient Olympics; Gutts-Mutts had suggested in 1973 the resumption of the Olympic Games; and major E.Tzapas (Bancialescu 1964) had, in 1859, organised the first "Greek Olympic Games". de Coubertin is not the founder of the Olympic movement. He only stimulated, directed, governed and gave a form to its development (Petrov 1981). Unlike his forerunners, he understood that in capitalist society objective conditions and prerequisites have already been created for wide economic, political and sporting relations between people. de Coubertin wanted to stop physical and spiritual degradation in society and created the contrasting, in some ways utopian, but attractive Olympic philosophy. He guaranteed the Olympic movement significant cultural, philosophical, sporting and scientific continuity and adopted many noble principles and ideas from the past (Petrov 1977,1981). Only a person with a Renaissance spirit could reform, through sport, interpersonal and international relations. At the very beginning de Coubertin wrote: "The resumption of the Olympic Games on the basis of and under conditions consistent with the requirements of modern life will allow the representatives of all nations in the world to meet every four years, and we want to believe that those peaceful and noble competitions are the purest internationalism". He eagerly desired that people come to know each other better, overcoming the hate and contradictions that lead to merciless war.

Being a devoted adherent of the ancient Olympic Games, de Coubertin drew the peace ideas from the Olympics. The Olympic armistice *("ekehairia")* began with the contract concluded between the owners Efitus from Hellas, Likurg from Sparta and

Kleosteos from Piza. The contents of the contract are characterised by a legend on a disc: "Olympus is a sacred place. One who dares to enter it with armed force will be anathemised before gods as a criminal". The armistice required all battles to be stopped during the games; the territory of Hellas was considered neutral, sacred and inviolable, and free access was assured to all participants. Although he showed a tendency to idealise the ancient Olympic Games, de Coubertin objectively analysed their history. He wrote: "The games had encountered great difficulties. The VIIIth Olympics were troubled with the discords between the organizers. Three centuries later, that holy armistice was broken down, which stopped the Olympic Games". He knew very well that in ancient Greece only a temporary peace had been achieved; however, he did discover the possibilities of sport in developing and strengthening friendship and peace:

> The Olympic idea breaks the fog of time like a ray of sun.... We are speaking about a movement which has sprung from deep and heartfelt human aspiration for peace and brotherhood. Peace has become a kind of religion whose altar gathers more and more believers.
>
> Solid democracy and correctly understood internationalism will enter the renewed stadium...

Sport at the Service of Peace

As an excellent pedagogue and an expert in sports, de Coubertin knew, that sporting exercises and competitions may be both useful and harmful:

> Sport can put into action the noblest and the meanest passions, to develop both the sense of honour and the pursuit of profit. It can be chivalrous or corrupt, bad or brutal, and finally it can be used both for stabilisation of peace and for preparation of war. However, nobleness and emotions, the sense of honour and unselfishness, the knightly spirit, energy and peace are primary necessities of modern democracies.

In the epoch of colonialism and imperialist aggressive wars, the problem of peace is of prime significance for people. The theoretical works of de Cooubertin on peace have an abstract-humanistic character, but his practical activity is remarkable for its realism, organisational talent and ability to realise in practice the most courageous ideas. The interrelation between sport, olympism and peace was expressed by de Coubertin in the introduction to the Olympic charter: "The purpose of the Olympic movement is to help the development of physical and spiritual qualities, which are the base of amateur sport, to gather all sportsmen in the world at the big sports festival every four years and in this way to promote international respect and goodwill, contributing to a better and peaceful world". In his famous *Ode to Sport*, de Coubertin expresses the main Olympic ideas. He believed passionately in the ability of sport to achieve peace:

> Oh, sport! You are peace! You establish good, friendly relations among people. You are agreement. You bring together people, desiring unity. You teach the youth, speaking different languages, respect and mutual trust. You are a source of noble, peaceful and friendly competition. You gather the youth- our future, our hope, under your peaceful banners. Oh,sport! You are peace!

One of de Coubertin's special merits is that he always associated the Olympic movement with the struggle for friendship, peace and understanding among people, although his hope that the Olympic Games would prevent wars was not realised. He greatly appreciated the idea that through the Olympic Games people would come to know each other better, and said with optimism: "We could not stop the war, but the war couldn't destruct everything". The Olympic movement is impossible without peace. It is an antipode of war and consequently it should be an active factor in the international movement for peace. It is true that some theoretical positions of de Coubertin are near to the ideological bases of pacifism, but in practise he actively fought against militarism, colonialism and all kinds of restriction and discrimination. His activity went beyond the scope of the biggest programmes of pacifists.

The passive negation of war in the Olympic movement is contradictory to the vital interests of mankind. In our troubled epoch, when the stored weapons can destruct life on this planet several times over, there is no place for hiding behind the mist of "a political sport", "neutrality" or pacifism.

The Olympic movement has a great role to play in peace, and it must replace the vain negation of war with a struggle for humanism and understanding among peoples. de Coubertin was fighting for "peace stronger than the balance based on fear". The necessity of trust, understanding and mutual co-operation among peoples has never been so great as it is today. de Coubertin's followers understand that his ideas mean an active struggle for disarmament and the discrediting of militaristic politics, for the uniting of people under the conditions of peaceful existence of states with different social systems. In 1967 the IOC accepted the appeal for defence and consolidation of peace and, after the tenth Olympic Congress in Varna (1973), the President of the IOC, Lord Killanin, declared: "Besides the motto *Citius, altius, fortius* , the Olympic movement has an additional motto - *Sport in a peaceful world*". The Olympic movement finds support from various public circles in the world. The statement of Urho Kekonen, the former President of Finland, is remarkable:

> World support must be ensured for the Olympic movement and the Olympic Games, which are the most important event in the field of international sporting co-operation. As a former sportsman and a sporting leader, I know that sport creates good premises for mutual understanding among people. In my speech on public security and co-operation in Europe, I cited a Finnish proverb: Security, that is not the building of barriers, but the opening of doors.

The peaceful role of sport can be increased by various means:

- Intensive development of interrelations and mutual aid among sportsmen, coaches, scientists and journalists from different countries
- Development of of sporting ethics and internationalism among both athletes and the public
- Clarification of the ideological and ethical inheritance of Pierre de Coubertin and emphasis on loyalty to his legacies
- Observation of the Olympic charter and an active struggle against all deformations in the Olympic movement.
- An active struggle *aigainst* all forms of militarism and *for* consolidation of humanism, democracy, peace and social progress

The appearance and the development of the Olympic movement can be considered an irreversible necessity in view of the state of international relations at the end of the nineteenth and during the twentieth century. Pierre de Coubertin is an interpreter of the ideas of, and an initiator of the organised struggle for, peace and understanding between peoples by means of sport. His life and deeds are full of a deep humanism, internationalism and belief in the integrative and peaceful function of physical culture and international sporting competitions. The modern Olympic movement continues the struggle for peace started by Pierre de Coubertin, following the example and observing the ideological and theoretical inheritance of this great humanist. In order to increase its peace-making role, it should substitute for vain negation, an active struggle for peace, humanism, democracy and social progress.

Finally, I would like to express my conviction that everyone who sincerely has respect for the ideas of Pierre de Coubertin, the Olympic charter, the oath and the flag with interwoven rings would never forget the legacy of de Coubertin: "It is necessary, in spite of everything, to direct our efforts to link the athletes in a lasting friendship. In their striving for peace they have to be indivisible, like the links of the chain". In our troubled epoch that legacy is a moral duty of everyone to all people and of every nation to the whole of mankind.

References

Bancialescu V (1964) Joocurille Olimpice de A. Lungul. Vercurilor. Editura unuinilde de Cultura Fizika si sports, Bucuresti
de Coubertin P (1975a) Olympic memoirs. Bulgarian Olympic Committee
de Coubertin P (1975b) Speeches and essays. Bulgarian Olympic Committee
de Coubertin P (1975c) Mutual respect. Bulgarian Olympic Committee
Diem C (1967) Weltgeschichte des Sports. Cotta
Petrova N (1981) Social-economic systems and development of the Olympic movement. Collection: Actual problems of the international Olympic movement. Medicine and Physical Culture, Sofia
Petrov R (1977) Purposes of the ancient Olympic Games. Collection: Problems of the Olympic movement. Bulgarian Olympic Committee
Petrov R (1981) Ideological and ethical inheritance of Pierre de Coubertin. Collection: Actual problems of the international Olympic movement. Medicine and Physical Culture, Sofia

The Role of the Olympic Games in International Understanding

G. Paulín and R. Jimenez

Olympiads as an Interactive and Communicative Process

Man naturally tends to live in society, because he is not self-sufficient enough to attend to the necessities of life; he needs the help of others and through this need he develops his communicative potential. Hence the history of man, in general terms, has been the history of his interaction and his communication.

Human interaction is the resultant of two polar processes, namely association and disassociation, between which a continuum of subprocesses tending towards one or the other pole is established. Amalgamation or mixture is the most complete process because it means the possibility of achieving cohesion between individuals in spite of their differences, and is only possible when man approach each other for co-operative purposes. *Co-operation* is possible due to the convergence of the elements that are involved in it, that is: emotion (which encourages sympathetic impulses), interests (which stress the identity of "I" and of "us" in relation to others), and situation (or the objective conditions that favour the association).

At the other end of the continuum of human interaction there is competition or the process through which persons tend towards an identical objective. In this process, as well as in the others, there can be tendencies for association as well as for disassociation; when associative tendencies are shown in the competitive process, thc attitudes of tolerance, commitment and adjustment make it possible for the competitors to achieve an understanding that puts up with union. By contrast, when in that same process disassociative tendencies prevail, the attitudes of rivalry and dispute stop or hinder understanding, thus resulting in disunion, disagreement and conflict. Extreme cases of disassociation in competition are rivalry or dispute. Rivalry centres completely on the competitor, while dispute centres on awareness of the scarcity of the objects being competed for.

The Olympiads, sporting events of an amateur character which from the end of the nineteenth century have been held every 4 years (except on two occasions, 1912 and 1936, during the two great conflicts of the twentieth century), have evidenced manifestations of both association and disassociation:

Firstly, there is a greater tendency to association when teams and national groups are adapted to an "us". Emotion, interests and situation then agree with the sense of co-operation that identifies them as an organised group "for itself", looking for the *attainment* of its goal; the *good* attainment (*performance*) and the acknowledgement of "others".

Secondly, either associative competition or disassociative competition arises during the games themselves. The former occurs when, in spite of differences, *interests* in the general or particular sporting activity that is being practised prevails, and *the natural desire for a human approach* predominates. Disassociative competition, on the other hand, occurs when the differences resulting from the individualist and nationalist feelings of honour, prestige and reward are aggravated.

Role of the Olympiads within the Framework of Contemporary International Relations

The contemporary world faces a paradoxical situation: On the one hand, there are countries that have attained a leading position in economic, technological and sporting development, and these countries have set the *patterns* to be followed by those that have been left behind. On the other hand, there is a hypertrophy of economy in relation to ethics, politics, culture, sport, art and other sectors of reality; this has led to, but has also been the result of, a tendency to invest all human efforts in gaining profits, power and prestige at the price of human impoverishment. The lack of proportion that exists between economic progress on the one hand and selflessness and charity on the other is the contemporary framework for the Olympic Games. For this reason a reality prevails in them that is without sense and human meaning. Hence, let us look for and try to give *human sense* to the Olympic Games.

The dehumanisation of the Olympic Games reflects the present historical juncture, when the entire global human society is split up into national societies grouped into two great blocs: societies in which an economy of liberal capitalism prevails, and societies in which there is communism or socialism of a Marxist type. Neither is capable of carrying out Olympic competitons that would lead to international understanding, and neither can contribute authentically to them.

In effect, with the individualism typical of the liberal capitalist societies, the relations between members of society are reduced to the adjustment of interests between individuals. This is the result of the attitude of opposition to the common good: individual interests is recognised as the only encouragement for action, ownership is seen as a natural right and there is freedom to dispose of and acquire property. When such nations are exalted if the Olympic Games, this distortion of reality promotes prejudice or attitudes of rejection on the basis of ethnicity, race and religion, blocking understanding and communication between participants.

With collectivism, private relations between exceptional men are denied owing to the identification of self-interest and common interest, to the identification of private property with the alienation of production goods in the immanent sense, to the submission of freedom to the authority of the state and to the complete integration of the individual with regard to public welfare. In the case of such nations that are exalted in the Olympic Games, this distortion of reality favours the obstruction of interaction and communication between participants.

As a result of the distortions of social reality which characterise either of these types of relations that restrain or avoid the development of the communicative and associative abilities of man, there will be national communities that will support progress in sport as far as the latter is perceived as being centered on material goods (medals) and non-material goods (honours) in which nationalism is exalted. This will only limit the development of the creative abilities that encourage the growth and progress of the social whole and of the individual.

In matters such as tourism and sport it is very easy to fall into wishful thinking. It is easy to claim, and apparently easy to substantiate, the statement that tourism and sport improve international relations. However, even if it is not easy to substantiate opposite claims, when facts are examined more closely it is possible to detect, under certain conditions, nagative consequences of tourism and sport for international relations and sometimes internal political stability.

Possibilities of the Olympiads as a Framework for Human Encounters

Modern Olympiads are carried out in a framework of international relations involving exaggerated nationalism. On the one hand, the developing nations require prestigious supports that will allow them to shape their national identity; on the other hand, the post-imperial states (those that have looked for political centralisation) and the "post-dynastic" states (those that have attained administrative centralisation) require the revitalisation of their prestige that may help them to retain their hegemonic position. Under these circumstances, the event sets up a forum of disassociative competition: (1) it places limits on human encounters; (2) it promotes the development of prejudices; and (3) it provokes the maintenance of existing conflicts and can lead to the appearance of others.

The manner of rewarding the individual for a sporting achievement places his personal effort in second place owing to the exaltation of two symbols: his national anthem and his flag. In addition the fact that the mass media give such prominence to attainments in quantitative terms, i.e. the number of medals acquired by each nation, leads to either a positive or a negative evaluation of ethnicity and to dispute and rivalry in events.

In summary, we propose: (1) the elimination of national barriers, i.e. anthems and flags; (2) instead of medals, expressive means that would allow the winner to convey his (her) techniques to others in an understandable way and (3) the use of an anthem that would symbolise the entire human effort, without artificial barriers that separate man from his fellow man.

References

García AL (1978) Filosofía de la Eficacia. Jus, México, pp 15-24
Millan PA (1978) Fundamentes de Filosofía. Rialp SA, Madrid, pp 389-394
von Wiese L (1959) Sistema de Sociología General, vol I. Cajica, Puebla (México), pp 273-381

Challenges Facing the Olympic Movement – The Outcome of the XIth Olympic Congress

P. Tallberg

The XIth Olympic Congress held in Baden-Baden, Germany, from 23rd to 28th September 1981 was the greatest gathering of Olympic and sports leaders ever held in the world. The list of participants was impressive: 82 members of the International Olympic Comittee, representatives of 26 International Olympic Federations, 9 International Federations recognised by the International Olympic Committee but not included in the Olympic Programme, 149 National Olympic Committees, 34 medal winner athletes (both men and women), 10 coaches, representatives of a number of other world sports organisations, both governmental and non-governmental, and 500 representatives of the mass media of the world.

The Aims of the Congress

The motto of the Congress was: "United by and for Sport". All participants agreed that it was mainly thanks to the leadership of the new President of the IOC and leader of world sports, Mr. Samaranch, that the congress turned out to be such a success and a great victory for the IOC. Contrary to certain expectations, the congress proved in a magnificent way that the capability and strength of the IOC are far beyond the level presented by the mass media and certain other outside forces. The boycotting of the Moscow Games by certain nations and federations was turned into a success for the IOC, and this was done in a way which appealed to most of those who were present, even the representatives of the boycotting countries themselves. The three main issues of the Congress were:

1. The future of the Olympic Games
2. International co-operation
3. The Olympic movement in prospective

Main Points of the Congress Declaration

Future Olympic Games programmes must more closely reflect modern tendencies in sport.

A new rule was adopted by the IOC at its session in Rome a month ago which stipulates that a review of the Olympic programme is to be made by the IOC after each Olympics, also covering the two preceding Games. In each review the IOC reserves the right to update standards for admission of sports, disciplines and events, and to eliminate sports, disciplines and events in which international interest is insufficient according to the standards for admission. The same applies if there is evidence of inadequate control according to the Olympic rules.

The IOC must keep up to date with modern tendencies in sport, thus creating a programme and an atmosphere that meets the requirements of athletes of various parts of the world on an equal basis. The programme of the Games shall not be tailored to suit only the top athletes of the "old" developed countries in Europe and the United States. New sports, popular in the developing countries, will surely be included in the programme of future Games.

There is no place in the Olympic Games for "professional" or "open" competition.

In his final speech in Baden-Baden, Sebastian Coe expressed the views of the participating athletes by saying:

> On Rule 26, the Eligibility Rule, it is illogical to expect one rule to be capable of attending to individual needs of all the sports in the Olympic Movement. We therefore echo the call in Congress for greater independence for International Federations in determining exactly what the needs of their sports are. The demand for a modern Olympian is considerable. Such a sacrifice to the cause of the movement should never be disregarded. It is therefore the moral obligation of the IOC to ensure that, within the framework of the Eligibility Rule, provision is made for the social consideration of the athlete.
> Open or "real" professional competition would widen the gap between athletes, both within the developed world and such nations as well as between rich and poor countries.

The Olympic Games should continue to be able to be held anywhere in the World.

It is of the utmost importance that the venue of the Olympic Games varies from one continent to another and from one country to another. In the late 1970s the games seemed to have expanded to an extent that would allow only the big and rich nations to bid for the hosting. However, the situation has changed rapidly. Two Asian countries fought hard for the 1988 Games and by now there are at least six countries which have shown interest in the 1992 Games. The tendency is in accord with the main purpose of the games and the whole movement, i.e. to spread olympism to all parts of the world, thus furthering international co-operation and peace.

The Olympic Games, the most important manifestation of international co-operation, must be supported by everyone.

The Olympic movement is open to all those who accept its principles and respect its charter. Everyone has his or her own place, and each place has a certain value. The principles express a particular way of acting in sport and via sport. Their influence on individual behaviour and everyday life becomes apparent in the form of fairness, friendship and respect of moral values. It is essential that advantage is taken of the success of the Olympic movement and the enthusiasm it has created, in order to spread the Olympic ideas further wherever and whenever possible.

All components of the Olympic movement must be integrated and in close interrelation with all parties concerned. A lot of commissions and working groups need to be set up in order to facilitate discussions, debates and interaction. A new opening was made in this respect at the Rome meeting of the IOC, which approved a draft resolution that will be examined and hopefully approved by the United Nations in the near future. The document binds nations of the whole world to respect the Games and the

Olympic movement, both of which are placed under the authority of the International Olympic Committee.

Everyone involved should persuade his or her organisation to assist developing countries to improve their sporting performances and to increase the general participation in sport. Olympic solidarity should provide the motivating force for this.

Olympic solidarity plays a leading role in the promoting of sport in the developing areas of the world. It has been created not only to strengthen the co-operation between the National Olympic Committees and the IOC, but to help the NOCs to overcome the imbalance and inequalities that may exist in sport.

The elimination of discrimination in sports is of the utmost importance.

Every now and then the IOC faces problems of very complicated nature, one of them being discrimination and apartheid in sports. The IOC has taken a very strict stand on this point and was the first organisation to ban South Africa in 1970, following its non-conformity with the Olympic charter and Olympic rules. The IOC will continue to pursue this policy and will not give up before discrimination in sports has been entirely eradicated.

In close co-operation with the International Federations, the National Olympic Committees and all supporting organisations, the IOC must lead the sports world in agreement with the principles of the Olympic Charter.

The IOC will endeavour to be worthy of this trust and responsibility. Mr. Samaranch is fully aware of the requirements set for the IOC and will, together with all members of the same, continue to undertake full responsibility in compliance with the Olympic Charter. The IOC will also fully respect the independence and autonomy of each party involved in the movement, i.e. the International Federations and the National Olympic Committees. However, one has to bear in mind that there are natural limits to this independence, as can easily be seen from the Olympic Charter. The Olympic movement has, since its foundation in 1894, been able to overcome a great many difficulties and I am convinced that it is, thanks to its new unity, now stronger than ever.

The Commission for the Olympic movement, consisting of members representing the IOC, the IFs and the NOCs should be enlarged to include representatives of other organisations.

This commission was set up after Baden-Baden, and it has met once. There are nine members from the IOC, the eight members of the Executive and the Chairman of the Athletes' Commission, nine members representing the IFs and nine members representing the NOCs. By establishing this commission, Mr. Samaranch has tried to avoid a certain friction which existed between the parties concerned in earlier years, when the number of members in the Tripartite Commission was very limited. It seems to have been the first step towards positive development, as an example of which a representative of the Athletes' Commission has been included in this body.

More opportunities should be provided for women in the administration of sports.

Miss Svetla Otzetova, Bulgarian rowing gold medalist, said in her speech in Baden-Baden:

> Women's sport is not yet adequately recognised in all countries - in some it is even discriminated against. The Olympic movement should contribute to overcoming these traditional ways of thinking. The athletes should welcome the fact that the IOC attributes special importance to the participation of women and that it promotes sport for women. This programme should, however, not only be limited to active sport, but should also extend to representation in the sports federations, in the NOCs, and last but not least, in the IOC.

Since Baden-Baden, three female members have entered the IOC, one representing the IOC in Finland, one in Venezuela and one in Great Britain. It has taken 88 years before the first lady attended a session of the IOC, the highest authority in world sports today. Let the development be more rapid from now on!

Education is of vital importance and should be organised on a governmental basis, stressing the beneficial aspects of practising sports.

It goes without saying that the governmental organisations bear the major responsibility for sports education in each nation. It is not the duty of the Olympic movement to interfere with the educational work carried out by the national authorities. The IOC, and especially the athletes linked to the Olympic movement, bear a certain responsibility towards the youth both ethically and morally. The IOC can and shall provide both cultural and educational training within its framework. The main responsibility, however, lies elsewhere. The Olympic Academy is of vital importance when it comes to spreading olympism throughout the world. The roles of UNESCO and the IOC were determined during the presidential mandate of Lord Killanin.

Work in order to achieve the goals and to fulfil the fundamental principles of the Olympic movement, quality of life, health and satisfaction will be much more successful if the independence and autonomy of non-governmental sports organisations are safeguarded and protected.

The IOC, the IFs and the NOCs are now regularly invited to attend the meetings of UNESCO, sports ministers and other governmental bodies. These organisations acknowledge officially the complete and necessary independence of the IOC. In most countries the clubs, federations and National Olympic Committees have to co-operate closely with their governments in order to survive and develop. It is therefore of the utmost importance to work at a respectful distance from, but to have good relations with, all parties concerned, not violating the complete autonomy and independence of the international sports organisations and without any subordination whatsoever.

It is obvious that the challenges facing international sporting links in the future are many, especially as far as the role of sports in promoting international understanding is concerned. The IOC is fully aware of its role in this process, and under the new President it has managed to consolidate and unify its resources in an outstanding way. Today the IOC stands strong and determined, ready to promote and spread Olympic principles among people, nations and world organisations, thus creating a fruitful atmosphere for mutual understanding on an international level and for peace in the world.

The Importance of the International Sports Movement in Promoting International Understanding - The Viewpoint of an Olympic Athlete

H. Kirvesniemi

In present-day society, more and more attention is devoted to top-level sport. Many reasons, such as the rise in the standard of living, the increase in leisure time and the development of the media have led to people today having greater opportunity to follow sport and have given sportsmen a far more fully developed possibility to train and to take part in international competition. This "professionalism" in sport brings with it a greater possibility of attaining the objectives, which are the major present-day principle of the Olympics - faster, higher, longer; but on the other hand the increased pressure caused by competitiveness has taken on many negative features. In spite of these problems sport can still be regarded in a favourable light as a profession or as a pastime, even though an often biased and contrary picture is conveyed to the public.

The Individual Uniting and Educative Effects of Sport

At least at the level of the individual, international sport is capable of furthering communication and by that means promoting a common understanding amongst the sportsmen of the world. Although top-level sport in itself involves the keen competition of one against another, there exists amongst sportsmen outside the sports arena a reciprocal understanding, remote from political, religious or even linguistic factors. The birth of contact between different ideologies surely helps to further the knowledge of the aspirations of the various peoples of the world and in that way helps in teaching man to understand his similarities and differences. Considering the present state of the world we live in today, this is without a doubt a very important step towards peaceful communication. The whole notion of sport does create a terrific driving force in forming a spirit of standing together.

In addition to this effect of drawing people together in a common cause, sport has always played a very noticeable role in education. At an early age in youth, sports games and matches help to bring up children to work in co-operation, and from the beginnings of active training the sportsman has to learn to develop stamina, to withstand continued stress and fatigue, to allocate time effectively and to be able to choose priorities concerning values in life. Forming these values into a way of life certainly assists the individual in his civilian life when his sporting career has come to an end.

A decisive factor in the challenge of reaching the top in sport is the ability to maximise one's performance. In aiming at this objective everyone realises that the chances of failing are very great. In spite of this a sportsman who has trained in the right way can enrich his life even in defeat. Defeat has to be learnt to be accepted equally as well as triumph, and an essential feature in sport is the ability to admit, at the moment of defeat, that another was better than you. The lack of this ability to accept defeat could be a leading factor in doping. The setting of high objectives, the uncertainty about being able to achieve them, the exaggerated excitement that surrounds sport and the pressures of publicity erode the sportsman's confidence in himself and, because of the real fear of defeat, drive him to forbidden substances.

Competition Between Nations

The Olympic Games represent, for most sports, the most outstanding, the most highly esteemed and the most demanding meeting of top-rated athletes. At its best the Olympics involve fair competition between athletes only, but today many outside influences, such as the competition between nations, commercialism and politics, have come to bear on these events. These factors need not necessarily break up the sporting spirit, but unfortunately they often do.

In my opinion competition between different nations is fully permissible if it occurs in the same spirit as between individuals and is free of any political objectives. It must not turn out to be a tug-of-war between different social groups whose goal in many cases is to achieve success at any price whatsoever. In this fashion the opportunities for working towards international understanding are completely destroyed. In the same way an individual sportsman's motives can deviate from national aims, resulting in a situation where these motives do not serve the same goal. Also the stress placed on individual performances in my opinion implies that the competition between nations in a single event should not be overemphasised. In spite of everything, performing under national banners and to the tune of national anthems suits the whole picture of the Olympics; it does after all provide some kind of advertising substitute for those sacrifices made by many states to support sport. It also cannot be denied that the motivation of some sportsmen to compete is increased simply by representing their country. Group events such as the relay even presuppose an official contest between various nations.

Sport and Politics

It is often said that politics has entered sport to stay, and this is probably the case, but surely within the bounds of sport and politics the rules of the game in sport still have to be observed. Everyone should have the opportunity to demonstrate his own ability independent of his own or his country's political viewpoint or activity. Bringing politics into the arena by boycotting and other similar political actions, at the expense of sport, affects most acutely those people who after years of work have to shelve their goals. It is quite a different matter if the individual sportsman's own decision is to follow his political convictions before his aspirations in sport, and he refuses to take part in a certain event. Politics in sport must not be used as a pawn for the affairs of others but must be preserved as an integral part of the matters concerning sport.

Commercialism in Sport

Commercialism has been blamed for bringing about the downfall of sport, and it does play a very visible role. In my opinion the magnitude of this particular problem cannot be compared with other issues, e.g. doping. The organisation of sporting events on the scale prevalent today costs a lot of money and advertising is needed to cover the great expenditure. On the other hand, a leading sportsman's work has become more and more a full-time job, or at the very least limits his ability to fulfil the demands of an ordinary job or to study. For this reason it has become necessary for the sportsman to look further afield than the public sector for sources of income to cover his sizeable expenses. In this way, as many sportsmen as possible can be assured the opportunity of full training.

The alternatives to the present situation would be to abandon commercialism, limiting the flow of funds from this source, or to create a situation where only professional sportsmen could participate. In the first case the number of sportsmen capable of taking part would certainly decrease and the standards would become much lower; at the same time it would put prospective sportsmen from various organisations in the society into a different class. Full professionalism, on the other hand, is pure utopia in many sporting events as the resources are in any case limited. To my mind the present situation is a good alternative and forms a basis for assured development. In this case the question would rather concern a more even allocation of funds from international sporting events in order that young aspiring sportsmen and trainers and coaches, who do not receiving their main income from these areas of activity, would be assured economic security. Although money is partly in conflict with the Olympic regulations, to may mind it only makes common sense that it should take first place and that the financial rewards a sportsman receives for his efforts be approved of. It is certainly a much healthier alternative for a sportsman to return at the end of his sporting career to civilian life on a firm financial basis, than to vainly attempt to struggle on when his life has already been restricted by the excessive ethical standards of a sporting career.

The Problem of Doping

The most adverse effect on the principles of sport has appeared in the use of artificial means to attempt to improve performance. This phenomenon, known as doping, is nowadays claimed by many to oppose the work carried out to promote sport, in spite of its everyday appearance on the track. I would like to make it quite clear that I am completely against doping and I try as best I can, with the means at my disposal, to work to eradicate it. I trust that I will have the opportunity to describe my experiences to young people in the sporting field, and to assure them that in spite of all the publicity that has been given to doping it is still possible to win even a gold medal cleanly and honestly by rigorous training. I am quite convinced that in very many events in top-level sport, a great number of sportsmen are competing honestly and fairly.

All in all, the whole discussion surrounding the doping issue has managed to create a very one-sided and biased picture of the extent of the use of drugs by exaggerating the whole thing. My point of view on this issue is that insufficient attention has been paid to those sportsmen who have succeeded in top-level sport without the use of drugs, or alternatively if they have been given an opportunity to speak and state their opinions, their claims have been held in doubt. This has had the effect of either frightening people away from sport altogether or creating a situation where sportsmen themselves believe that the only way to improve performance is by using drugs - they may even accept their use on the grounds that others have resorted to them.

The reasons for abolishing doping are many. From the viewpoint of sports in general, the most important is the fact that those who use drugs are no longer at the same starting point as those who do not. This is based on the assumption that doping is, in fact, capable of improving results. The health-risk factors, too, are significant. From the viewpoint of training the biggest drawback is that when attempting to maximise performance by developing training methods, the effects of the training itself on the body become masked. Investigating the methods used in training either becomes more difficult, or the areas in which doping could be used to advantage are one-sidedly stressed. In this respect certain factors, such as the influence of the psyche on performance, are completely overlooked. Fortunately this situation can work against the sportsman using drugs, when the one who has trained in a fair and honest fashion can attain, within the limits of the approved methods, a certain element from his improved performance that the drug user does not even take into account. In general, research shows that there is good reason to place more stress on the physiological and biomechanical phenomena connected with training, which will in turn improve training methods.

Measures to Prevent Doping

Although the doping problem has received widespread public attention only during this decade, I am quite sure that, considering the present controls and bans employed in the Olympics, the situation has been improved for the present. However, the work on behalf of international enlightenment has not achieved completely satisfactory results, as the problem still exists. In order to achieve better results, the controls imposed should be extended to include sporting events on a national scale and to ensure parity in the control of international events. In addition to this, the punitive measures could be intensified and extended to include not only the sportsmen involved but also those persons who are indirectly responsible, bearing in mind, of course, that nobody is threatened legally. This presupposes a real willingness to cooperate on an international scale, but it would be a step in the right direction. My own personal wish is for a much greater reserve (money, methods, facilities, experts etc.) to be directed towards solving the doping problem.

One difficulty concerning banned drugs has been the definition of their suitability and keeping the list up-to-date. As far as the stimulants are concerned, the situation seems to be in hand, as the methods of inspection are reliable; but as far as hormone preparations are concerned, the situation is more difficult. An attempt has to be made to prevent the transference to more dangerous drugs which cannot be effectively controlled because the methods employed in testing are not sufficiently comprehensive. On the other hand, the dependence on the former should be eliminated. I am certainly no expert to say which is a dangerous substance and which is not, but in my opinion a sufficient basis for banning a certain drug is if the use of such a drug could improve one's performance. Taking this into consideration, it should not be possible to deviate from the present policy by, for example, allowing the use of anabolic steriods, under a doctor's supervision, in order to compensate for a hormone deficiency due to training. This is an often heard argument in favour of the use of anabolic steriods, but it would make monitoring even more difficult, the health risks would become even greater and at the same time matters such as the position of sportsmen from the developing countries would be complicated. Faith in sport would suffer an even harder blow and more and more mothers and fathers would be reluctant to allow their children to pursue a sporting career. In addition to this, one of the finest features - the fine balance between rest and exertion - would lose its meaning if a return to a normal state were to be accelerated by medical means.

Mass Media and Sport

The power of the media in sports is very great indeed, and a lot of attention is certainly devoted in the press, on television, and on the radio to top-level sports and other forms of gymnastics. This indicates that in spite of the attacks made against top-level sport, the interest of the peoples of the world is still very apparent. At the same time it presents to all of us involved in the sporting field a true challenge to maintain this great popularity and requires that solutions to the problems be found. Everyone has to recognise their responsibility on behalf of sport when the question concerns information or publicity, whether it concerns sports writers or the people who give them information. The education of sports writers should ensure that they become qualified enough to enable them to become experts in their own field. In the same way sportsmen and all personnel working in the sport should be made to realise that they do not only speak on their own behalf. By this I mean that it is not correct to give a false picture that affects the very spirit of sport, by giving observations or by quoting individual incidents without genuine facts to back them up. As already mentioned, doping is certainly a problem in sport, but just on that basis it would not be correct to come to the conclusion that it is the only way to the top. The information that is presented to the public must be closer to the truth - that only through rigorous training can one reach the top - and it is unfortunate that the exposure given to the doping problem and the investigation surrounding it indicates that some sportsmen who have resorted to the use of drugs have also resorted to other banned methods. A picture has been created in which the sportsman, at suitable intervals, pops pills into his mouth from a variety of pill-boxes, leaps onto the track and creates a new world record. In making a public statement of this nature, I am, of course, attacking only a small group of writers, perhaps equal in number to the group of drug users amongst sportsmen, but just as it is advantageous for us sportsmen to bring about an end to the distortion of facts, it is equally advantageous for sports writers to work to eradicate this kind of ignorance in order that their own jobs can be secured for the future. The problems and trials in sport must certainly be given space, but in accordance with the truth and on the right scale.

Conclusion

The Olympic movement and the field of sport in its totality have survived well together, sharing their joys and sorrows. Ensuring a secure future assumes that sport can be allotted its rightful place in such a way that it can preserve its backbone and allow a full opportunity for fair competition amongst the best in the world, support sports in other sectors of the society and above all play a role in furthering the peaceful development between the nations of the world.

Great Britain and the 1980 Olympics: A Victory for Olympism

J. Riordan

This paper, written in conjunction with Prof. Cantelon's Canadian paper, traces the course of events and the conflicts surrounding the British Government's attempted boycott of the 1980 Olympic Games; it examines the forces engaged in the controversy and the implications for international and British sport.

Introduction

A study of the course of events leading up to the British participation in the 1980 Olympics reveals manifest tensions within British society for which the attempted boycott acted as a catalyst. It also sheds light on the changing structure and ethos of British sport, and indicates possible implications for future sports development at home and abroad.

A century or so ago, individual enthusiasts from among the British leisured class pioneered the development of organised sports, gave them their rules and conventions, and initially made them exclusive to their social, racial and sexual group. There were thus established in Britain single-sport clubs, governing bodies for individual sports separate from one another, based on their members for purposes of control and for most of their financial support. What resulted were voluntary independent organisations based on a particular social group with a particular *'amateur-elitist'* outlook (which became enshrined in the Olympic Charter) based on fair play, the spontaneous enjoyment of games, and the notions of sport being the garden of human activities (albeit a private garden) and of it being the playing, not the winning, that counts. It also included a hostility to government interference, professionalism and commercialism. Over the last half century this ethos has been challenged by that of another social group, espousing a *'commercial-professional'* ethos, based largely on profit making, money values, and a single-minded commitment to record setting and winning; this group advocates the professional and commercial manipulation of sport, and government involvement to help it both financially and in the pursuit of its objectives internationally. The conflict between these two trends came to a head in Britain over the attempted boycott.

Sports Structure

Government involvement in sport has steadily increased over the past 20 years. Central government is involved in sport through the Department of the Environment.

An Under-Secretary of State has special responsibilities for sport and recreation and heads a Sport Division within the Department for the Environment; this 'Minister for Sport' has responsibility, in addition, for the countryside, historic buildings, ancient monuments and royal palaces.

In 1972 the Sports Council was set up by Royal Charter with the task of co-ordinating sport in Britain. It is the supreme body for sport and constitutionally independent, although in practice it is entirely dependent on the government for its budget and must "have regard to any general statements on the policy of our Government that may from time to time be issued to it by Our Secretary of State" (Parliamentary Report 1980). In the 1980-81 fiscal year it received the relatively paltry sum of £19.5 million. It has considerable interest in the Olympic Games because it normally supports financially the preparation and training of British teams.

Outside this government and quasi-government structure are the various sports federations, the British Olympic Association and the Central Council of Physical Recreation. The BOA constitutes the National Olympic Committee of Great Britain and Northern Ireland, which is entirely independent of government and raises its own funds to send British teams to the Olympics. All of these bodies are autonomous of government control and none were consulted, for example, when the British Government signed the Gleneagles Agreement on Sport and Apartheid in June 1977, or the UK-USSR Sports Agreement of 1978 - even though it is, of course, the sports bodies that are expected to carry out these agreements. Typical of the pre-boycott government attitude to British sport was the letter sent by Peter Blaker of the Foreign and Commonwealth Office in 1979 in response to a request from the BOA Chairman, Sir Denis Follows, for government help in establishing headquarters for an international sports organisation in London. The letter included the clear-cut policy statement: "As you will know, the Government has never attempted to emulate other countries by giving assistance to international sport for political or other purposes" (Palmer 1981, unpublished paper).

The Olympic Boycott Campaign

When the IOC chose Moscow in 1974 as venue for the 22nd Olympiad, it was the first time in the history of the modern Olympics that a communist country had been selected to host the Games. At the time, many felt the USSR to be worthy of the honour; not only was it the most successful and versatile nation in Olympic history, but it had done much in Olympic forums to enhance the pre-eminent role of sport and the Olympic movement in moral leadership in world politics, and in employing sport for peace, goodwill and understanding. However, the distaste in some British circles for communism and the USSR began to find increasing publicity in the media as the Games approached. As the BOA General Secretary, Richard Palmer (1981, unpublished paper), attests: "By May 1979, leaflets and letters, particularly from organisations such as the Women's Campaign for Soviet Jewry, the National British Women's Total Abstinence Union and the Board of Deputies of British Jews, and from a number of M.P.s, began appearing in the BOA office." In July 1979, the Women's Campaign for Soviet Jewry launched publicly a "Campaign to Remove the Olympics from Moscow" (Palmer 1981, unpublished paper). On 1 August, the Liberal Party launched a campaign "to harass the Soviet Government over the 1980 Olympics" (Guardian, 1 Aug). On 24 August, David Owen, then British (Labour Party) Foreign Secretary, said in a TV news interview (ITN) that "The Russians should not take it for granted that the 1980 Games would take place in Moscow." Reports began to appear in the British press that the Soviet authorities were planning to remove all schoolchildren from Moscow for fear of contamination by Westerners, and that all political dissidents were to be shifted from the capital. As *The Guardian* reported (15 Sept): "The Moscow Olympics chistka, or purge, is gathering momentum in the capital as the authorities ready themselves for the 1980 Games."

In September 1979 "the BOA felt it necessary to take the unusual step of discussing its participation in the Games, which, in normal circumstances, would have been taken for granted" (Palmer 1981, unpublished paper). It passed the following resolution:

> Throughout the history of the Olympic Games and in accordance with the established principles of the Olympic movement emphasis has always been placed on the participation of the individual competitor in the Games. The BOA therefore is of the opinion that subject to the laws of each participating nation, and in accordance with the regulations of the International Federation concerned, any competitor, if selected, should not be denied the privilege of participating in the Olympic Games. (Palmer 1981, unpublished paper)

The BOA was in no doubt that "there was a concerted campaign, orchestrated mainly from the right, from religious and human rights groups and particularly from some M.P.s who found easy publicity in furthering an anti-Olympic issue" (Palmer 1981, unpublished paper). For example, ever since 1978 the Conservative M.P. Sir Frederick Bennett had made several forays into the media as Chairman of the National Campaign, Olympic Games Moscow Objectors (NOGO), backed by the extreme right-wing Freedom Association. However, as a NOGO member put it in late 1979, "Until Afghanistan we did not have a peg to hang the coat on" (Palmer 1981, unpublished paper).

Afghanistan

A new period in the anti-Moscow Games campaign began with the entry of Soviet troops into Afghanistan on 27 December 1979. It provided the campaigners with precisely the ammunition they needed, and they used it with gusto. As Richard Palmer testified: "It was the most intensive pressure that had ever been applied to sport."

The idea that the British Government should throw its weight behind the campaign to boycott the Moscow Olympics began to be canvassed early in 1980. A Hands Off Afghanistan Committee of M.P.s was formed and wrote to Sir Denis Follows urging a boycott. In the House of Commons on 14 January, Douglas Hurd, Minister of State for Foreign Affairs, hinted that Britain would back the USA if it attempted to boycott the Olympics. And on 17 February, following President Carter's lead, the Prime Minister, Mrs. Margaret Thatcher, called on the BOA to "approach the IOC urgently and propose that the Summer Games be moved from the Soviet Union." She offered three site in Britain: the Crystal Palace, Earl's Court and the Albert Hall, and offered £50 million for the purpose; but she was immediatety rebuffed by

Monique Berlioux, director of the IOC, who stated categorically that "there would be no change of veneu." Sir Denis Follows pointed out that the only body qualified to act for Britain on Olympic matters was the British Olympic Committee. At that, on 14 February, the Prime Minister appealed to British athletes, over the heads of their national federations and the BOA, to boycott the Games if they were to take place in Moscow, declaring that athletes had the same responsibilitiy for the defence and preservation of freedom as any other citizens. On 27 February, Prince Philip, President of the International Equestrian Federation, made a bitter attack on countries (obviously communist states) that saw success in world sport "as an advertisement for political ideology." A few days later, the right-wing columnist Bernard Levin wrote in *The Times* on 1 March that our athletes might witn medals in Moscow, but that "not all the skills of alchemy will ever transmute their prizes into anything but tarnished badges of shame." This was a mild statement (but one to be taken up frequently) beside the hysteria being whipped up by the 'popular' press.

For all that, it was revealed in *The Guardian* on 14 March that "78 out of 108 Olympic possible indicated yesterday that they wanted to compete in the Games of Moscow."

The Fightback

Clearly these were difficult days. As the BOA Secretary states

> The whole of Fleet Street was against us, and the debate was being kept perpetually in people's minds by carefully planted questions in the House and by a near hysteria in the Press who were seizing upon anything remotely to tdo with Afganistan and the Games. These were dark days and the voice of sport was clearly not being heard. (Palmer 1981, unpublished paper)

As the establishment withdrew its support from the Games, the ordinary people came forward to take its place. The main problem now was money to finance the Moscow trip. As early as 9 March, *The Observer* had quoted George Nicholson, Secretary of the British Olympic Appeal, as ssaying that "The Government's decision not to support us has resulted in a flood of small donations from individuals." More money now began to come in from Co-operative Societies, Peace Councils, trade unions, Labour and Communist party branches, the British-Soviet Friendship Society and ordinary working people and pensioners. Five local Scottish authorities donated a total of £2700 to the British Olympic Appeal; this was followed by some 35 other Labour councils subscribing money to the Appeal. Yorkshire Miners donated £500 and organised individual pit collections; the Manchester branch of the British-Soviet Friendship Society raised £1000.

In the end, as Sir Denis Follows put it in the *Official BOA Report of the Games:*

> Thanks to the support given by the British public, local authorities, trade unions and (though to a lesser extent than ever before) industry and commerce, the Olympic Appeal raised more than £800,000 – a record total given by twice as many contributors a on the occasion of any other Appeal. But most of the traditional money-raising activities had to be cancelled because of the attitude of the Government.... The crisis, for financial crisis it was, showed what could be done, and that the heart of the country is sound in its support for the Olympic Games.

In fact, the involvement of the people of Britain in the Olympic movement gave it a new dimension. The Olympic Games in Moscow began to take on the character of a festival of peace in a world that was preparing for war, and the campaign to raise money became a demonstration against the Thatcher Government and all that it stood for. As Nobel Peace Prizewinner and ex-Olympic silver-medal winner, the late Lord Philip Noel-Baker said in a letter to *The Guardian* on May 8:

> I feel a sense of outrage at the continued persecution by the British and US governments of their sports leaders and athletes who are loyal to the Olympic movement, and who therefore want to go to the Games in Moscow... (the Games) have given the whole world a vision of all-embracing international friendship and co-operation, which was in sharp contrast to the folly and wastes of the arms race and of war... The Games in Moscow will serve the short-time and the long-time cause of peace.

On 27 May, the IOC announced in Lausanne that 85 countries had accepted invitations to compete in Moscow. Of the 22 nations that had won two or more gold medals in the 1972 or 1976 Olympics, only five had decided not to compete in Moscow: the USA, West Germany, Norway, Kenya and Japan. As *The Times* editorial stated on 26 May, "The most conspicuous hole in the boycott has paradoxically been Western Europe, nations closely allied to the United States." In fact, the British Olympic team, consisting of 326 persons, was the fourth biggest at the Games.

By the end of the Games, the mood of the nation was so strong, with millions of British people extremely proud of their athletes, that the would-be boycotters cut their losses and let the matter rest. As the Daily Mail sportswriter Ian Wooldridge put it, "They had burned their fingers in a futile exercise" (Official BOA Games Report 1981). Of course, there was no official Government welcome home for the athletes, and no recognition for Coe, Ovett, Wells, Thompson, Goodhew and the rest in the traditional Honours List (though there were CBEs, MBEs etc. for several non-Olympic sportsmen).

Conclusions

In many ways, the boycott controversy brought to a head some of the tensions that had long been latent in British sport and society.

The first is the action of right-wing anti-communist groups in Britain who wish to see the total destruction of the Olympic Games as they are at present constituted. As long as the West was winning and could dictate sports policy, of course, there was never a suggestion that the Olympics were too big, political, nationalistic or unworthy of a particular country (including Nazi Germany in 1936). The loss of this supremacy in sports arenas and forums has caused such groups to conclude that the time has come to sever links with the Olympic movement and to form a West-oriented grouping of sports nations. Although these goups have for the moment been defeated, the danger still exists of them seizing upon other international incidents to destroy the Olympic Games and fragment the structure of world sport. How cynically such politicians and media used the Moscow Olympic Games, and thus sport, for their own ends can now be seen in retrospect; since the Games, not one statement has been made in the British House of Commons or by the Prime Minister or any other member of the Government on the subject of Afganistan - nor has there been one leading press article.

A second tension that the boycott controversy made manifest was that between the traditional amateur-elitist and the ascendant commercial-professional ethos. In many areas of British sport it is the latter which is at present predominant; and yet it was the former that won the day with the participation of the British team in the Moscow Olympics. For such traditional (and conservative) figures as Sir Denis Follows and the late Marquis of Exeter (as well as Lord Killanin), the dominant credo in regard to sport has always been that it should be divorced from politics, government interference and commercialism, as also a firm commitment to the Olympic ideal. British governments have tended to espouse this philosophy, too, particularly since it absolved them of any financial commitment to sport. The year 1980 changed all that. As the Sports Council Chairman, Dick Jeeps, put it:

> The year under review will be remembered above all as the period when the governments of the Western democracies became involved in the government of sport. Never again can it be said that sport can have a separate existence, independent of politics. Following the Olympic Games in Moscow, governing bodies and Government will have to look anew at their respective positions. The relationship is bound to be different; it is hoped it will be better. But one thing is certain – it can never be the same again. (Palmer 1981, unpublished paper)

It may well be that, henceforth, the commercial-professional ethos will permeate and dominate even in the erstwhile 'amateur' sports (indeed, the process has been developing for some time) and that governments will increasingly attempt to use sport as an instrument of foreign policy (having learned the lesson of their 'failure' over the boycott). Whether this occurs or not may well depend on the third and last major actor in British sport: the British people.

Although it is largely ordinary men and women, increasingly from the working class, who are involved in the playing of sport, including within the Olympic team (any comparison of the social composition of prewar British Olympic teams – as in the 1924 team portrayed in the film *Chariots of Fire* – with that of 1980 demonstrates the radical change that has occurred), it is not working men and women who *govern* British sport. However, the boycott controversy presented examples of what *can* be achieved given popular will, purpose and unity. To take the athletes: despite the hardships, the blackmail and the taunts of 'traitors', they stood up for the right to compete in the Olympics in peace and friendship, faithful to the Olympic ideal. It was not easy. Let me cite the example of the oarsmen. The Amateur Rowing Association decided to boycott Moscow. But the oarsmen can count too. They lobbied MPs, they met ATA officials, they wrote letters to *The Times* and other newspapers, and 40 potential Olympic oarsmen came out in favour of going to Moscow. The ARA was forced to change its line, and the dichotomy of it all could well echo around other sports as an example of what the athletes themselves can achieve.

A glimpse into the future may also have been gained by the many thousands of people in factories and offices who had to step into the breach and organise fund-raising events when big business withdrew its support. It may be that, in joining the national Olympic movement, they will now fight for a greater measure of democracy within the movement. Some of the trade unions, co-operatives and town councils that made the sending of an Olympic team to Moscow possible are beginning to realise the need for greater involvement in running their country's sport if the Olympic spirit and movement are to survive. Having saved the Olympic movement from destruction once, they are becoming aware that it may be their efforts and even control that are needed to ensure that the Olympics continue to be such a unique occasion in bringing people from all over the world together in peace and concord. In the extremely dangerous world in which we live, there may be, indeed, precious few such opportunities left to mankind.

References

Official British Olympic Association Report of the 1980 Games (1981). Epic Publishing, London
Parliamentary Report (1980) House of Commons Report from the Foreign Affairs Committee, 1979–80. Olympic Games 1980. Ordered by the House of Commons to be printed 12th March 1980

The Canadian Absence from the XXIInd Olympiad - Some Plausible Explanations

H. Cantelon

This paper, written in conjunction with Dr. Riordan's British paper, will argue that the underlying structure of the Canadian state explains the decision of the Canadian Olympic Association to boycott the XXIInd Olympiad, and that the strong federal government presence in Canadian amateur sport, along with an underlying ideology hostile to the USSR, influenced the COA to make the decision it did.

Introduction

On 1980 April 22, Canada's Minister of External Affairs, Mark MacGuigan stood in the House of Commons and announced that "the Soviet action in Afghanistan makes it wholly inappropriate to hold the (Olympic) Games in Moscow." MacGuigan went on to assert that although the federal government would not revoke the passports of athletes, spectators or the Canadian Olympic Association (COA) members who wished to travel to the Moscow Games, any traveller would journey without the moral or financial support of the Canadian government. In effect, MacGuigan sounded the death knell for Canadian participation in Moscow. Four days later, on 1980 April 26, the Canadian Olympic Association voted to accept the government decision in spite of the condemnation levelled at the government by COA President, Richard Pound. Not mincing his words, Pound accused the government of practising "Mickey Mouse" politics (Dawson 1980 p 3). One way well wonder why, if the COA was so vehemently opposed to the government decision, did Canada not follow the British example (see Riordan 1982). Had not the COA voted 25-5 in favour of attending the XXII Olympiad on 30 March 1980 (Globe and Mail 1980a)? Had the Committee not also refused to impose sanctions on individual sports federations who sent representatives or officials to the Games despite the government decision (Globe and Mail 1980b)? A discussion of the reasons for the acceptance of the boycott on the part of Canadian officials is the topic of this paper. I wish to suggest some possible explanations for the Canadian decision to boycott the XXIInd Olympiad.

Ideological Explanations

The Canadian state is steeped in the ideology of meritocratic liberalism, in keeping with modern capitalism (Parkin 1972). Such an ideology may emphasise the desirability of providing social services, welfare provisions and equal opportunity for all citizens to attain the scarce rewards of the society. But, as Miliband points out (Miliband 1973 p 66), the ideology does not question the validity of the 'free enterprise' system. Any policy or proposal is meant to ensure the greater strength and stability of the capitalist system, not to erode or supplant it. Thus, Miliband attests:

> Bourgeois politicians and governments view the system... as most closely congruent with 'human nature', as uniquely capable of combining efficiency, welfare and freedom, as the best means of releasing human initiative and energy in socially beneficient directions, and as providing the necessary and only possible basis for a satisfactory social order (Miliband 1973 p 68).

The consequence of such an ideology has profound implications for sport and for the Canadian government's position regarding the Moscow Olympiad in particular. Given that the USSR, in 1917, embarked on an experiment in planned economic activity, it is not surprising that capitalist politicians and governments view such attempts as aberrations to the 'natural order' of economic life and as very real threats to the capitalist system. Thus, although it was never clearly articulated until the Afghanistan crisis, the Canadian government and state interests were always uneasy about the decision to award Moscow the 1980 Olympic Games (see Hansard 1978).

The uneasiness was articulated in many ways. By way of illustration consider the following. In 1979 an official Canadian sports delegation attended the USSR's All-Union Spartakiad. The Canadian group was firmly convinced that the Soviets would deliberately attempt to intimidate their opponents and use every psychological device possible to gain and advantage in the 1980 Olympic competition. This was so strongly believed that Sport Canada officials made detailed plans to hold a pre-Olympic psychological training camp in West Germany (Barr 1980 p 4).

In March 1980, several weeks before any official government position on the American boycott, I was in the USSR on a pre-Olympic fact-finding tour. We had spent seven hectic but worthwhile days viewing Olympic facilities and meeting sports officials, and were generally satisfied that Moscow would not have the technical or construction problems which plagued Montreal in 1976. Further, we were guardedly optimistic that the Canadian government might actually refuse to join the Carter administration it its boycott. On the eve of our scheduled departure from Moscow, a colleague and I contacted a member of the Canadian Embassy, responsible for assisting any visiting Canadian team. The discussion with 'our' official representative in Moscow quickly dissipated any aptimism we may have felt. I was shocked to listen to a representative of the government utter libellous and utterly false statements about the USSR. When my colleague, Bruce Kidd, a former Olympic athlete, tried to defend the ideals of the Olympic movement, he was dismissed as "sounding like Pravda" (see Kidd 1980 p 32).

After this experience it was not surprising to learn that when James Lawton, a sports reporter for the *Vancouver Sun,* attended the Games his instructions (like those of the majority of his western counterparts) were to provide "no up-beat stories from Moscow. Newsmen were told they needn't bother filing anything which reflected well on the Olympic organisers" (Lawton 1980 p 35). Nor was I surprised to read in the official publication of Sport Canada, *Champion,* the following synopsis of the Olympiad:

> *From the very moment the Olympics were awarded to Moscow they have been in danger of collapse.* Long before the invasion of Afghanistan the USSR busied its arrogant propaganda machine in the construction of moral and political traps for its guests, who, after all, seemed more than willing not to notice what was happening. *From the beginning the groundrules for attendance at the Moscow Olympics have been untenable* – that by merely showing up for the Games any visitor automatically akcnowledge the 'correctness' of Soviet foreign and domestic policy. Even Hitler in 1936 was not so blatant.

> If the Olympic movement dies in Moscow - and who at this point would bet against it? - then the Soviet Union must bear the brunt of the blame. *The rest of the world, however, will have to ask itself why it allowed it to happen. (McDonald 1980 7; emphasis added)*

I would argue that the above examples illustrate the ideological statements which advocates of meritocratic capitalism utilise to undermine alternative economic projects.

But ideology alone cannot account for the difference. As Riordan (1982) has demonstrated, meritocratic capitalist ideology is as strong in Britain as it is in Canada. Why then, did the British Olympic Team participate in Moscow while the Canadians stayed home? The reason, I believe, lies in a question of power. There is a fundamental difference between the degree and kind of government involvement in sport in the two countries. This involvement, coupled with the meritocratic ideology, resulted in Canada's boycott of the XIInd Olympiad.

Power and Its Relationship to State Involvement in Sport

Historically, in Canada there has been a long tradition of state intervention in sport, recreation and leisure activity (Metcalfe 1976, 1978; Kidd 1981; Gruneau 1979). Initially this was an indirect involvement and coincided with the strong government prescence in economic affairs generally (see Kidd 1981). Until 1961, the idealist notions of sport and politics not mixing, at least not *directly,* was a major aspect of Canadian sport. In 1961 the Fitness and Amateur Sport Act (Bill C-131) was passed, the first step towards direct government involvement. Since that time, the federal government has become a dominant factor in Canadian sport, particularly at the national and international levels (Campagnolo 1977, 1979a, 1979b; Regan 1981; Rhea 1969; Munro 1969, 1971).

The federal government has steadily usurped the autonomous authority of the amateur Sports Governing Bodies (SGBS). When Iona Campagnolo, the first Minister of State for Fitness and Amateur Sport, called for discussion on her proposed policy of sport (Campagnolo 1977), she constantly heard complaints that the volunter, 'the backbone' of Canadian sport, was being squeezed out; that the government was committed to a policy of significant control over the future direction of amateur sport; that there was an excessive emphasis on the pursuit of excellence; and that ultimately "too much government control would destroy the drive and enthusiasm of amateurs" (McCabe 1978b). The government countered with the argument that federal presence was essential of amateur sport in Canada was to become more efficient and productive. To quote the oft-repeated phrase of federal officials, "We have moved the operation of amateur sport off the kitchen table, into the boardroom." The government made it perfectly clear that its involvement would continue, regardless of the criticism of various and sundry interest groups.

> What it comes down to is this: when all criticisms of government action in the field of sport and recreation are taken into account, there remains *a national public interest to be protected and the federal government is the only entity, given the present state of our sporting community, that can carry out this responsibility effectively.* And, in the ultimate sense, only the federal government can coordinate existing programs to meet national goals and international challenges. (Campagnolo 1979a p 9).

The effect of this involvement in high performance sport has been profound. With the introduction of "Game Plan" in 1973, our amateur athletes have been able to train and compete with substantially less hardship than they had experienced in the past. But the negative must also be considered along with the positive. Here again, Miliband offers some appropriate insights. In *The State in Capitalist Society,* Miliband argues that political leaders and governments of capitalist societies are strongly committed to the belief that very govern 'in the national interest', that somehow they are universal men and women who have the pulse of the nation in focus on each and every decision that is made. And, Miliband goes on to argue:

> ... if the national interest is in fact inextricably bound up with the fortunes of capitalist enterprise, apparent partiality towards it is not really partiality at all. On the contrary, in serving the interests of business and in helping capitalist enterprise to thrive, governments are really fulfilling their exalted role as guardians of the good of all. (Miliband 1973 p 69)

The relevance for sport in Canada is obvious. The participation/administration of amateur sport represents a strong class bias in Canada; specifically, a class bias that is most committed to the ideology of meritocratic capitalism (Beamish 1978; Hollands and Gruneau 1979; Bray 1981). Consequently, we find a reproductive capacity in the organisation of amateur sport, i. e. a reproduction of the rationalised business enterprise. The increased government involvement has meant that, in effect, amateur sport is now comparable to a business enterprise, i. e. the Fitness and Amateur Sport Branch is the parent company while the associated sports and recreation groups, dependent on federal funding, are the 'wholly owned subsidiaries' (McCabe 1978a). With the steady influx of tax dollars into amateur sport, the athletes and SPGs have become increasingly dependent on this form of support. The percentage of government funding is enormous. In 1981, it was estimated at 90% (Regan 1981). Of the remaining 10%, almost all comes from donations from the private business sector, which, since 1972, has been able to claim generous tax deductions for contributing to amateur sport (McKelvey 1972 p 6). It follows that those most committed to meritocratic capitalism are now also instrumental in deciding the direction sports policy will take in Canada. They also exert an enormous influence in making decisions about the sporting competitions in which Candadian athletes will participate. But even more crucial, since the majority of administrators and athletes operate with similar class perspectives as those making the ultimate decisions, these decisions are not seen as discriminatory, but legitimate. The government can be seen as operating on democratic principles as well, since it is confident that ultimately its policy decisions will be carried out. This was very apparent in the boycott issue. Most athletes merely accepted without question the government decision to boycott. Those who did not accept this position were given the opportunity to criticise, even in Sports Canada's own publication *(Champion).* The President of the COA was not censored for accusing the government of 'Mickey Mouse' politics and others were permitted to bemoan the demise of the Olympic ideal. In the end, the government, acting in 'the national interest' made the decision it had originally intended: boycott.

As mentioned above, the amount of the government funding is substantial and all but 10% of the SGBs would collapse without this money (McCabe 1978a). Any additional funding comes from private donations and memership fees. In the case of the COA, federal funding and private corporate donations account for all but 1% of money received.

The private donations to the COA are handled by a unique entity known as the Olympic Trust. The Trust represents the most powerful sectors of indigenous and multinational capital in Canada: All the country's banks, Inco, Imperial Oil, Alcan, Dome Petroleum, Stelco, Noranda, Weston's Bakeries, Bell Canada, Eaton's Hudson Bay Company, McCain's Foods, Canada Packers, Molson's Breweries, Seagrams Distilleries. It is not surprising that this bastion of meritocratic capitalism is, on the one hand, hostile to the state socialist economic system and, on the other, strongly influenced by the position taken by parent companies and competitors in the United States. Thus, when J. Paul Austin, chairman and chief executive officer of Coca-Cola Ltd. (U. S. A.), accounced that his company would comply with the Carter administration's call for a boycott (Whig-Standard 1980), it was not long before Canada's Olympic Trust announced "that a government boycott would be supported" and that the Trust executive "were receiving negative responses from corporate donors who did not want to contribute to athletes going to Russia" (Dawson 1980 p 3).

But the Thatcher government also withheld funds from the BOA as well as revoking the special leaves for civil servants or military personnel who were members of the Olympic teams. In spite of this the BOA still voted to travel to Moskcow. Why did this not occur in Canada? The answer ultimately resides with the pressure the government exerted on the COA.

Using the terminology Riordan (1982) has introduced, the present COA membership can be broken down as follows: amateur-elite, 20 %; commercial-professional interests, 20 %; SGB representation, 60 %. The consequence of this structure is that the SGBs control the vote on any decision taken by the COA.

In the case of the Olympic boycott the COA was divided on two issues: the political pressures being exerted in the Olympic movement and the latent hostility towards the USSR. The amateur-elite with their strong sense of Olympic idealism voted against the boycott; the commercial-professional interest voted against Canadian representation in Moscow. This left the deciding votes to be cast by the SGBs. Individually some representatives favoured going to the Games. The athletes had trained long and hard for the opportunity to compete and there was a suspicion that amateur sport was being made a 'scapegoat' for the government position. (It was widely publicised in the Canadian press, for example, that at the same time our amateur athletes were being told to stay away from Moscow, grain sales to the USSR were being increased and Hockey Canada officials were seriously negotiating with the USSR Hockey Federation to send a team to the 1981 Canada Cup; see Globe and Mail 1980c, d; Cobden 1980 p 6; Hill 1980). In spite of these misgivings the SGBs voted to boycott. The reason should now be obvious from my discussion. Amateur sport relies almost totally on federal funding to operate its programmes. The government can place great pressure on the athletes, administrators and voting members of organisations like the COA to carry out the preferred policy. The SGBs did not wish to risk their major source of funding simply for the sake of thise athletes who wishes to compete. Moreover, some SGB administrators are not sportsmen per se but career civil servants. For these individuals, personal career takes precedence over Olympic competation. Overall the attitude of Canadian athletes was (and continues to be) surprisingly passive. Most simply accepted both the boycott call and the compromise for missing the Moscow Games: a special concert in their honour featuring several of Canada's top performers (e.g. Gordon Lightfoot), special uniforms, and awards banquet, commemorative medals and alternative competitions (Champion 1980).

Ramifications of the Boycott

Bruce Kidd, former international athlete and long-time advocate of Olympic reform has just completed a detailed document dealing with athlete's rights (Kidd and Eberts to be published). Kidd's investigations indicate that the agreements which carded Canadian athletes sign in order to receive federal assistance conform to standard labour contracts. As athletes become more aware of this similarity they may also utilise the legal system to fight against human rights violations and to ensure proper labour practices. It is also possible that future boycott attempts could be challenged in the courts. Kidd maintains that if Canadian athletes are serious about protecting their individual and collective rights they should consider unionisation.

One should be cautious about believing that unionisation would eradicate all the problems concerning government intervention in sports. Government foreign policy is rarely consistent or logical; rather it is based upon vested interest (cf. Canada's boycott of the USSR Olympics over Afghanistan but no such action against the USA over Vietnam). Unionised athletes can pursue vested interests just as easily as governments. They could just as easily vote to compete in Moscow as they could to compete in South Africa or any of the many countries Amnesty International cites as the worst violators of human rights. Kidd's suggestion of unionisation is only one step in a long process of consciousnessraising in sport. When the UNESCO recommendations (1978) for physical education and sport are a reality in all countries then we will see an indestructible Olympic Movement.

Acknowledgement. I wish to acknowledge the generous financial support I have received from the Faculty of Arts and Science and the School of Graduate Studies and Research.

References

Barr G (1980) More than competition on their minds. Champion 4:(1):2, 4
Beamish RB (1978) Socioeconomic and demographic characteristics of the National Executives of selected amateur sports in Canada (1975). Working papers in the sociological study of sports and leisure 1 (1). Centre for the Study of Sport and Leisure, Queen's University, Kingston
Bray C (1981) Social class and the coaching association of Canada: A study of the readability of Coaching Review magazine 1978-1981. Unpublished M.A. Thesis, Queen's University
Campagnolo I (1977) Toward a national policy of amateur sport: a working paper. Government of Canada
Campagnolo I (1979a) Toward a national policy on fitness and recreation. Government of Canada
Campagnolo I (1979b) Partners in pursuit of excellence: a national policy on amateur sport. Government of Canada
Cantelon H, Gruneau R (eds) (1982) Sport, culture and the modern state. University of Toronto Press, Toronto
Champion (1980 Lightfoot and friends in Olympic team tribute. Champion 4 (3) August 1980, p 21
Cobden M (1980) Olympic boycott: a nice, easy way to avoid the test of our principles. The Whig-Standard 24.4.80, p 6
Dawson B (1980) Olympic financing likely to dry up. The Whig-Standard 23.4.80, pp 2–3
Globe and Mail (1980a) Canadian officials say athletes will go to Moscow Games. Globe and Mail 31.3.80, p 1

Globe and Mail (1980b) Federation posts a Games chance. Globe and Mail 3.5.1980, p 8
Globe and Mail (1980c) Letters to the Editor: the boycott. Globe and Mail 19.4.1980, p 7
Globe and Mail (1980d) Olympic boycott bid berated. Globe and Mail 19.4.1980, p 5
Gruneau S (1979) Power and play in Canadian social development. Working papers in the sociological study of sports and leisure 2 (no 1). Centre for the Study of Sport and Leisure, Queen's University, Kingston
Hansard (1978) The Official Report of the House of Commons Debates. 14.12.1978. Canadian Government Publishing Centre, Ottawa, p 2162
Hill B (1980) The Olympic boycott: letter to the Whig-Standard Editor. The Whig Standard May, 1980
Hollands R, Gruneau RS (1979) Social class and voluntary action in the administration of Canadian amateur sport. Working papers in the sociological study of sports and leisure 2 (no 3). Centre for the Study of Sport and leisure, Queen's University, Kingston
Kidd B (1980) Teaching prejudice. This Magazine 14 (no 3), May–June 1980, pp 31–33
Kidd B (1981) Sport and the Canadian state. Proceedings: National Association for P.E. in Higher Education. Human Kinetic Publishers, Champaign, Ill.
Kidd B, Eberts M (to be published) Athletes' rights in Canada. Ministry of Tourism and Recreation, Toronto
Lawton J (1980) Moscow Olympics lacked a soul. Champion 4 (no 4), November 1980, pp 3, 16, 35
McCabe N (1978a) Federal funds going only after medals. The Globe and Mail 9.5.78, p 36
McCabe N (1978b) Less bureaucracy in amateur sport urged by volunteers. The Globe and Mail 16.1.78, p S6
McDonald D (1980) Conflicting emotions revealed in opinion study. Champion 4 (no 3) August 1980, pp 6–7
McKelvey G (1972) Sport and politics in Canada. A paper presented at the Symposium on sports, man and contemporary society. Queens College, New York: March 10-11, 1972
Metcalfe A (1976) Organized sport and social stratification in Montreal. In: Gruneau RS, Albinson JG (eds) Canadian sport: sociological perspectives. Addison-Wesley, Canada
Metcalfe A (1978) "Working class physical recreation in Montreal 1860–1895." Working papers in the sociological study of sports and leisure 1 (no 2). Centre for the Study of Sport and Leisure, Queen's University, Kingston
Miliband R (1973) The state in capitalist society: the analysis of the Western system of power. Quartet Books, London
Munro J (1969) Speech to the Canadian Amateur Sports Federation (1971) Jan 1969
Munro J (1971) Sport Canada/Recreation Canada. Government of Canada
Parkin F (1972) Class inequality and political order: social stratification in capitalist and communist societies. Paladin Books, St. Albans, England, p 123
Regan GA (1981) A challenge to thc nation: fitness and amateur sport in the 80's. Government of Canada
Rhea W (chairman) (1969) Report of the task force on sports for Canadians. Government of Canada
Riordan J (1982) Great Britain and the 1980 Olympics: victory for olympism. Paper presented at the Congress on Sport and International Understanding, Helsinki, 1982
UNESCO (1978) Developments in physical education and sport in the Canadian Commission for UNESCO, Ottawa
Whig-Standard (1980) Coca-Cola worit ship to Moscow. The Whig Standard 22.3.1980, p 82

The New Role of the 1988 Olympic Games in Seoul

Y.S. Han

Historical Background of the Olympic Games

As readers may know, the first ancient Olympic Games were held at Olympia, Greece, in 776 B.C. From that year on the Olympic Games were held every 4 years for nearly 1200 years without interruption until they were halted by the decree of Emperor Theodosius I of Rome in 394 A.D. The Games were suspended for 15 centuries; However, during this time many philosophers, writers and educators contemplated a revival of the Olympic Games. In 1882 the Frenchman Baron Pierre de Coubertin, commissioned to study physical education by the government, became convinced that athletics combined with education could improve international understanding and he publicly set out to establish a modern Olympic Games. His wish was "to promote the development of those fine physical and moral qualities which are the basis of amateur sport and to bring together the athletes of the world in a great quadrennial festival of sports, thereby creating international respect and goodwill and a more peaceful world."

When Baron Pierre de Coubertin revived the Olympic Games 1896 he sincerely hoped that the Games would represent the ancient concept of *ARETE* (striving and contesting for excellence) at its finest. He was opposed to the idea of the Games being held only at Olympia and firmly believed that the Olympic Games should be celebrated in cities in various parts of the world; he further believed that the modern Games should not be held under any national and/or political influence.

The 1988 Olympic Games will be the first in Olympic history to be staged in a middle developed country. The honour of hosting the 1988 Olympic Games is in recognition of the strong efforts of the Republic of Korea for the cause of peace. The Organising Committee of the 1988 Olympic Games in Seoul has already begun the groundwork and has budgeted about 22 billion U.S. dollars for the Games. The universal significance of the Games is evident when one considers that they help to develop friendships, encourage mutual understanding, foster goodwill, promote active co-operation and contribute to world peace. According to Lord Killanin, "the Olympic Games are not only for Olympians. They spread the spirit and principles of friendly games to the youth of the world, thus creating international trust and goodwill leading to peace in the world." The IOC Fundamental Principle I clearly states that "the education of young people through sport in the spirit of a better mutual understanding helps to build a better and more peaceful world."

Clearly, the ultimate aim of the Olympic Games lies not in determining winners and losers but in enhancing and promoting worldwide peaceful co-existence. Unfortunately, because of international political differences this principle of developing world peace is not readily adhered to by all. In the strictest sense, no country wins in the Olympic Games, but, regretfully, since the 1896 Games most countries have rated Olympic perfomance in terms of national units. Historically, we know that since 1936 the Olympic Games have become a place for the display of nationalism, especially when the Olympic movement accelerated toward gigantism during the 1960s. The emphasis and stress placed on nationalism in the Games has been further exaggerated by the strong emphasis placed on athletic perfomance and success and the equation of Olympic success with political and ideological superiority. In addition to successful performance, the publication of records and medal tables, governmental and business sponsorship of team sports, and the use of national anthems, uniforms and flags have all contributed to the strengthening of nationalism in the Games rather than the ideal of friendly internationalism for a peaceful world. Of course, there have been incidents, such as the founding, structuring and staging of the Olympic Games, which have contributed to their politicisation. A well-known example was the use of the Games as an instrument of ideological and nationalistic propaganda by Nazi Germany. Other influential factors have been the growth of sports since World War II, the growth and advancement of television and the exploitation of athletic accomplishment by governments.

Nations and their respective news medias must become aware that continued emphasis on nationalism may well damage the future of the Olympic Games. We all know that the Olympic Games are among the fastest growing and most important social phenomenon of modern times and that the Olympic movement has become a vital part of modern civilisation around the world. We must remember that the Origin of olympism lies in the love of athletic training and competition displayed by the Greeks in the pre-Hellenistic era. That the earlist ancient Olympic Games had been associated with religious festivals is a well-established fact, as is a historical continuity between ancient and modern olympism. The hope that world peace and co-existence will be achieved through Olympic competition is a basic element of olympism; therefore, we must remember that the Olympic Games are not a place for servants of ideology or commerce from any nation.

Problems Related to the Olympic Games

Today the Olympic Games strongly attract the close attention of tens of millions of people around the world. The amateur and Olympic code of athletics profoundly affects millions of young mend and women in our world. Olympism has three main characteristics, namely, equality (regardless of race, religion or ideology), peace and beauty, and Coubertin's lifelong adherence to the Hellenic trinity of mind, body and spirit. These are the Olympic idea and ideal; therefore they should be emphasised when educating our young men and women.

At this point I would like to list some problems and issues related to the Olympic Games:

1. Political problems - most notably the dissension engendered by the 1936 Berlin Games and the boycott of the 1980 Moscow Games by the U.S.A. and other national teams

2. The use of the Olympic movement and Games as a political instrument
3. Amateur/professional controversy
4. The selection and protection of Olympic emblems, symbols and protocol
5. Conflicts over racial discrimination
6. The use of drugs
7. The commercialisation of the Games
8. The economics of staging and hosting the Games

Suggestions for Solving the Problems of the Olympic Games

It is our task to solve these problems as soon as possible; however, obviously they cannot be solved without preparation. Keeping these problems in mind I would like to make the following suggestions:

1. A more effective idea bank should be established for the Olympics.
2. A scientific forum should be set up to discuss future Olympic matters. Members should be one or two representative(s) from each NOC and results should be considered by the IOC.
3. A World Olympic Bank should be established to deal with Olympic business and commerce and to give financial support to the city hosting the forthcoming Olympic Games.
4. If any member nation chooses not to participate in the Games, they should be barred from the next Games, so as to discourage boycotting of the Olympic.
5. The International Olympic Academy of Greece should be upgraded and promoted to college level standards so as to produce world sports leaders.

The goals of the Olympic Games must correlate with those of modern international physical education in schools. The Olympic Games must play a key role in promoting physical education and recreation at all levels.

The Games should minimise the addition of new sports and economise on expenses in order to aid the staging of and participation in the Olympics by underdeveloped countries. The Olympic Games should also provide opportunities for research and/or study in a variety of academic disciplines, e.g. history, sociology, psychology, medicine and health and physical education. Players, facilities and all game related activities should be available to the approved body of researchers. An important fact to be pointed out is that the Olympic Games are not supported by a single culture as they were in ancient Greece; therefore it is necessary to study the effects of this cultural mix before, during and after the Games on understanding among participating nations.

Acceptable social philosophies of the Games should be developed and definitions of olympism and other related matters should be redefined. Female athletes, sports administrators and coaches will be increasingly involved in Olympic sports and therefore more qualified women should become IOC members.

The most outstanding athletes from participating nations compete in the games for athletic records, but the Games should provide equal opportunities to participate. For example, a certain ball game may have an inherent handicap of player height (Asian vs American players).

An economically unsound nation may be able to field only a small team while an advanced nation can afford to send a large number of players. These situations present a problem of unfair participation. The staging expenses for the Games should be shared by IOC members so that middle developed nations can also host the Olympic Games.

Questionnaire on Attitudes Towards the Olympic Games

As a matter of interest I conducted a poll in reference to the Olympic Games to be held in Korea, using 200 randomly selected male and female subjects. Questionnaire were constructed and distributed to the subjects. Of the 200, 130 (65%) responded to the poll (62 men, 68 women).

Some selected major questions were:

1. Do you think the Olympics promote international understanding, co-operation and goodwill?

Strongly agree	56 or 43.1%
Agree	70 or 53.8%
No opinion	2 or 1.5%
Disagree	1 or 0.8%
Strongly disagree	1 or 0.8%

2. Is it unjustifiable that the host nation must alon pay all the expenses of staging the Olympic Games?

Strongly agree	30 or 23.0%
Agree	50 or 38.5%
No opinion	11 or 8.5%
Disagree	19 or 14.6%
Strongly disagree	20 or 15.4%

3. Should the Olympic Games be used as a political instrument?

Strongly agree	5 or 3.9%
Agree	15 or 11.5%
No opinion	20 or 15.4%
Disagree	50 or 38.5%
Strongly disagree	40 or 30.8%

4. Should the best man or woman from his or her country participate in the Olympic Games regardless of their amateur or professional status?

Strongly agree	19 or 14.6%
Agree	54 or 40.9%
No opinion	11 or 8.5%
Disagree	20 or 15.4%
Strongly disagree	26 or 20.0%

5. Do you think the ideal of the modern Olympic Games has been negated by excessive chauvinism and commercialism?

Strongly agree	42 or 32.3%
Agree	38 or 29.2%
No opinion	13 or 10.0%
Disagree	17 or 13.1%
Strongly disagree	20 or 15.0%

6. Do you think we should build a permanent site for the Olympic Games?

Strongly agree	46 or 35.3%
Agree	14 or 10.8%
No opinion	5 or 4.0%
Disagree	26 or 20.0%
Strongly disagree	39 or 30.0%

7. Do you think the size of the Olympic Games should be reduced?

Strongly agree	11 or 8.5%
Agree	19 or 14.6%
No opinion	42 or 32.3%
Disagree	28 or 21.5%
Strongly disagree	30 or 23.0%

8. Do you think the elimination of national uniform, anthem and flag at the Olympic Games is needed?

Strongly agree	14 or 10.8%
Agree	26 oir 20.0%
No opinion	19 or 14.6%
Disagree	32 or 24.6%
Strongly disagree	39 or 30.0%

9. Do you think the team sport programme at the Olympic Games should be eliminated?

Strongly agree	13 or 10.0%
Agree	26 or 20.0%
No opinion	21 or 16.2%
Disagree	57 or 43.8%
Strongly disagree	13 or 10.0%

10. Do you think nationalism in the Olympic Games will have disappeared within the next 10 years?

Yes	19 or 14.6%
No opinion	32 or 24.6%
No	79 or 60.8%

Conclusion

After Studying the poll I reached the following conclusions:

1. Nearly all the subjects (97%) believed that the Olympic Games promote international understanding, co-operation and goodwill.
2. Nearly 62% of the subjects felt the Games are of value and should continue regardless of cost.
3. Over 69% of the subjects were against the use of the Olympic Games as a political instrument.
4. Of those questioned, 56% strongly agreed that the best athletes should represent their country regardless of athletic status. However, a strong 35% disagreed.
5. Of the subjects, 61% thought the ideal of the modern Games has indeed been negated by excessive chauvinism and commercialism.
6. On the subject of building a permanent site for the Games the subjects were equally divided: 46% for and 50% against.
7. Nearly half of the subjects, 45% did not want to reduce the size of the games; however, a large percentage, 32%, had no opinion.
8. Of those questioned, 55% felt there is no need to eliminate the national uniform, anthem and flag while 30% felt there is.
9. More than half, 54% were against eliminating the team sports programme, while 30% were for its elimination.
10. More than half, i.e. 60%, of the subjects felt that nationalism will still be present in the Olympic Games even 10 years from now.

Since the revival of the Olympic Games in 1896, many related problems have arisen. Over the years many have been solved but on the other hand many still exist. The 1988 Olympic Games will definitely set new standards for the Olympic movement and Games. The Organising Committee for the 1988 Olympic Games in Seoul is confident that the Games will play a new and beneficial role:

1. The 1988 Olympic Games in Seoul will set a new precedent for subsequent Olympic Games.
2. The Seoul Games will not be a showcase for any nation, society or ideology.
3. The Seoul Games will not only serve as a site of physical and moral competition among all Olympic family members, but will also provide cultural and educational exchange and competition for the Olympians and spectators.
4. The Games in Seoul will play a vital role in upgrading glorious Olympic history by promoting human relations and providing every possible co-operation and hospitality.
5. The Seoul Games will promote and strengthen friendships between sportsmen and women of all countries, regardless of race, religion or political ideology, in the quest for world peace.
6. The 1988 Olympic Games in Seoul will be staged as an educational enterprise for elite athletes and for mass participation in sport.

In conclusion I wish to reiterate the Olympic motto, *"Citius, Altius, Fortius"; "Faster, Higher, Stronger"* for health, happiness and a peaceful world. "Remember, the most important thing is not to win but to take part."

References

Chester D (1971) The Olympic Games handbook. New York
Crafts V (ed)(1980) Proceedings. National Association for Physical Education in Higher Education, vol II (5-8 June 1980)
Durant J (1973) Highlights of the Olympics. Hasting House, New York
Harris HA (1966) Greek athletes and athletics. Indiana University Press, Bloomington
Kieran J, Daley A, Jordon P (1977) The story of the Olympic Games, 776 B.C. to 1976. J.B. Lippincott, Philadelphia
Lenk H (1979) Social philosophy of athletics. Stipes, Champaign
Maitre HJC (1980) The 1980 Moscow Olympics: Politics and policy. Hoover Institution, Stanford University
Mandell RD (1976) The first modern Olympics. University of California Press, Berkeley
Maier KV (ed) (1979) J Phil Sport VI
Seagrave J, Chu D (eds) (1980) Olympism. Human Kinetics Publishers, Champaign
Shin HJ (ed) (1981) History of physical education. University Press, Seoul
Spears B, Swanson RA (1978) History of sport and physical activity in the United States. In: Smith ET (ed) Wm. C. Brown, Dubuque
Ziegler EF (1975) Personalizing physical education and sport philosophy. Stipes, Champaign

4. The Role of International Organisations

UNESCO's Role in the Field of Sport and Physical Education and the Challenges Facing International Sporting Links in the Future

Z. Zachariev

Main Goals of UNESCO

Since its creation, UNESCO has always endeavoured to use education, science and culture to strengthen relations between men and between countries and to promote "collaboration among the nations... in order to further universal respect for justice, for the rule of law and for the human rights and fundamental freedoms which are affirmed for the peoples of the world, without distinction of race, sex, language or religion, by the Charter of the United Nations".

In its spheres of competence, UNESCO has the important mission of "assisting all societies to acquire the ability to clarify and analyse their own problems, so as to be capable of unimpeded self-determination in full knowledge of the facts". UNESCO's approach to this mission is defined in the light of the fundamental and related aspirations of each individual and of each people to freedom, dignity, respect, solidarity and progress shared with all other men. In the long-term, its goal is a just and lasting peace, and the means to that end is education, in the broadest sense of the word:

> Through education, through the spread of culture and through the broadest possible dissemination of information, UNESCO's fundamental task is to work for peace, more especially by seeking to bring its influence to bear on the conscience and intelligence of individuals and peoples so that they may overcome prejudice, misconceptions and the feelings of hatred and intolerance which give rise to aggressiveness and war.

We must pursue this action in all areas, including that of physical education and sport, against everything that helps to maintain injustice, inequality and the other evils that undermine human dignity and are undeniably so many obstacles to understanding between individuals, peoples and nations, and hence so many challenges to us.

The First International UNESCO Conference on Physical Education and Sport

Since it convened the first International Conference of Ministers and Senior Officials Responsible for Physical Education and Sport in Paris in 1976, UNESCO has always been concerned - working in harmony with governments and specialised organisations in the field of physical education and sport - to seek ways both of enabling every individual in every member state to engage in physical and sporting activities and of elucidating the problems which arise in connection with the establishment of understanding between men and between countries through the development of sporting links based on ethical, aesthetic, cultural and physical ideals and values similar to those of the Olympic movement.

International Charter and Intergovernmental Committee

Following this first International Conference, which expressed the wish that a committee should be created "to draft the guidelines of international sporting events", the UNESCO General Conference at its twentieth session adopted both the International Charter which proclaims the fundamental right of every human being to free access to physical education and sport, and the Statutes of the Intergovernmental Committee for Physical Education and Sport, whose mission is to promote international co-operation in the sphere of physical education and sport, with a view to strengthening peace, friendship and mutual understanding and respect between peoples, in particular by helping member states, at their request, to co-ordinate their programmes and activities in this sphere [Art. 4, paragraph 1 (b)].

This vocation includes, among other things, analysing the difficulties which increasingly beset the organisation and staging of international sporting competitions throughout the world, and studying, in co-operation with the international sporting organisations concerned, the principles on the basis of which these difficulties might be smoothed out by concerted intergovernmental action. In so doing, the General Conference bore in mind the major aims assigned to the Organisation in its different spheres of competence, in accordance with its Constitution.

During the 1979 and 1981 sessions of the Intergovernmental Committee several recommendations were approved, some concerning the need to elaborate programmes of physical education and sporting activities for special groups of the population (in this case the handicapped) and to encourage the development of physical education and sport in various countries with a view to allowing all free access to physical and sporting activities. Other recommendations adopted concerned the dissemination of the International Charter of Physical Education and Sport. The Intergovernmental Committee also set up an ad hoc committee to direct priority attention to urgent problems such as: efforts to eliminate all forms of radial, political and religious discrimination in the field of physical education and sport, and in particular the condemnation of apartheid; the commercial influences which run counter to the interests of sports and sporting organisations; increased participation by developing countries in international competitions; the increasing cost of installations and excessively frequent alternations ot technical standards; medical problems and all forms of drug-taking.

The problems that were closely studied by the ad hoc committee constitute an undeniable challenge. Mindful of their importance, the Intergovernmental Committee had already recommended, in March 1981, that collaboration between member states, non-governmental organisations and other public and private bodies should be developed in order to seek solutions to the problems and find sources of financing to assist member states in establishing centres for the training and advanced training of personnel in the field of physical education and sport. In the same spirit, it pressed strongly for the establishment of technical co-operation among developing countries in order to help such countries to identify means of reinforcing the mobilisation of human, technical and fincancial resources in support of actions in the field of physical education and sport, just as it expressed its desire that the information flow should be intensified. Furthermore, it entrusted the ad hoc committee with the elaboration of guidelines for the organisation of a World Week for Physical Education and Sport and recommended that UNESCO immediately invite the member states to take action on the proposal to encourage the inclusion of the Olympic idea, as defined by the International Olympic Committee, in school curricula.

International Fund for the Development of Physical Education and Sport

While restating the priority attention that UNESCO could give to the development of physical education and sport throughout the world, as part of its contribution to lifelong education for all, the Intergovernmental Committee made a number of decisions - in relation to the International Fund for the Development of Physical Education and Sport, set up in 1976 - concerning the definition of more precise criteria for the activities of the Fund and the use of its resources. It may be helpful if I recall that this Fund was constituted within the framework of UNESCO to ensure intellectual, technical and financial collaboration aiming particularly at:

- The formulation of strategies, policies and programmes for the development of physical education and sport at national, regional and international level
- The creation or strengthening of institutions, structures and facilities whose purpose is the development or practice of physical education and sport
- The training of specialists
- The fostering of public awareness of the importance of physical education and sport for all
- The promotion of study, research and experimentation on all aspects of physical education and sport (scientific, educational, physical, medical, social, economic, infrastructure and equipment etc.), including new methods and ideas, special attention being given to operations which may have multiplier effects
- The organisation of meetings and of exchanges of persons concerned with physical education and sport
- The encouragement of the exchange of experience and the development of information and documentation facilities

Thus, through the Intergovernmental Committee and the Fund, and by means of programmes of physical education and sport, UNESCO has equipped itself with the means to contribute to the improvement of relations between men, peoples and nations, based on mutual respect, reciprocal understanding, co-operation and fundamental human rights, without which the promotion of international understanding is neither conceivable nor possible.

This re-statement of the objectives of the Intergovernmental Committee and of the Fund provides me with the opportunity to summarise once more the problems facing us today to which the correct solutions must be found if international goodwill and co-operation are to be strengthened.

Major Ethical Problems in International Sport

In the first category of problems of an ethical nature, there are three types of major difficulties, each one a contradiction, and a challenge. The *disparities,* which have become entrenched between, on the one hand, *the principles* laid down in the International Charter of Physical Education and Sport and the International Olympic Charter and, a fortiori, the intentions expressed by sports officials and those responsible for physical education and sport and, on the other, the *real conditions* in which the promotion and practice of physical and sporting activities and the preparation and staging of major international competitions take place.

Then there is the persistence of *limitations on the participation of athletes* who should all have free access to sporting events: these limitations are based on various types of discrimination, according to race, sex, religion or ideology, or other criteria, be they implicit or explicit, concerning the number of affiliated athletes in a particular country, the representativeness of a particular continent, history etc. The ad hoc committee, having given the matter long consideration, recommended that the Intergovernmental Committee appeal both to governments and to specialised non-governmental organisations, whether national or international, to the sportsmen and women themselves, to the officials and to trainers, to disseminate the substance of such official documents as the Universal Declaration of Human Rights, the International Charter on Physical Education and Sport, the Convention Against Discrimination in Education (1960), the International Declaration Against Apartheid in Sports (1977) and the final declaration adopted by the Olympic Congress at Baden-Baden, and to contribute to the application of these texts by bringing home to these sportmen and women that *apartheid* is one of the most serious violations of human rights.

Lastly, to be deplored is the *tendency of certain sports officials* to consider that the attainment of the goal they have set themselves or set their athletes, namely, obtaining the best possible results at any price, justifies resorting to certain procedures or methods hardly compatible with sporting ethics. Fortunately, such cases are few. Nevertheless, such behaviour cannot fail to be worrying insofar as it may set an example if it is not roundly condemned by the authorities.

Need for Greater Democratisation

As regards increasing the involvement of developing countries in international sports competitions and bodies, note must be taken of the urgent plea of many states, particularly from the Third World, for greater democratisation of international sport and more equitable representation of the different nations. This problem, which is essentially concerned with the principles of equality between peoples and nations, of dignity and of justice, must be resolved as well and as quickly as possible, for it represents an undeniable challenge and obstacle to the development of international relations based on understanding between peoples and nations.

In an age when one of whose outstanding features is the de facto interdependence linking nations and peoples, it may seem contradictory that sometimes the participation of certain nations or the representation of certain continents in major international competitions is based on choices made according to criteria which only aggravate frustration and bitterness, and existing imbalances and inequalities. It may well be objected that the most deprived nations, lacking the material resources and techniques needed to prepare their athletes methodically for these competitions, are condemned to play the even more frustrating role of 'also-rans'.

The Economic Problems

The economic importance of sport, which is tending to increase, is admittedly a significant factor. But co-operation and mutual assistance, which are at the heart of sport, should make it possible to correct these disparities and enable developing countries, even the poorest, to equip themselves with the infrastructure, equipment and staffing structures necessary to forge a sporting *élite* which is sufficiently representative and to acquit themselves honourably in the major sporting events, while at the same time developing physical education and sport for all. If there is a genuine desire to promote international understanding, is it not proper that all countries in the world, whatever their financial resources, should be able to take part freely in international sporting events and develop friendly and solid relations with other countries which will contribute to spreading tolerance, respect and understanding?

Would it not be appropriate for the Olympic Charter - whose fundamental aims are to encourage respect and goodwill among nations and thereby contribute to the creation of a better and a more peaceful world, to bring together Olympic competitors from all nations in honest and fair competition and to forbid all forms of discrimination against a country or an individual for reasons of race, religion or political opinion, in competitions - to serve, like the international charter adopted by UNESCO, as a conceptual framework for international action making it possible to secure the presence, in the major international competitions, of countries which cannot as yet take part, because of the complexity and excessive cost of these events?

Promotion of Mass Sport

The subject of the democratisation of sport and the participation of all countries leads us to re-examine the possibility of all individuals taking an active part in physical and sporting activities. The promotion of mass sport is one of the essential concerns of UNESCO in this particular field of its competence since it is exactly in line with its underlying moral principles. Anxious as it is put into practice the International Charter of Physical Education and Sport, the Organisation cannot but support endeavours which enable each human being to make effective use of his acknowledged right freely to develop and preserve his physical, intellectual and moral resources through the practice of character-forming physical and sporting activities which encourage not only the harmonious self-fulfilment of individuals, but access to the fundamental human values which are the basis for the full development of peoples.

The promotion of mass sport therefore calls for an even closer link between all forms of educational life and sporting life. Education *through* sport should exist alongside education *for* sport. In order that it should be complete and fully effective, it is essential to persuade all those in charge of educational systems in the world, political leaders, educationists, parents, pupils and students, that physical and sporting activities have an important part to play in encouraging international understanding as well as physical growth and the development of individuals from the cognitive, moral, aesthetic, emotional, social and cultural standpoint and that they are an indispensable element for academic success and, hence, for success in life.

Possibilities of the Media

If the Olympic ideal and the spirit of fair play are fostered and taught as part of physical education and sport, if they are instilled in the child from the earliest age, if educationists pay attention to the way sport is practised throughout a student's school career, and indeed outside school, there should be grounds for hope that those taking part in sporting activities may be freed from the concern to be first at any price from the feelig that one must win whatever the cost, whatever the means used. But in order to achieve this, would it not be desirable for the media to stop giving top-level competitive sport pride of place, to the detriment of sports for all? Should the activity of the media not be turned towards seeking a type of education and information tending to bring about an evolution in behaviour patterns which would arouse, within the various sections of the population, the desire for a more sporting approach to life, and attitudes of understanding and goodwill towards the competitors, to be seen as partners rather than as opponents?

Inadequacies have, however, been noted in the educational activity of the media in this sphere, either because there is not enough information, or because they tend to focus on outstanding facts or events which do not pay sufficient attention to the social importance of the humanistic goals and the moral value which physical education and sport transmit. The educational activity of the media should therefore be developed, with a view fostering more trusting, friendly and egalitarian relations between spectators, sportsmen and women, and peoples in order to promote understanding between nations.

Doping Problems

The use of chemically produced substances with a stimulant action and of procedures applied in order to increase the athletes' potential or resistance is also to be considered. This is a challenge which deserves consideration inasmuch as the constant striving to surpass oneself and the systematic pursuit of the best possible performances are increasingly leading to the violation of sporting ethics and to excesses, no doubt varying from one sport to another, in accepted procedures for athletes' training programmes. Even if it not in the long run harmful for the organism - which has not been proved - the over-training imposed upon sportsmen nevertheless forces them to live a life of *'conditioning'* completely centred around their sport, with an obsessive concern for the result, and develops an extreme form of selfishness which distorts normal conditions of existance and makes their future reinsertion in society more difficult. Experience increasingly indicates that these practices are ushering in a new form of individual alienation.

Even though the essential function of flourishing mass sport is not to produce sportsmen of a very high calibre, it still makes it possible by assuring healthy rivalry at all levels of the 'pyramid' and by providing a favourable atmosphere for physical activity for the most talented athletes to make an impression and for the best to receive a more functional training; at all events, it helps to create conditions which discourage the use of drugs and of procedures which are, at the very least, artificial and dangerous, not only for the individuals concerned but also for the establishment of relations based on loyalty, dignity and a respect for human integrity.

UNESCO, through its educational activities, will no doubt have an important role to play in this field in the future. This action will doubtless be directed towards preventive action and reinforcing information and educational courses in order to encourage moral and ethical qualities, including the development of sportsmanship and fair play.

Commercialisation

Lastly, the involvement of commercial firms in the organisation and staging of major sporting events and, increasingly, in the careers of high-level sportsmen, either using their reputation for advertising purposes or playing them on a more or less regular basis, sharpens the disparities between nations and disturbs good relations between them inasmuch as the commercial exploitation of sport is practised only by certain countries and tends to favour their great industrial and commercial concerns.

It is well known that the scale of the financial interests connected with the major international competitions has given rise to a trend towards the large-scale and extravagant, which doubtless varies from one sport to another, but which is reflected in the scale and the proliferation of events, the increasing cost of equipment charges in technical standards, and athletes who are increasingly finely tuned and overstrained.

Conclusion

The present conference, for its part, is proof of the interest shown by non-governmental organisations in understanding and solving the problems discussed above.

There is unanimity within the international sporting movement on the need for a common front to face the challenges of the future and the obstacles impeding the development of international sporting relations in order to reject, in complete agreement with the United Nations and with its Specialised Agencies, all forms of discrimination and to ensure respect for human rights, together with the promotion of international sporting relations based on *a new sporting order,* which will make it possible to strengthen understanding between men, whether performers or spectators, between peoples and between nations. This will enable sport once more to serve its essential purpose, which is to free man from prejudices, to develop all his abilities and to make him receptive to a humanist view, to the basic values of self-respect and respect for others, respect for dignity, equality, mutual understanding and concern for equity, friendship and brotherhood, without which it is not possible to prepare a better future for the community of man.

Organisations for Sport Sciences: Developments and Perspectives

M. Hebbelinck

Introduction

For more than 30 years, since the end of World War II, almost continuous expansion of research in physical education and sport has been going on and a vast body of knowledge has been accumulated. Today by conservative estimates some 25 000 books and journal articles are published every year in the broad area of physical education and sport. This explosion of documentation and information as a problem in itself worthy of in-depth study and analysis (Broekhoff 1980). Before the 1960s there existed only a few countries where research workers in the area of sports were organised, and most information was scattered in various professional and scientific journals. Attempts has been made to rally sport scientists, but no permanent result has been obtained.

One such effort was the establishment in 1928 of the "Wissenschaftliche Gesellschaft für körperliche Erziehung" in Berlin, which has an international membership with sport scientists such as F. Buytendijk (The Netherlands), C. Diem (Germany), K. Gaulkofer (Austria and later The Netherlands), W. Kohlrausch (Germany), K. Lindhard (Denmark), T. McKenzie (U. S. A.) and P. de Coubertin (France). The purpose of this society was "to scientifically work in the field of physical education and also to promote and to encourage such (scientific) work in broader circles". In order to fulfil this task it was permitted to use research procedures from both the natural and the human sciences; special emphasis was laid on "the pursuit of fruitful collaboration between both fundamental directions" ("ein fruchtbares Zusammenarbeiten beider Grundrichtungen") (Bernett 1980). This first multidisciplinary international organisation of sport sciences held scientific meetings in Hamburg (1929), Vienna (1930), Berlin (1939) and Amsterdam (1939). Lectures were presented in German, English and French. The Second World War as well as the death of Gaulkofer (28 October 1941) put an end to this scientific organisation of physical education.

Another international professional and scientific organisation which had an early start and is still very much alive, is the International Federation of Sports Medicine: this, too, was founded in 1928 ("Association Internationale Medico-Sportive"), on the occasion of the second Winter Olympics in St. Moritz. This federation held its first congress in Amsterdam (1–4 August 1928), with the participation of 281 sport physicians from 20 countries, and for the first time systematic scientific studies were carried out on athletes (those competing in the ninth Summer Olympic Games). It is interesting that by 1933 (Turin, 2nd International Sports Medicine Congress) the name had been changed to "Fédération Internationale Medico-Sportive et Scientifique", and as early as 1934 the present name of "Fédération Internationale de Médecine Sportive" (FIMS) was chosen (Tittel 1980). It is beyond doubt that the activities of FIMS have not only contributed greatly to the international contacts between sport physicians all over the world but have also given impetus to the international development of other sport sciences.

Present Situation

It was not until the 1960s, however, that sport science gained its full momentum. In many respects, the development of sport science organisations was a logical outcome of the trend towards "scientification"[1] (Grupe 1981) which occurred in industrialised society as a response to a series of complex changes and which induced the following developments: (1) the creation of employment opportunities capable of sustaining lifetime careers, (2) the development of scientific conferences and (3) the founding of organisations devoted to the promotion of the scientific needs of the professional community. These changes, however, did not occur simultaneously, but developed gradually over the last three decades. There were, in fact, several factors impeding the early advancement of autonomous sport science organisations. One was that the context of sport science overlapped to various degrees with a number of well-established disciplines such as anatomy, physiology, biochemistry, psychology, philisophy, sociology, education and history. This application to other academic disciplines made it difficult for the sport sciences to gain an independent identity. Moreover, before the 1950s physical education and sport had largely been a field of study in education (e.g. scientific section of FIEP) and in some instances a biomedical topic (e.g. FIMS).

This configuration changed, however, because of the growing interest in sport as an important sociocultural phenomenon which attracted funds for sport science research in both the private and the public sectors in several countries. During the period 1950 to 1960 several departments or institutions for higher learning began to expand their curricula and programmes with specific topics in sport science.

It was not until the 1960s that specific organisations of sport science came into being. A clear definition of an organisation is provided by Lüschen (1981):

> Organizations are social units which delimit membership and have an internal differentiation of roles. Organizations are oriented toward the fulfilment of specific goals and purposes. Organizations incorporate bureaucratization and rational procedures to realize these goals and purposes.

Most international sport science organisations were established on the occasion of an international meeting (congress, conference, symposium or seminar) where scientists within a certain field presented their research work and found an interested audience of fellow scientists engaged in the same area of research. The need for exchange of information was felt and sometimes joint research ventures were planned. Very often the formation of sport science organisations was a logical outgrowth of developing scientific interests in other academic disciplines (e.g. psychology of sport, history of sport, biochemistry of exercise; see Table 1). In some instances a remarkable develop-

1 In the English translation of Grupe's article, the German word "Verwissenschaftlichung" has been translated as "the subjection" of sport to science. I think, however, that in analogy with other terms which designate a form of transformation into an object of study for science and scientists, the word "scientification" can be used.

ment took place in the shaping of the scientific organisation. For example, the first international seminar on the biomechanics of sport took place in 1967 in Zurich and was primarily organised by and intended for scientists working in the area of biomechanics applied to sports. This seminar was the start of a series of international congresses on biomechanics and on the occasion of the third international seminar at Pennsylvania State University (1973), the International Society of Biomechanics was constituted. Ever since, the ISB has been expanding its field of interest far beyond the topic of sports. Recently (1982) some sport scientists felt the need to create an International Society of Biomechanics of Sports, independent of the ISB.

Table 1. Discipline-oriented organisations of sport sciences

Discipline	Sport science oragnisation	ICSPE – specialised committee
Medicine	FIMS (St. Moritz, 1928)	–
Psychology	ISSP (Rome, 1965)	–
Sociology	ICSS (Cologne, 1965)	Committee
Ergometry		Research committee, working group (Berlin, 1965)
History	ICOHS (Prague, 1967) HISPA (Zurich, 1973)	Committee
Biochemistry		Research committee, working group (Brussels, 1968)
Philosophy	PSSS (Boston, 1972)	–
Biomechnics	ISB (Penn. State, 1973)	Research committee, working group (Zurich, 1967) Working Group of Biomechanics of Sports (1982 ISB/ICSPE)
Kinanthropometry		Research committee, working group (Brasilia, 1978)
Orthopedagogy	IFAPA (Qucbcc, 1973)	–
Comparative education	ISCPES (Halifax, 1980)	–
Pedagogy	(Scientific Commission of FIEP[a] (Brussels, 1923) Research Committee of ICHPER (Rome, 1958) AIESEP (Lisbon, 1962) IAPESGW (Copenhagen, 1949)	

[a] 1923, FIGE (Fédération Internationale de Gymnastique Educative); 1930–1953, FIGL (Fédération Internationale de Gymnastique Ling); 1953, FIEP

From Table 1 it can also be seen that the International Council of Sport and Physical Education (ICSPE) and particularly its Research Committee, founded at Rome in 1960, played a major role as a catalyst and promoter of the creation of international sport science organisations. The Research Committee was established in order to achieve the aims of ICSPE in terms of the provisions of Article 28 of the Statutes:

1. Promote and support scientific work in sport and physical education in different countries

2. Obtaining and communication of concise information on research activities in various parts of the world
3. Constitute a forum for the integrative study of cultural, humanistic and scientific aspects of sport and physical education
4. Sponsoring of international congresses, seminars and colloquia in the field of research in sport and physical education
5. Co-operation with the Bureau of Documentation and Information (now IASI) as well as integration of the work of other bodies of the International Council
6. Co-operation with national and international organisations working in the field of research in sport and physical education

Perhaps this programme was too ambitious, too much for one body to achieve. Nevertheless, over the years the Research Committee did assist directly or indirectly in many ways in the establishment and development of international sport science organisations (e.g. the International Society of Sport Psychology, the International Committee of History of Sport and the International Society of Biomechanics). Moreover, the Research Committee has several working groups in such areas as exercise biochemistry, ergometry, biomechanics of swimming and kinanthropometry. Other specialised committees of ICSPE have chosen a more autonomous constitution, e.g. the International Committee of Sport Sociology, the International Association for Sport Information (formerly the Bureau of Documentation and Information, a permanent committee of ICSPE) and the International Committee on Sports Facilities and Equipment (IAKS - Internationaler Arbeitkskreis für Sport und Freizeiteinrichtungen), all of which still have the status of a special committee at ICSPE. Still others started independently from their very beginning, e.g. the International Society of the History of Sport (HISPA, Zürich, 1973), the International Society of Sport Psychology (ISSP, Rome, 1965), the International Federation on Adapted Physical Activities (IFAPA, Quebec, 1973), the Philosophical Society for the Study of Sport (PSSS, Boston, 1972) and the International Society on Comparative Physical Education and Sport (ISCPES, Halifax, 1980). One may wonder why no specific organisation has been created in such an important fields as education. This may be explained by the fact that several international organisations whose members are mostly teachers of physical education have been working for many years (FIEP since 1923, ICHPER since 1958, IAPESGW since 1956 and AIESEP since 1962) in this domain and have always promoted the scientific study of the teaching and educational processes.

While these organisations for sport science are, for academic purposes, organised for the scientific aspects of research and study connected with sports and physical activity (Table 1), other organisations are problem or theme oriented (Table 2). These latter organisations are of a multi- or interdisciplinary type (i.e. with a membership of scientists stemming from different disciplines, very often working on a topic of common interest) and are a reflection of contemporary topical interests, e.g. the International Society of Physical Fitness Research (formerly the International Committee for the Standardization of Physical Fitness Tests, established on Tokyo in 1965), the International Committee on Fair Play (Gauting 1964), and the ICSPE committees on "Leisure and Sport", "Sport and Development", , "Sport, Mass Media and International Understanding", "Teacher training and programmes" and "Sport and Tourism" (Table 2).

Table 2. Theme-oriented organisations of sport sciences

Theme	Organisation	ICSPE – specialised committee
Physicial fitness	ICPFR	-
Leisure	WLRA	+ Committee
Mass media and international understanding		Committee
Teacher training and programmes	AIESEP	+ Committee
Facilities and equipment	IAKS	= Committee
Development		Committee
Tourism		Committee
Fair play	ICFP	= Committee
Biomechanics of swimming		Research committee, working group
Ageing		Research committee, working group
Aesthetics		Research committee, working group

International sport science organisations are also often a reflection of personal endeavours, the ambitions of historical constellations and international developments, and they have interaction with national and regional organisations and structures. National professional organisations for sport sciences have been created in many countries of the world, and governmental bodies co-ordinating and developing sport scientific policies and programmes have also been established. In addition, intergovernmental organisations have been created, such as the Sports Research Committee of the Committee for Sports Development of the Council of Europe or the Committee for International Scientific Cooperation in the field of sport and physical culture in the socialist countries.

Moreover, UNESCO has recommended that member organisations and the collaborating non-governmental organisations prepare a programme of international co-operation with regard to scientific and educational research on the problems of physical education and sport (cf. UNESCO Final Report 1976, p 19). In October 1980 an international panel of experts met in Paris with the aim of identifying "the steps which must be taken to organize the exchange of data and the findings of fundamental and applied research on physical education and sport". At this meeting the experts suggested 25 lines of research to be of world-wide importance, taking into account the needs of and implications for developing countries. In this respect the recommendation was made to make funds for research available through the UNESCO International Fund for the Development of Physical Education and Sport, in agreement with Article 2.2 of this Fund, which stipulates "... the Fund's resources will be used to provide intellectual, technical and financial collaboration in areas such as:...(e) the promotion of study, research and experimentation on all aspects of physical education and sport (scientific, educational, physical, medical, social, economic, infrastructure and equipment, etc.) including new methods and ideas, special attention being given to operations which may have multiplier effects".

Final Remarks and Recommendations

In a discussion paper on the role of science and sports science organisations, Buggel (1980) quite rightly points out:

> There will and must exist such organizations bringing together scientists of the individual branches for an exchange of experience, facilitating the arrangement of the various individual results into the complex theoretical building of sport science and promoting an effective use of the existing scientific potential. The complex scientific investigation into the phenomena of physical education and sport, their position in society and their significance for the development of mankind opens up the possibility and underlines the necessity for ICSPE/CIEPS to shape its character as a world-wide body of sport science and to complete its general and co-ordinating roof-function with other international organizations of sport science. The main subject for ICSPE/CIEPS is to initiate and support the setting-up of new and the stabilization of existing bodies of various branches and fields of sport science as an expression of its further development by a *process of systematic differentiation.*

At the same time it is ICSPE/CIEPS's function to *integrate* the branches of sport science as well as to integrate the fields of sport science. The main task is to bring together by integration the differential special knowlege and potential to a highly efficient total in such a way that it will meet the practical needs and requirements of sport.

The study of organisations of sport science is at an early stage of development and has to be carried on in the coming years, taking into account possible co-ordination and integration, as well further differentiation. It is striking that, for instance, no international scientific organisation for sport physiology and sport pedagogy has been created. It is also to be noted that quite recently a first International Seminar on the History of Sports Science (Wonneberger and Liebold 1980) took place in Berlin (G. D. R.), and a second in June 1982 at Macolin (Switzerland).

This growing interest in the history and development of sports science is a reflection of the rapid increase in scientific research in the domain of sport. The multiplication of the institutions of local and national sport science and research centres with a consecutive high number and mulitplicity of national and international organisations will pose a challenge for the coming years with regard to obtaining better co-ordination and co-operation among the international organisations for sport science. Such an effort supported by governmental and inter-governmental organisations, as well as by private institutions, may be the task of the International Council of Sport (Sciences) and Physical Education, thus contributing to the improvement of scientific research in sports, to the enhancement of the understanding of the phenomenon "sport in modern society" and to the quality of life of all human beings.

List of Abbreviations of Organisations

FIMS	Fédération Internationale de Médecine Sportive
ISSP	International Society of Sport Psychology
ICSS	International Committee for Sociology of Sport
ICOHS	International Committee for History of Sport and Physical Education
HISPA	International Association for the History of Physical Education and Sport
PSSS	Philosophical Society for the Study of Sport
ISB	International Society of Biomechanics
IFAPA	International Federation on Adapted Physical Activities
ISCPES	International Society on Comparative Physical Education and Sport

FIEP	Fédération Internationale d'Education
ICHPER	International Council for Health, Physical Education, and Recreation
AIESEP	Association Internationale des Ecoles Supérieures d'Education Physique
IAPESGW	International Association of Physical Education and Sports for Girls and Women
ICPFR	International Council for Physical Fitness Research
WLRA	World Leisure and Recreation Association
IAKS	Internationaler Arbeitskreis Sport- und Freizeiteinrichtungen
ICFP/CIFP	International Committee of Fair Play/Comité International pour le Fair Play
ICSPE/CIEPS	International Council of Sport and Physical Education/Conseil International pour l'Education Physique et le Sport

References

Bernett H (1980) Anfänge sportwissenschaftlicher Vereinigungen. In: Wonneberger G, Liebold K (eds) History of sports science. International Seminar, Berlin (DDR), Protocol, vol II, pp 246–255

Broekhoff J (1980) Ways and means of organizing a system for the standardized collection of documentation in physical education and sport. ICHPER-UNESCO report (contract 207-547), ED-80/WS/68, Paris

Buggel E (1980) Basic orientation for the work of ICSPE. Working Document, 33rd Executive Board Meeting of ICSPE, 9–10 Oct 1980. Sofia

Grupe O (1981) Die Rolle der Wissenschaft im Sport. In: Olympische Leistung, Ideal, Bedingungen, Grenzen. Begegnungen zwischen Sport und Wissenschaft. Bundesinstitut für Sportwissenschaft, Cologne, 1981. (Olympic performance. Ideal, conditions, limits. Meetings between sport and science) pp 13–22 (German Text); pp 288–397 (English text)

Lüschen G (1981) The analysis of sport organizations. In: Lüschen G, Sage GH (eds) Handbook of social science in sport. Stipes, Champaign, pp 316–329

Tittel K (1980) Entwicklungsetappen der Fédération Internationale de Médecine Sportive (F.I.M.S.). In: Wonneberger G, Liebold K (eds) History of sports science. International Seminar, Berlin (DDR), Protocol, vol I, kpp 254–258

UNESCO Final Report (1976) First International Conference of Ministers and Senior Officials responsible for Physical Education and Sport. UNESCO House, Paris

Wonneberger G, Liebold K (eds) (1980) History of sports science. International Seminar, Berlin (DDR), vol I and II

On Some Essential Tasks of and Prospects for International Co-operation in Sport Science

E. Buggel

Progress in the development of the physical education of the young, of the sporting activities of the population and of the results achieved in top-level sport at both national and international levels is increasingly dependent on scientific activities and research. The need for scientific solutions requires a differentiated disciplinary approach to detailed questions; such an approach always places new demands on the various fileds of science and initiates the formation of new fields of science. Simultaneously the complexity of the problems to be solved demands integrative interdisciplinary research. The productiveness of such research depends on the efficiency of the individual fields of science and on continual elaboration of the basic theoretical positions of physical education and sport from an integrative point of view. These two aspects have to be reflected in international organisations of sport science too. Thus there are and must be organisations uniting scientists from the different fields of science for an exchange of experience as well as organisations surveying the whole of sport science (thus facilitating integration of the manifold scientific findings into the complex building of sport science) and promoting the effective application of existing scientific knowledge by means of co-ordination. Considering the aims and tasks of international scientific organisations in the field of physical culture and sport from this point of view, we can see that these distinctions are indeed implemented in practice. But this principle has not been absolutely accepted, for under the concrete historical conditions of our time and as a result of the personal engagement of internationally prominent sport scientists and sport officials in several fields, co-operation at different levels has developed.

International Bodies

A number of international bodies make an essential contribution to the development of various fields of sport science, e.g. the International Society of Sport Psychology, the International Committee of Sport Sociology of ICSPE, the International Association for Sports Information, and the working groups of the ICSPE Research Committee on Biochemistry, Biomechanics and Ergometrics. Furthermore, international bodies have developed that primarily deal with the practical implementation and utilisation of results obtained in sport science, e.g. the Fédération Internationale d'Education Physique (FIEP), the International Association of Physical Education and Sport for Girls and Women, and the International Association of Physical Education Colleges (AIESEP). Within this ensemble of international organisations dealing with questions of sport science in a narrow sense or with the utilisation of its results, the International

Council of Sport and Physical Education (ICSPE) is of the nature of a world-wide association of sport science. The new statutes of ICSPE adopted at the Xth General Assembly reflect this tendency more than ever before. ICSPE initiates and supports the formation of new or the consolidation of existing boards of specialists in different fields of sport science. This reflects the fact that there is an objective need for further shaping and specialisation in sport science in order to make, by means of diverse and specialised knowledge, a contribution to the solution of the complex problems that exist in sport. Parallel to this it is ICSPE's aim to act for an integrative concentration of scientific results. Here the primary task is to bring together the differentiated special knowledge and potential in such a way that they will be highly effective and uniform, meeting the needs and requirements of sporting activities and thus being of advantage to them.

Taking the scientific results and practical experience of national and international institutions of sport science, ICSPE wants to generalise theoretically and to process them for practical application. Another aim of ICSPE is to help to disseminate these results in the interest of the development of physical education and sport in all countries of the world and to promote the independent measures of the different international organisations of sport science by means of co-ordination, avoiding unnecessary repetition of work.

Co-ordination of International Sport Science

The complex character of scientific and social problems and of interaction between scientists makes co-operation between sport science and conterminous fields of science and their institutions of special importance. On the one hand, recognition of and esteem for sport science is internationally promoted by the integration of sport science into the system of science. On the other hand, knowledge in other fields of science is made utilisable for the development of sport science and to improve the effectiveness of sporting activities for all those interested in them. This implies that it would be beneficial to develop co-operation with these international scientific institutions and organisations, and it seems worth striving for contacts between ICSPE and the International Council for Scientific Associations.

In the interests of better co-ordination of scientific work and of greater access to scientific knowledge in sport, longt-term co-ordination of the activities of all international organisations in sport science and extension of the relations that exist with conterminous sciences seem desirable. This will involve thoroughly thinking over the present international structure of sport science. We can start from the fact that it is possible to divide the contents and forms of expression in sport science into three major domains:

The first domain includes the individual fields of sport science and their interaction. Apart from fields of investigation into sporting methods, this covers socal science, natural science, sports medicine and sports technology. The interaction of these scientific fields follows logically from the inseparable connection between social and biological factors in nature and society.

The second domain covers the contents and forms of practical application os sport-scientific findings in the different areas of physical education and sport: compulsory sport in schools and the services, organised and private sports for the masses, top class sport, sport for women, sport for the elderly, sport for the handicapped, fitness sport, sport in the factory, sport in the residential area and sport during holidays. In this second domain are to be found the formation and training of sports cadres, research, treatment by sports medicine as well as the technical and economic tasks.

A third domain concerns information on and documentation of sport science as well as the dissemination of the value of sporting activities via the mass media, sports and scientific publications for the general public, belletristic publications, films, speeches, exhibitions, conferences etc.

In all three domains a variety of problems are being or could be tackled by existing international bodies of sport science. On the grounds that it is necessary to strive especially for qualitative progress at the international level, we have to study in which fields the international progress in knowledge can and must be promoted by existing or by new organisations or committees. Here new possibilities could be opened up for many countries - especially for the young nationally liberated states - to the benefit of the world-wide development of physical culture and sport. These countries could acquire the abundant and manifold treasure of knowledge and experience in sport science and adapt it to their own particular needs.

Sport and Health: An Outline of the World Health Organization's Position

M. J. Karvonen

Introduction

The nations of the world have established a series of organisations for international collaboration. Of world-wide coverage and of particular significance are the organisations of the United Nations's family, where sovereign states are the members. Two of these organisations are actively concerned with sports: UNESCO (the United Nations Educational, Scientific and Cultural Organization) with sports and culture and the WHO (the World Health Organization) with sports and health.

Historical Background

The World Health Organization was established in 1948. In the preamble of its constitution, health was defined as a state of complete physical, mental and social well-being, and not merely absence of illness or infirmity. In a world still suffering from hunger and malnutrition, from appalling infant mortality, from a multitude of infectious diseases and on three continents from all the ravages of the war, this was a revolutionary target, held by many to be quite unrealistic. We all now know the tremendous progress made over the last 35 years in health. Well-being has become a realistic goal but, meanwhile, many nations have already learned that wealth is not automatically accompanied by well-being. What this really is, and how to achieve it, has to be learned.

WHO Activities

During its first 20 years of existence the WHO was committed to fighting hunger and disease. Sports entered in a visible way into its programme for the first time in 1967, when a group of experts convened in Geneva to discuss exercise tests in relation to cardiovascular function (WHO Technical Report 1968). The following year a scientific group considered the optimum physical performance capacity in adults (WHO Technical Report 1969); the recommendations have been a stimulus for a spectrum of studies relating to sport and health. Furthermore, the group proposed that the study of physiological and medical aspects of physical activity and various aspects of physical performance capacity should be introduced into the curricula of medical schools and of the appropriate schools for paramedical personnel. Nine years later, a joint workshop was organised with the Commission of European Communities in Luxembourg to discuss physical activity in the primary prevention of ischaemic heart disease (Joint EEC/WHO Workshop 1978).

The WHO also has either itself published or sponsored several books in this field. A manual *Fundamentals of Exercise Testing* came out under the joint authorship of experts from eight countries (Lange Andersen et al. 1971). Another handbook *Habitual Physical Activity and Health* had a team of authors from seven countries and has become a standard source for both the principles and the methods (Lange Andersen et al. 1978). A further volume is to complete this series of pioneering guides: *Physical Activity in Disease Prevention and Treatment,* a joint venture by the WHO, the International Society and Federation of Cardiology (ISFC) and the International Federation of Sport Medicine (FIMS) (WHO, in press); its 26 authors represent 17 countries. Undoubtedly, the collective efforts of experts from several countries contribute to international understanding in regard to objectives, concepts, methods and terminology. Such an approach should be regarded as an asset to any new science and discipline.

While all the above publications have been written for the medical professions and sports scientists, the WHO adopted a new approach to reach a wider audience. In collaboration with some well-known publishers it launched a 10-volume *Encyclopedia of Health;* one of the volumes is devoted to physical activity and health (Salvat 1980; Favre 1981). The Encyclopedia aims essentially at health promotion rather than prevention and treatment, and in this sense is indeed a pioneering venture. The Scientific Director of each volume had been closely involved in the activities of WHO, and the group of collaborators were international; in the volume physical activity and health they came from ten countries.

Sports and health can interact through other channels too. At its sixty-ninth session on 26 January 1982 the "government" of the WHO, its Executive Board, made history in health education with regard to smoking. Stressing the key role of cigarette smoking in the causation of lung cancer, it: (a) commended the Scottish association football team for its participation as a non-smoking team in the 1982 World Cup competition, thus setting an excellent example to their supporters and to all participants in sport; (b) hoped that other teams might wish to emulate this initiative; and (c) requested that the Director-General take appropriate action to support this important health education opportunity in relation to the World Cup competition.

The slogan of the WHO today is Health for All by the Year 2000 (WHO 1979; 1981). The emphasis is on the grass roots level, in active community participation. Sports for All will have its natural place together with health for all.

References

Favre R (ed) (1981) La Santé. L'encyclopédie pour vivre mieux, 1-10. Editions Grammont SA, Lausanne, Alpha Editions SA, Paris, Editions Erasme, Brussels/Antwerp

Joint EEC/WHO Workshop (1978) On physical activity in primary prevention of ischaemic heart disease. Luxembourg 22-24 February 1977, Commission of the European Communities, Luxembourg

Lange Andersen K, Masivoni R, Rutenfranz J, Seliger V (1978) Habitual Physical Activity and Health, World Health Organization, Regional Office for Europe, Copenhagen

Lange Andersen K, Shephard RJ, Denolin H, Varnauskas E, Masironi R (1971) Fundamentals of exercise testing. World Health Organization, Geneva

Salvat J (ed) (1980) Enciclopedia Salvat de la salud, 1-10. Salvat S. A. de Ediciones, Pamplona

World Health Organization (1979) Formulating strategies for health for all by the year 200. WHO, Geneva

World Health Organization (1981) Global strategy for health for all by the year 200. WHO, Geneva
World Health Organization Technical Report Series No. 388 (1968) Exercise tests in relation to cardiovascular function. Report of a WHO Meeting, WHO, Geneva
World Health Organization Technical Report Series No. 436 (1969) Optimum physical performance capacity in adults. Report of a WHO Scientific Group, WHO, Geneva

International Workers' Sport as a Means of Bringing Peoples Together

M. Ahde

Background

The process of organising the culture of physical exercise for working people can be divided into three major historical phases: (1) the birth of worker-supported sports as part of the bourgeois national sports movement in the latter half of the nineteenth century, (2) the development of an autonomous worker's sports movement as part of the working class movement in the period between the world wars and (3) the joint activity of the workers' sports movement with the bourgeois sports movement following World War II. Although salient differences exist in the organising process and ideology of workers' sports from country to country, we can nevertheless consider the above-mentioned breakdown to be quite generally applicable. The basis of the breakdown into periods is the question that had dominated the history, present stage and future of workers' sport: *the relationship of workers' sport to the bourgeois sports movement.* In all periods the forms of organisation of workers' sport have been determined in terms of the solution at any given time to to this key question. An examination of the history of international workers' sports shows this quite convincingly.

The workers' sports movement got going in the leading industrial countries a little over a hundred years ago when wage earners began to strive to participate in the culture of physical exercise. At first this occurred in the sports movement that had been formed under the leadership of the bourgeoisie. In most countries the sports associations founded by working people also joined the national sports organisations. Quite soon the timely question arose as to whether or not the working class could achieve its physical culture aims within the framework of the bourgeois organisations. The linking of working class sports policy aims with the general political objectives of the socialist workers' movement led to the formation of an autonomous workers' sports movement. In a number of European countries, nationwide workers' sports organisations sprang up around the turn of the century and thereafter (in Germany as early as 1892).

Even before World War I, the working class sports movement grew into a wide mass movement. This meant a splitting in two of the bourgeois sports organisations having a nationwide orientation. The working class sports movement set itself the goal of *bringing about a socialist physical culture as part of the workers' movement.* Worker-supported sports thus constituted a significant part of the working class culture. Its central task was taken as the bringing up of socialist youth, in both mind and body, to be balanced socialist human beings who would have the maturity to realise the social aims of the working class movement.

Since the aims of the working class sports movement were complementary to the goals of the international working class movement, it is clear that the efforts of the international worker-supported sports movement, too, were antithetical to those of the Olympic movement and international sports organisations. These international aims of the worker-supported sports movement, which concerned sport in itself, did not really differ from the idealism of the Olympic movement in the Coubertinian sense. But the gist of the movement was that the workers' movement did not believe that the ideals of sport (the amateur spirit, impartiality and international understanding) could be realised under middle-class leadership. That is why it strove to shake itself free from the signs of the degeneracy (commercialism, chauvinism, overemphasis on setting records) that it had observed in bourgeois sports life. The worker-supported sports movement wanted to bring up the worlds' working class youth in the spirit of *peace and international solidarity,* separate from the middle class sports movement, so that the above-mentioned fringe phenomena in sports life would not also spread to the domain of the working class sports movement.

Organisation of the Working Class Sports Movement

It was on the basis of this separation that the international working class sports movement developed. As early as 1913 an international workers' sports organisation was established in Ghent, Belgium, but its activity had hardly started when World War I broke out. The experiences of the war intensified the bifurcation within the international sports movement. In Finland, the Civil War which was waged in 1918 gave decisive impetus to the founding of the Workers' Sports Union, which occurred in January 1919.

In the autumn of 1920 the Socialist Workers' Sports International was formed in Lucerne, Switzerland; its founding organisations came from Germany, Belgium, Switzerland, England, France, Czechoslovakia and Finland. In addition to these countries, workers sports activity also had wide support in Austria. The total membership of the international's member organisations reached the two million mark during the 1920s, though more than half of the membership was from Germany's ATSB alone. In any event, the international was a significant international organisation in the 1920s and 1930s.

The international working class sports movement endeavours to realise the aims of socialist physical culture outlined above. Keeping to the essentials, we can observe that the central ideological starting points of worker-supported sports were:

1. A balance between intellectual and physical education
2. The priority of mass sports over competitive athletics (competitive athletics were deemed valuable as an ennobling and exemplary activity, but when carried to the extreme, competition would lead to the degeneration of sports)
3. The building of peace and international solidarity
4. Linkage with the goals of the rest of the workers' movement "To be an athlete is good but to be an athlete and a socialist is better still" was the declaration of the Workers' Sports International heard from the Vienna Workers' Olympics in 1931.

The Period of Isolation

The efforts of the worker-supported sports movement to create a socialist physical culture distinct from the bourgeois sports movement were reflected in the fact that workers' sports organisations in different countries refused to take part in all joint activity with national organisations. In the Nordic countries, an important exception was Sweden, for Swedish Social Democracy right from the start took the view that in sports policy the workers' movement should try to achieve a leading position within the nationswide union.

The international workers' sports movement also became isolated from the Olympic movement. A reflection of the aim of retaining cultural integrity was *the working class's own Olympic movement,* which organised three summer and winter games (1925, 1931 and 1937). Besides competitive athletics, these games placed great emphasis on mass performances. An effort was made to turn *physical exercise* - as the German Fritz Wildung emphasised - into the working class's *new international language,* which would be capable of breaking down all language barriers and increasing the international solidarity of the working class.

In point of fact, the 1920s remained the golden age of the international worker-supported sports movement. At the end of the 1920s, the exacerbated disagreements and power struggle between the Social Democrats and the Communists sapped the movement's forces. In 1927 relations between the Red Sports International, which was founded in Moscow in 1921, and the Socialist Sports International were broken off completely. Outside the Soviet Union, the Communist sports movement had support in Norway, Germany, France and some other countries.

Weakened by internal conflicts, worker-supported sports suffered a heavy defeat when fascism almost completely destroyed workers' sports organisations in the 1930s and during World War II. With the demise of the German, Austrian and Czechoslovak organisations, the Social Democrats and Communists began to carry out popular front tactics in sports policy, too. Towards the end of the 1930s, nationwide sports unions were indeed formed in a number of those countries in which fascism did not come to power (e. g. Switzerland and the Nordic countries). With a view to ensuring parliamentary democracy, both the Social Democrats and the Communists strove to support the national sports front. An important facet of their activity was the criticism of the 1936 Berlin Olympics for their unscrupulous use of sports in the service of Nazi propaganda.

In the international solutions taken by worker-supported sports in the 1930s, Finland's TUL became an important exception: it flatly refused to join the nationwide union that had been proposed in 1936. The first step towards Finnish sports reconciliation was taken in the spring of 1939 when arrangements were being made for the Helsinki Olympics. It was not until after the Winter War, in August 1940, that a joint agreement between TUL and SVUL (Finnish National Sports Union) was reached concerning co-operation in organising competitions. Thereafter an agreement procedure of this kind has been the main model in Finnish sports policy, and on the international level TUL is the only significant workers' sports organisation that has for more than 60 years without interruption upheld the principles of Lucerne.

The Period of Collaboration

In any event, World War II meant for workers' sports the beginning of a new epoch: a shift was made from uncompromising isolation to joint activity, a policy which has been carried out in different countries either in nationwide unions or by separate agreements (cf. TUL in Finland). This turning point was ultimately sealed and approved when worker-supported sports were virtually driven to the brink of destruction under the heel of fascism. On the other hand, the struggle against fascism and the result of World War II promoted the international integration of the sports movement. *A belief in the significance of sports in building peace and democracy was strong immediately following World War II.*

In the years 1945–1948, the workers' sports organisations in Western Europe eagerly sought to re-establish the Workers' Sports International. The Soviet Union, however, was reluctant to go along with this for it wanted to join international special unions. It did not take part in the activity of the International Workers' Sports Committee CSIT (Comité sportif international di travail), the body established in London in 1946, which was originally supposed to form an international.

In the post-World War II period, the picture of international worker-supported sports has changed significantly from what it was during the years of isolation in the 1920s and 1930s. It can be said that the international channels of influence open to workers' sports have become diversified, though, again, there is a multiplicity of fringe phenomena and political pressures which threaten the original ideals of sport.

Roughly speaking, there are three channels of organisation and activity open to international workers' sports: (1) activity within the nationwide national sports unions and the exercising through them of influence in the Olympic movement and international special unions, (2) the sports movement of the socialist countries and (3) CSIT with its national member unions (a total of 16 organisations in 13 countries, in Western Europe and Israel). All of these channels aim to develop international joint activity in sports and renounce the tactics of isolation once adopted by worker-supported sports. Beyond a doubt, *the contribution of the socialist countries in the international sports movement has in recent decades become very sizeable.* It bears noting that it was during the Cold War years that the socialist countries for the most part joined the international Olympic movement. In addition we must remember that the international sports policy pressures which have increased of late have been caused almost completely by factors beyond the control of the sports movement.

On the other hand, in both international sports and workers' sports there continue to be certain unsolved problems which continually weaken the potential of worker-supported sports as a means of bringing peoples closer together. From the standpoint of workers' sports organisations, a solution has yet to be found regarding their *representation in international special unions* in which national sports organisations represent their respective countries. Again, worker-supported sports have in recent decades been able to strengthen their international significance in the nationwide unions of different countries and in their national Olympic committees.

One of the central problems facing the independent workers' sports movement is also the tole of CSIT, since this organisation throughout the entire period of its activity has not been able to achieve the significance which its 2.2 million strong organisation would be expected to have. This is chiefly due to two factors: first, the member organisations of CSIT are - perhaps with the exception of TUL and Austria's ASKÖ (Arbeiter Sport-und Kulturbund Österreichs) - rather weak in their own countries, and, secondly, for all its positive stands on programme orientations, CSIT has not been able to establish an autonomous international sports policy. This became apparent, for example, 2 years ago when CSIT did not as an organisation give its joint support to the Moscow Games.

The Future of the Working-Class Sports Movement

Despite the problems outlined above, the prospects for workers' sports are, as I see it, mainly bright. The international sports movement needs both independent workers' sports organisations and workers' physical culture policy that takes the form of joint activity. Nothing can be stated categorically regarding the superiority of one or the other model, for the conditions in different countries dictate to a large degree the terms according to which worker-centred physical culture policy can be practised. Yet it seems to me that workers' sports have a number of fields of activity and modes of international co-operation which have so far not been tried to any mentionable degree. Traditionally, indeed, the workers' sports movement has *a strong link with the rest of the workers' movement* and thereby, for example, the sports movement and the trade union movement can in the future have most important points of co-operation, say, in the promoting of mass and employee sports. On the other hand, the fundamental aims of workers' sports have always tended in the direction of exercising a physical culture policy that is in harmony with the needs of the nation at large. Here we see a continual convergence of the aims of the workers' movement and the worker-supported sports movement.

In international sports policy, the connections of workers' sports with the socialist countries are especially important. TUL is in a key position internationally to play a role - to cite a notable example - in improving the relations between CSIT and the socialist countries. The same applies on a wider scale to East-West sports policy relations, in which TUL has worked to open up the way ever since 1922.

The traditions and timely sports policy aims of workers' sports in the wider international sports movement offer novel solutions in the struggle against the continual encroachment of fringe phenomena. If we think of the theme of this presentation, the paramount consideration is the observation that *the workers' sports movement has from its inception worked to achieve the ideals which, for example, the Olympic movement strives for.* It is just that the history of workers' sports has so far been studied so little that the public is not sufficiently aware of this fact. It is nevertheless true that sports as a means of bringing peoples closer together have never been the sole possession of the Olympic movement. In fact, the whole post-World War II evolution shows that the bourgeois sports movement has had to recognise that the representatives of the workers' sports movement were correct in the criticism they have been making for decades: sport is a social phenomenon and its ideals are not realised by themselves, without political will and effort. To cite a case in point: the signs of the modernisation of the Olympic movement have of late provided a clear-cut indication that these facts must be recognised.

The goals of peace and solidarity declared by the international workers' sports movement have remained timely from one decade to the next. The workers' sports movement fulfils a central task within the international sports movement in carrying these banners and in acting as a representative of the organised workers' movement. This role becomes all the more important, the firmer the foothold which democratic principles gain within the national sports unions and in international sports policy.

Nordic Co-operation in Sports

M. Ståhlberg

Introduction

The Nordic countries - Iceland, Norway, Sweden, Denmark and Finland - form an area within which co-operation is naturally and sensibly pursued in relation to culture, science and attitudes. Should sports constitute an exception to the successful collaboration in other fields? The answer is an emphatically "non". The motives behind sporting activity and management are certainly the same in all five countries; both priorities and the structure of sports life are similar. Thus the Nordic countries are closely interconnected through extensive and beneficial exchange in the field of sports and physical education. The Faroe Islands and Greenland have also made a contribution in some sectors of co-operation in this field.

Collaboration has traditionally been practised in the field of sports and physical education between National Olympic Committees, between special sports federations and between central federations for sports and physical education in various countries.

This paper seeks to describe the existing forms of co-operation between the central federations for sports and physical education within the framework of the work done by the Faelles Joint Committee.

The Role of the Faelles Committee

The Faelles Committee, established by the central sport federations in the Nordic countries, has assumed a considerably closer and more official role in co-operation than, for instance, the Olympic Committees and special federations. The activity of the Faelles Committee, initiated as early as the second decade of this century, is based on provisions that can be amended when necessary. The Committee convenes every second year in each member country in turn. In accordance with the Committee provisions, five representatives from each country, i.e. from each central federation, and, additionally, the required number of experts, participate in sessions. As a founder and an official member, the Finnish Central Sports Federation has, to the benefit of active co-operation in sports and physical education in Finland, customarily invited participants from two other central federations in Finland, the Workers' Sports Federation and the Central Federation of Swedish Sports Organisations, to represent the Finnish delegation. Each organisation individually covers the expense incurred by sending these representatives.

As prescribed in the provisions, the Faelles Committee acts as a consultative sports body for the Nordic countries with the aim of achieving a consistent Nordic position on matters pertaining to sports and physical education. The Committee also represents the Nordic countries in international sports organisations. The Committee does not attempt to make decisions for its members but instead submits comments and recommendations upon which each central federation bases its official decisions.

The Committee's Sphere of Competence

A great number of items always appear on the agenda of the Faelles Committee. It naturally deals with issues related to sports ideology, but mainly it deliberates on current every-day problems. The following serve as examples of the topics dealt with:

- In-depth reports, including information on activities and their development
- Organisational issues, such as fluctuation in membership, measures required due to the age structure of the membership, new organisations and organisational changes
- The finance, staff and other operational resources required
- Competitive sports and the problems they create, like doping and its control, the status of amateurs and ultranationalism
- Sports for women as a distinct and significant sector of sporting activities
- Contacts with political decision-making and interest groups as well as with radio and television, industry and commerce, the Nordic Council and the Nordic Cultural Fund
- Legislation, insurance and environmental issues involving sports
- Sports for the handicapped
- International topics, such as the establishment of the International Assembly of National Confederations of Sport and the activity of the European Sports Conference, the Ministerial Conference and the Sports Committee of the Council of Europe

A Joint Youth Committee of Nordic central organisations for sports and physical education and a Joint Committee for Scientific Research in Sports have been set up to function alongside the Faelles Committee. The Youth Committee is charged with consulting, drawing up recommendations, laying down policy lines for youth sports and physical education for children, and promoting collaboration between the youth organisations in different countries. In 1985 in the United Nations' Year of the Child, Finland will arrange a physical education camp for children.

The Committee for Sports Sciences is to promote research by arranging scientific seminars and congresses on the problems confronted in sports and physical education, launch international research projects, work for the dissemination of information and provide information and documentation services.

Other Areas of Co-operation

As mentioned earlier, co-operation has traditionally occurred between the individual National Olympic Committees and special federations for sports and physical education. This co-operation mainly involves only the specific issues in the Olympic movement and in different sports, whereas all areas and issues in sports and physical education are dealt with in exchange between the federations for sports and physical education.

Co-operation between officials working in the field of sports and physical education, which is by its nature unofficial and outside the jurisdiction of the Nordic Council, deserves mention in order to give a complete picture. These unofficial meetings with official representatives are convened two or three times a year to consider questions of mutual interest and to find solutions to problems that frequently concern a specific theme. Discussions related to activities of sports institutes are also held annually.

Prospects for the Future

Co-operation is always of value irrespective of the field or the mode in which it is practised. Although co-operative endeavours may not always have a concrete result, this is no indication of failure. Exchange of opinions stimulates the participating parties, opens up new views and contributes to mutual understanding. The increasingly complex structure and content of sport and solutions to the problems arising in this context, the availability of resources required by large-scale projects, and the support of common regional interests are other motives for further co-operation.

Joint efforts usually lead to rapid and decisive results - without detracting from any one party's decision-making authority - in solving common problems and resolving current issues in a manner satisfactory to all parties involved. For these reasons, great expectations must be held of the future. On behalf of all representatives of the Nordic countries, I firmly believe that co-operation will continue to progress in the same positive spirit witnessed to date.

School Sport Across Borders - Education in Internationalism

A. Sastamala

Establishment of the International School Sport Federation (ISF)

The exact date of birth of international school sporting events could be the year 1963, when a teacher of physical education, Mr. Jan Kloen from the Netherlands, organised an international handball tournament for school teams in his school in Doetinchem. Before this tournament some private contacts had already taken place between some European countries as well as between countries in other continents. Until 1967 these handball tournaments were held in Doetinchem. This was the beginning of the regular organisation of tournaments by some active persons in Central Europe.

In 1968 the handball tournament took place for the first time outside of the Netherlands: in Wiesbaden in the Federal Republic of Germany and in Eisenstadt in Austria in 1969. Also in 1969 the first basketball tournament was held in Zagreb in Yugoslavia, and the first football tournament in Kaiserslautern in the Federal Republic of Germany. At this time an organising body was founded, representatives coming from participating countries. This unofficial board has formulated the directives for international extra-curricular school sport work (Andrecs 1977).

More and more interest began to be shown in these tournaments. Therefore it seemed most necessary to form a permanent coordinative organisation and to draw up statutes for international school sport work. One very important reason why the organised international school sport work had proved necessary was that pupils began to be capable of entering competitions at a much earlier age. Even the top level sportsmen and women were of a lower age. Moreover the raising of the school-leaving age in many European countries required that schools took over an ever-increasing number of tasks which had formerly been performed by other institutions. It was obvious that the schools and the teachers had to bear many responsibilities which had formerly been fulfilled by sports associations. It also seemed important to bring the educational aspect of intracurricular physical education into the competitive sport of school-aged young people, even at the international level. Because the basis for the establishment of a supranational school sports organisation had been created, the Austrian Ministry of Education and Culture held an international conference at Raach in Austria from 16 to 18 September 1971. Twenty-two countries participated and it was decided to found the International Federation of School Sport. This conference prepared the 1st General Assembly, where the International School Sport Federation (ISF) became a reality. The 1st General Assembly of ISF took place in Beaufort in Luxembourg on 4 and 5 June 1972 (Minutes of the Conference ..., 1971).

Philosophy of the ISF

Objectives and Limits

The ISF tries to encourage sport at school and to co-ordinate school championships at international level. As a school organisation, the ISF gives priority to educational objectives in all its activities. As an umbrella federation it does not wish to influence school sport at national level, but it is ready to accede to any request for assistance by giving information and support. The ISF organises international school sporting events in various sports among various countries and encourages international contacts between school-going young people, to promote better mutual understanding.

The ISF seeks close co-operation with the school authorities of its member countries, with the international sports federations and with international organisations that pursue similar aims. It restricts its activities to primary and secondary schools. It is free from political, religious or racial considerations (International School Sport Federation 1979).

The Olympic Movement and the ISF

In many areas of life the vital influences occur during childhood or adolescence. Various experiences are accumulated and a great many skills and abilities acquired during that formative stage, but above all judgement ripens and the established patterns of behaviour are consolidated.

The ISF is conscious of the great responsibility entailed by the organisation and co-ordination of international school championships. Since its foundation it has constantly been attempting to reconcile its educational aims with the organisational requirements of modern sporting events. Its priority has been to establish good social contacts, to comply with existing age regulations, to avoid excessive competition, to promote the idea of fair play, and to incorporate to championships into a cultural programme which offers many opportunities to meet other young people, both inside and outside the framework of the sporting competitions.

By emphasising team spirit through the school team serving as the sole representative of a country, by giving priority to educational objectives, and by insisting that the competitors be accompanied by teachers, the ISF (International School Sport Federation 1979) hopes to achieve full realisation of the Olympic ideal within the framework of its activities, namely:

- Value participation more than victory
- Defend the cause of honesty and fairness
- Fight self-centredness and encourage spontaneity
- Emphasise community spirit
- Integrate sport into the cultural entity

Education in Internationalism

School-aged young people are curious, unprejudiced, honest and unable to feel deeply unsympathetic towards other people. To a young person friendship is an inviolable, highly valued matter, in which he or she is willing to trust. If we succeed in building friendship between our young people, I believe this will promote mutual understanding and peace in the world.

It is obvious that sport is a common denominator, in the framework of which there are many possibilities for educating school-aged people towards the kind of internationalism that would be more encouraging to peace and friendship than are the attitudes prevalent in many parts of the world of today.

The ISF wants to offer young people from various countries, societies and school systems opportunities of coming together. In this way they become acquainted with new nations, new societies, new cultures and new persons, have many new experiences and acquire knowledge of other countries and their inhabitants. With such knowledge and experiences it is easier to build a picture of life and a set of values on which to base behaviour.

As already mentioned, in ISF activities the social and cultural programme plays a very important role. Apart from the official championships the ISF also organises contests with mixed teams and it seems that our school-aged young people enjoy competing as much and even more with mixed teams. One reason might be that there is no stress whether they win or lose; rather there is only the fascinating spirit of competition and movement. They accept each other, joke, laugh and are in interaction.

Increasing the interaction of young people at international level increases the mutual understanding in the world, and that is a very necessary premise for building world peace. School sport across borders is education towards internationalism in practice.

Past Results and the Future

Our tasks have been to lay emphasis on ethical and educational values and to broaden the picture of life of school-going people in the framework of international sporting activities and in this way to educate them in internationalism. Have we achieved our tasks? According to my understanding, ISF is on the right track and has made some forward steps during the 10 years of its existence.

During this time we have met with interference on a number of occasions. Some have concerned the security of teams, some have been based on the world political situation and some have even involved national and international sports federations. The latter problems have been resolved through consultation and by supplying more information on the tasks of the ISF. The ISF works very hard to solve the political confusions that arise.

The third item of the European Conference on Security and Co-operation, being held in Helsinki, is dealing with co-operation in the area of humanistic questions. In this item one task is to increase the contacts between young people in the world. It is this aim which ISF has tried to achieve when organising school sports events.

In emphasising the educational aspects that are involved even in extracurricular school sport, it has been natural to involve teachers of physical education in the ISF's work. This entails international interaction between teachers and communication on pedagogic and didactic questions.

Next year ISF is widening its work to alternative and leisure sports. In the future this kind of course will concern both pupils and teachers involved in extracurricular school sport (ISF 1981).

The ISF is growing. We have 33 full members and two associate members. The discussion of regional events has already begun. More important is the increasing influence of our work and the achievement of our objectives. For me this means:

to give every child a possibility to run,
not because she has to escape or
because he feels fear,
but to run voluntarily
only because she has a need to run
and because he enjoys the movement.

References

Andrecs H (1977) Fünf Jahre Internationale Schulsport-Föderation (ISF). Leibesübungen - Leibeserziehung 7:149-151

International School Sport Federation (1979) Statutes, Rules of Procedure, General Rules of Competition. ISF, Vienna, pp 3-41

ISF (1981) Symposium IN-TER-SCHOOL. Bloso, Brussels

Minutes of the conference for the establishment of a European school sport federation (1971) Vienna/Raach 16-18 Sept 1971, pp 1-3

The Finnish Student Sports Federation as a Promoter of International Understanding

H. Mäki-Reinikka

Students and young people generally have, in recent decades, become known for their active participation in promoting international understanding and working for peace and disarmament. In many cases they have also functioned as the conscience of the nation in questions of creating greater international equality and working for solidarity with (and providing aid to) the developing countries. On the other hand, sport is a major factor in international relations, its importance lying in the large amount of international sporting competition and the publicity and interest it awakens within the nations of the world. One can also say that sport is an important educator and former of opinion in nearly every country.

By means of sporting activity, the Finnish Student Sports Federation is working for international understanding, peace and detente, and for greater co-operation with the developing countries. I would like to stress that these aims have become an integral part of our activity, and that we pursue them both at an international and at a national level.

International Activities

The Finnish Student Sports Federation (OLL) is working through a network of international relations, the most important bodies involved being the International University Sports Federation (FISU), the International Union of Students (IUS) and the Academic Sports Federation of the Nordic countries (NAIF). Also worth mentioning is the bilateral co-operation with the *Burevestnik* from the Soviet Union and SAIF in Sweden.

We naturally see our co-operation and work with FISU, which has 67 national member federations and even more nations participating in its major events, as very important. FISU has also played an active role in international sporting life in many questions of political impact, being a kind of avant-garde. Thus FISU was the first body to accept the GDR as a member, the Peoples' Republic of China has been participating actively in FISU activities, and so on. The question of the developing countries was also taken up by FISU before the discussions on "olympic solidarity" started in the IOK. Recently, at their last meeting in Edmonton, the FISU executive committee accepted a plea for disarmament, directed to the participants in the United Nations' 2nd special session on disarmament.

The OLL strives to make an independent contribution to FISU's work: in 1970 we arranged complete winter games, the "Polar Universiades", in 1974 a CESU (the scientific conference of FISU) congress, in 1978 Student World Championships in orienteering and in 1982 Student World Championships in judo. We feel that these events, like all FISU events, are exceptionally good forums for promoting international understanding owing to their character as great international sport meetings, while at the same time they are more purely in the spirit of amateur sport than other events at the same level.

If the co-operation within FISU is focused mainly on top-level sporting collaboration (not forgetting its work in the scientific field), the co-operation between OLL and the Department of Physical Education and Sport of the IUS basically concerns the so-called normal students. IUS arranges international sport camps for students, which are an excellent opportunity for students from different countries and representing different social systems to overcome their prejudices. Their common sporting activities serve as a natural basis for getting to know each other, and thus also each others' peoples and life-style.

Together with IUS and the National Union of Finnish Students (SYL), OLL has been arranging both winter and summer sport camps for students in Finland. The slogan of these camps has been "Through Sports Towards Peace and Friendship". IUS also has plans for an international seminar on student sports and developing countries.

The NAIF, which is an organisation for regional co-operation among the Nordic countries, provides several means for close connections, generally at what could be called the grass-root level. I wish to mention only one aspect of this co-operation, but it is something that we in OLL look upon with great satisfaction – namely the co-operation between the NAIF member organisations on providing aid to student sports in the developing countries. This is a very new area within the work of NAIF, and there are certainly still many questions to be solved, but the important thing is that the idea has received serious support in all member countries.

In close connection with this I would like to mention OLL's bilateral relations with SAIF (our sister organisation in Sweden). SAIF is running a project whereby they gather sporting material for the students of Tanzania, and we have discussed the possibility of co-operating with them in this venture.

The other bilateral partner of OLL with which we have regular co-operation is the student sports federation of the USSR, *Burevestnik*. This co-operation has traditionally taken the form of exchange visits by sports teams, but in connection with this we have, of course, also had the possibility of carrying out discussions. Also worth mentioning is that Vice-president Sharov visited Finland and lectured at a seminar arranged by OLL on the "Olympic Movement and International Politics". As a new form of co-operation a delegation from *Burevestnik* visited OLL in the autumn of 1983, and one of the topics of discussion was promoting peace and disarmament through student sports. The programme for developmental aid currently being worked upon in FISU will also be discussed, and we shall be searching for possible mutual efforts in this field.

National Activities

Above I have tried to give a brief picture of the means and channels that the Finnish Student Sports Federation uses at the international level in order to promote international understanding and co-operation. The other side of the coin is OLL's work at the national level. This means spreading and promoting internationalism and solidarity among Finnish students. We try to achieve this through the international student sport camps mentioned above, and, of course, also through competitive international exchange. Here, however, I would especially like to describe one, or, more precisely, two activities: the so-called Academic Quarter and the seminars held in connection with it. The Academic Quarter is a yearly street relay for students arranged by OLL. Together with the preliminary local relays it attracted 6000 participants in 1982, thus being a major mass sporting activity in Finland. The point I want to make is that the theme or slogan of the race traditionally refers to some international question. So, this year it was "Speed to Disarmament and Permanent Peace in Europe". Last year it was "For a Non-nuclear Zone in the Nordic Countries", and the year before it was a plea for the Moscow Olympics, against the boycott. In connection with the Academic Quarter relay in 1980 we also arranged a seminar, as I mentioned above, on the Olympic movement and international politics. In 1982 we renewed the idea of a seminar in connection with the race, the topic being "Sports - Developing Countries - National Identity", and we hope to make this a tradition in order to awaken and strengthen the discussion among Finnish students and others involved in sport about the different connections between sport and vital international problems. The purpose of the seminar is twofold: Firstly, to stimulate nationwide discussion about aid to developing countries. (In this work students have been pioneers in Finland.) Secondly, to stimulate discussion among sporting people. It was also our purpose to get all sport organisations to develop some concrete plans/projects about such aid.

In this seminar OLL pointed out that the values of sport at present largely centre around competition, commercialism and chauvinism. OLL stressed that it is time to influence development, not to be subjected to it. OLL views the present situation as such that neither students nor the sporting community has a right to abstain from international responsibility. Considering the significance of sport, aid to developing countries rapidly turns into an obligation. We have to encourage those sporting values that protect and construct life.

In the statute of UNESCO it is mentioned that sport has to be included in development programmes because of its importance in helping developing countries in many ways. It is very important that this point of the statute is adhered to closely. In the spirit of the UNESCO statute, OLL tries to create positive attitudes to this challenge at the national level. The purpose is to broaden the discussion to small sport clubs and so on, in the same way as has been achieved in other national movements (especially the student movement). Through sport we can ensure that ever more people will work for a better world.

In co-operation with the national student movement other projects involving sport will be developed; for example, in conjunction with plans to sponsor universities in developing countries there can be projects to assist with constructing sports sites and obtaining sports equipment. We hope that such plans will serve as an example to the whole sporting world.

The Prerequisites for the Improvement of International Understanding by Sports Organisations

T. Niwa

Purpose

When we consider what types of organisation are necessary in order to improve international understanding, the present situation of sport and sports organisations deserves priority. By identifying its problems I want to reflect upon what would be the ideal practice of sports in Japan, and to offer ideas on how to create and maintain an organisation that would promote international understanding.

The principles by which we create sports organisations vary according to the organisers' point of view. But whatever organisations are created, they are, in the long run, strongly affected by (i) the aim of the people who control sports, (ii) the logic of sports inherent in the sports themselves, and (iii) social needs etc. Taking this into consideration, I think it is possible to approach more essential problems by dwelling upon these points rather than by analysing various organisations.

Present Situation and Problems of Sport and Sports Organisations in Japan

Level of Participation in Sports

Sports in Japan have developed in two directions, that is, mass sports (everyday sports) and elite sports. Mass sports have become popular among women, children and the aged, both at the place of work and in the home. For example, in 1979, 76% men and 62% of women played sports. A difference is noticed between the sexes. However, counting the 1965 participation as 100, the male index in 1979 was 131 and the female 175, which shows that women's participation increased more quickly during this period (The Prime Minister's Office 1965, 1979). The percentage of participation by age group increased especially in the case of the aged and women above 40 years old (Table 1).

Participation in Three Different Types of Sport

Light sports and field sports are popular among every age group of both sexes, while competitive sports are popular among men uner 40 years old (Table 2).

Reasons for Participation in Sport

Table 3 shows that most people play sports for pleasure and that the number of those who play sports for reasons of health increases with age.

Table 1. Changes in participation in sport by age group

	Age group	1965 (%)	1979 (%)	Index in 1979, counting the 1965 participation as 100
Men	20–24	90.5	94.8	105
	25–29	79.4	96.0	121
	30–39	67.9	91.2	134
	40–49	58.0	76.3	132
	50–59	40.7	58.2	143
	60	20.9	49.0	234
Women	20–24	71.2	89.3	125
	25–29	43.7	70.2	161
	30–39	41.5	76.9	185
	40–49	30.6	63.2	207
	50–59	19.0	45.3	238
	60	6.4	31.1	486

Source: Prime Minister's Office (1965, 1979)

Table 2. Change of rate of participation in each type of sport [a]

Sex and age group		Light sport			Field sport			Competitive sport		
		1965 (%)	1979 (%)	Index (1979/1965)	1965 (%)	1979 (%)	Index (1979/1965)	1965 (%)	1979 (%)	Index (1979/1965)
Men		38.6	64.3	167	37.4	53.9	144	31.2	43.4	139
Women		24.7	55.1	223	20.4	29.7	146	10.7	21.7	203
Men	20–24	72.2	88.5	123	67.5	85.4	127	64.3	76.0	118
	25–29	60.8	86.1	142	62.9	79.2	126	60.8	79.2	130
	30–39	42.6	78.8	185	40.9	67.5	165	40.2	63.6	158
	40–49	33.3	61.8	186	39.3	58.2	148	20.5	41.8	204
	50–59	26.6	43.9	165	22.0	37.2	169	18.1	17.9	99
	60+	14.7	43.3	295	9.0	16.5	183	2.8	7.2	257
Women	20–24	50.9	81.6	160	61.3	66.0	108	30.1	55.3	184
	25–29	27.8	59.6	214	26.7	40.4	151	14.8	29.2	197
	30–39	28.3	69.5	246	22.5	45.9	204	12.0	35.0	292
	40–49	23.4	53.5	229	13.5	24.1	179	7.7	18.4	239
	50–59	13.6	43.1	317	7.2	12.9	179	3.2	4.4	138
	60+	6.4	29.7	464	0.6	2.8	467	-	0.5	-

[a] Light sport – catchball, casual badminton, circle pass of volleyball, bowling, jogging, folk dancing and others
Field sport – skiing, golf, hiking, angling, camping, cycling, swimming, boating, yachting and others
Competitive sport – baseball, volleyball, softball, tennis, table tennis, judo, Japanese archery, kendo (Japanese fencing), soccer, track and field events, and others

Source: The Prime Minister's Office (1965, 1979)

Table 3. Reasons for participation in sports (%)

Sex and age groups		Promotion of health	Pleasure	Shortage of physical activities	Mental training	Others	Did not understand
Total		20.3	44.5	21.8	3.0	3.5	6.9
Men		22.1	46.5	18.6	3.9	3.1	5.8
Women		18.5	42.5	25.1	2.0	3.8	7.9
Men	20–24	19.8	59.3	14.3	3.3	1.1	2.2
	25–29	15.5	51.5	18.6	6.3	6.2	2.1
	30–39	17.1	51.9	19.4	3.9	3.1	4.7
	40–49	22.6	46.3	17.9	3.2	4.2	5.8
	50–59	23.7	40.4	25.4	3.5	2.6	4.4
	60–	42.1	22.1	13.7	4.2	-	17.9
Women	20–24	8.7	66.3	16.3	3.3	1.1	4.3
	25–29	8.0	54.9	25.7	0.9	4.4	6.2
	30–39	15.6	43.3	29.3	1.1	5.2	5.6
	40–49	19.6	37.0	24.9	4.2	5.8	8.5
	50–59	30.4	30.4	26.5	2.0	-	10.8
	60–	40.9	19.7	18.2	-	1.5	19.7

Source: The Prime Minister's Office (1979)

Social Conditions Leading to the Promotion of Mass Sports

Social conditions which have promoted general and everyday sporting activity are (i) economic factors (increase of income shown in Table 4), (ii) time factor (increase of free time shown in Table 5) and (iii) change in the philosophy of life (from logic of austerity to that of satisfaction).

Table 4. Estimates of per capita national income and national disposable income (US $, per year)

	1960	1963	1970	1973	1974
Japan	417	625	1636	3275	3546

Source: Statistical Office of the United Nations (1976), statistical yearbook: twenty-eight issue

Table 5. Actual weekly hours of work per worker (manufacturing industry)

	1966	1967	1968	1969	1970	1971	1972	1973	1974	1975
Japan	44.6	44.8	44.6	43.9	43.3	42.6	42.3	42.0	40.0	38.8

Source: Statistical Office of the United Nations (1976), statistical yearbook: twenty-eight issue

Problems of Sports in Japan

Present Situation Regarding Championship Sports

In spite of the increaase in (a) children, women and the aged who participate in sports, (b) those who participate in light sports and field sports and (c) those who participate for pleasure and health, the majority of Japanese, including sports club members, still think that nothing but victory matters. The typical characteristics of their sports philosophy are as follows (Niwa 1982): (i) a "nothing-but-victory" spirit controls training as well as contest, (ii) vertical human relations of director, coach and captain prevail everywhere, (iii) in order to succeed in becoming the best team, training of excellent players is most important and the team members are forced to bear hard training, and (iv) the "nothing-but-victory" spirit controls the whole club – there is no room for individual freedom and it is accordingly taken for granted that the team has priority over individuals.

We can list the following reasons for the popularity of championship sports and the "nothing-but-victory" spirit:

1. In the Meiji era, 1867-1912, when sports were imported to Japan, people had no background history of sports, and the imported sports were therefore developed as championship sports by the sports clubs of higher education institutions; moreover, the nothing-but-victory spirit conditioned by the Bushido spirit controlled sports.
2. Japanese sportsmen who were sent to Olympic Games and other international sporting events went with this spirit and philosophy. In order to select the Japanese delegation, a preliminary system had been organised first in local prefectures, then in area prefectures and finally on a nationwide scale; today this system is applied even to junior high schools and it is feared that the system might even penetrate elementary schools.
3. People who controlled these sports organisations had been famous in championship sports; also people within organisations encouraged sportsmen to train themselves for victory and created new organisations.
4. The mass media inform us repeatedly of championship sports, and everyday sporting activities by general people are seldom heard of; people are very strongly influenced by this, as seen in live broadcasts of such professional sports as baseball and golf.
5. Championship sports broadcasts by the mass media have increased the number of people who prefer watching and listening to games rather than playing sports themselves (Table 6); this functions as a substitutional satisfaction for the general public's desires.
6. Victories in sports that have a large new value bring lots of political, economical and social benefits, and many people want to make use of such sports. For example, big enterprises plan sporting events and sponsor them for propaganda, and nations hold Olympic Games and other international events in order to elevate their prestige. It is a fact that Olympic Games are events for peace, but we can witness a substitutional war of nations for prestige, e.g. secret techniques may be developed for victory, international espionage may be undertaken to gather information about opponents, and doping may be employed. Why do we go such extremes in order to win? Here is the most critical problem of championship sports today.

Table 6. Likes and dislikes towards sport (%, Juni 1972)

Sex and age	Total number of persons	Likes				No preference	Dislike
		Prefer playing sports	Prefer watching games	Like both (playing and watching)	Total		
Total	2529	20	24	18	62	31	7
Men	1114	23	26	20	69	25	6
Women	1415	17	23	16	56	36	8
20–29	547	36	16	28	80	17	3
30–39	655	27	20	24	71	25	4
40–49	607	15	27	15	57	35	8
50–59	363	6	33	11	50	42	8
60–	357	3	31	4	38	46	16

Source: The Information Unit of the Prime Minister's Secretariat (1972)

Problems of Championship Sports

Victory Controls Everything

In championship sports, only one team or person wins; all others are losers. Unstinted praise is given to the victor, whose victory is eulogised as the symbol of the great union of man's body and will, whereas the weaker contestants are neglected.

Victory itself is indeed wonderful, but it is extremely difficult for one to be a victor by dint of one's individual efforts, because with our present high standard of sporting ability and our social situation, systematic and scientific training is almost indispensable in winning. Accordingly, the present development of athletic ability has resulted in demanding victory from players who are excellent as motor machines, just as good products depend upon excellent machines in an industrial society with a supervised organisational system.

At the basis of this situation lies the idea "Victory as Almighty", which basically supports the logic of productivity. This slogan divides players into the strong and the weak, imposes victory as the impetus to prove the superiority of one's own race, nation and group, or conforms people ideologically to the establishment. Therefore, in effect sports become inevitably associated with nationalism. In the championship sports of present-day Japan, sporting technique is related basically to victory, and this victory strengthens the ideological control of the establishment. And so, the weak and the non-conformists must be outsiders in championship sports. Such a gap as is recognised between the insider and the outsider has resulted in a bipolar disintegration of elite sports (championship sports) and mass sports (recreation). Therefore, players of championship sports are given spiritual and material aid from the establishment as sponsors and must receive strenuous training as a major part of their daily routine. We do not blame the players for this professionalism; we blame the social mechanism which works beyond the individual will of players.

Commercialisation

On the other hand, what about mass sports? The present-day mass complex without personality and individuality was born out of our post-World War II mass society. We feel anxiety and loneliness as outsiders of megalo-society, and seek for dependable values and norms. Large enterprises take advantage of this mass psychology and begin to make use of the masses for profit. Such enterprises have created new fashions through the mass media, and have also created new desires by giving only temporary satisfaction and substitutional fulfilment. Accordingly, they have made vast profits by selling products utilising these consumer desires.

It is common for sportswear and sporting equipment to carry the trade marks and names of the sponsoring enterprises and manufacturers. It is ultimately so contrived that the more popular the players become, the more advertised the enterprises are. This is an aspect of fashionable "massification" of sports controlled by large enterprises. Even in recreation and mass sports, where people participate in order to enjoy a full life, it must be confessed that people are being used by these enterprises.

In this system of sport – the system operating in Japan today – people are manipulated through the arousal of desires; a mechanism of social control has been established by granting people temporary emotional satisfaction through commercialised sports.

What kind of sports, then, should be pursued? In order to answer this question, it is necessary firstly to examine our sports today, which have come to be commercialised or to serve as an agency for nationalism. It is then necessary for us to change the sports logic, dominated by its essentially competitive character, and to consider a new sports logic that will provide the enjoyment of a full life; i. e. a sports logic based on humanity and solidarity must be created. Sport based on this logic can provide the pleasures of self-actualisation and co-operation. Players can therefore enjoy it with contentment and satisfaction, and they will be able to understand and be friendly with each other. We cannot, however, deal with the problem of the ideal way of sport without prior knowledge of the mechanism of sports and society.

Search for the Ideal Way of Sport

Logics of Sport

Man must struggle for the survival of his body, but at the same time may act freely and spontaneously in search of meaning in a world beyond his utilitarian activities. The two logics, that of nature and that of freedom, are in a competitive and co-existing relation as far as man is concerned. For example, with healthy young people the logic of freedom is predominant, whereas the logic of nature predominates with people who worry about their health and physical fitness.

In our present generation the logic of freedom in the field of sport has been tied up with the "principle of competition", and moreover it has been manipulated by nationalism and commercialism; these factors have brought about dysfunction of sport, stimulating the spirit that nothing but victory matters and disturbing international understanding.

People today, especially when human behavioural patterns have been standardised through the mass media, thirst for something exciting because they have begun to feel the helplessness that they are nothing but parts of huge organisations. Taking advantage of such psychology, the various nations and enterprises dramatise sports so subtly that this permeates the entire sporting world. The popularity of spectator sports is the result. Table 7 shows this phenomenon: in 1975, about 10% of the whole population of Japan watched professional baseball games. Those baseball watchers are active people who can practise sports themselves.

Table 7. The number of spectators at professional baseball games (thousand units)

Year	The Central League	The Pacific League	Total
1960	5304	2800	8104
1965	6252	2501	8753
1970	6543	3069	9612
1975	9480	3200	12680

Source: The Tax Administration Agency (1976)

Search for a New Way of Sport

It is recognised that the Japanese people acquire attitudes and understanding towards sports through the mass media, and that physical educators also play an important role. For example, in 1972 in Japan, the number of radio receivers per 1000 inhabitants was 658, and the number of television sets, 229 (In 1979, 81.8% of households had a television set - The Statistical Bureau of Prime Minister's Office 1981.) The number of published newspapers was 519 per 1000 inhabitants (Statistical Office of United Nations 1977). Everybody aged 6 to 20 takes physical education classes more than once a week.

Mass media and education have become so well organised that the information diffuses is extremely influential. The principle of sports should be restored from "nothing but victory matters" to "do your best". Every participant can do his best on his own, and both winner and loser can be satisfied that they have done their best.

The "victory controls everything" principle, where only one wins and all others are worthless, improves sporting technique greatly and changes the effectiveness of sports as a means of drama. However, the same principle makes many participants subject to chagrin. Thus we have come to decide that the kind of sport which gives contentment and satisfaction to the handicapped, the weak, the aged and those of low ability as well as to those of excellent ability is the principle that emphasises "do your best". This principle could be important in correcting an inhuman tendency, i. e. the bipolar disintegration of challenge (competition) and solidarity (co-operation - a serious defect of human sports. Such a defect is a mirror of modern society and life.

As is shown by team games, there are a number of cases where competition is impossible without the premise of co-operation. Therefore, sports have the ability to integrate competition and co-operation or challenge and solidarity. This dialectical integration is the very starting point of a new theory of sport. It is attainable when the fundamental principle changes from "nothing but victory matters" to "do your best". The curriculum of physical education in our educational system has begun to change direction considerably. The tendency is towards the restoration of play in sports, but the mass media still have "nothing but victory" as their principle. Herein lies the greatest problem. On the other hand, it is a fact, too, that easy and light sports have become more and more popular (Fig. 1). Sports should move from the stage where the effect and result matter to the stage where meaningful participation and experiences matter.

In 1981 Niwa and Muramatsu clarified that the cultural characteristics of sports affect the attitides of participants: that club members of English, American and Japanese sports have come to reflect the cultural characteristics of each sport. This causes us to conclude that it is important to produce sports with unique cultural characteristics.

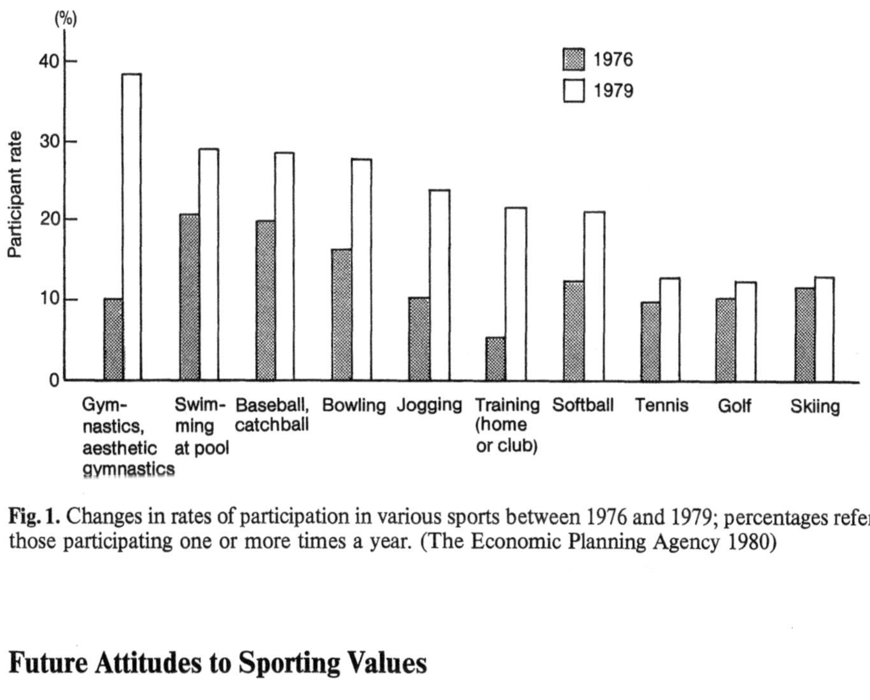

Fig. 1. Changes in rates of participation in various sports between 1976 and 1979; percentages refer to those participating one or more times a year. (The Economic Planning Agency 1980)

Future Attitudes to Sporting Values

Tension Created by Highly Developed Technology

The more developed scientific technology is, the greater people's anxiety about and criticism of it; yet on the other hand they feel that they profit by it. This is one characteristic of modern tension.

The two kinds of spirit supporting sports, especially competitive sports, are the spirit of play and the spirit of science. But as the society has put more emphasis on science, the spirit of science has come to overpower that of play, and freedom, creativity and spontaneity, which are fundamental elements of play, have decreased.

Championship sports have changed from private play as personal culture to a huge social phenomenon standardised and supported by establishments. This change has been brought out by scientism and industrialism, which are encouraged by progressivistic ideas. Sportsmen have been trying to jump higher, to run faster and to throw farther, and they have come to win by 1/100 second, which is a shade of difference not affecting people in their daily life. Advanced scientific technology measures such slight differences, gathers statistics and applies them to players in order that they can be trained scientifically. Ranking of players by measurement is done ruthlessly. Competition among players has also become very keen; friends have become enemies, and their tension in everyday sporting activities has increased greatly.

In the post-atomic bomb world, the belief in science has begun to weaken, but it has not lost its vigour in the world of sport. People usually feel uneasy and anxious if something artificial is applied to them. Therefore, it is natural that people show great anxiety and criticism towards the future of sport when it is becoming too public, too administrative and too scientific, losing the spirit of play.

The Situation in Post-industrial Society

In industrial society, sporting techniques have been improved, and the further the past records are broken, the more social praise is received by the players. This, on the other hand, has given rise to a bipolar disintegration which, in turn, has made it difficult for the general public to participate in elite sports, with spectator sports becoming more and more popular. In industrial society, individual man in organisations is treated materially for the sake of creating new records. But if successful, he is given rewards in money, kind and status, which are barometers of wealth and success.

In post-industrial society, independence and self-actualisation will be regarded as more important, and personal human relationships in communities and health, culture and pleasures in daily life will be sought after.

In democratic society, as the values people seek are diversified, so their desire for sports will increase. Sports in themselves will become more diversified, and people will thus have more choice when selecting their sports. More emphasis should be put on the identity of participants. In Japan, as in England 100 years ago, one organisation of new sports after another has been established (Tables 8, 9).

Table 8. The organisation of new sport in Japan

Organisation of new sport	Date
Japan Esci Tennis League	1951
Japan Roller-Skating Federation	1953
Japan Surfing Federation	1965
Japan Auto-Camping Association	1968
Japan Orienteering Commission	1969
Japan Parachute Sport League	1971
All Japan Diving League	1972
Japan Field Athletic Association	1973
Japan Wind Surfing Association	1974
Japan Kendama (Cup and Ball) Association	1974
Japan Frisbee Association	1975
Japan Hang Gliding Committee	1978
Japan Indiaca Association	1980
All Japan Association of Gate Ball League	1981

Table 9. The earliest national organisations of sport in Britain

Sport	Earliest national organisation	Date
Horse-racing	Jockey Club	1750
Golf	Royal and Ancient Golf Club	1754
Cricket	Marylebone Cricket Club	1788
Mountaineering	Alpine Club	1857
Association football	Football Association	1863
Athletics	Amateur Athletic Club	1866
	Amatuer Athletic Association	1880
Swimming	Amateur Metropolitan Swimming Association	1869
Rugby football	Rugby Football Union	1871
Sailing	Yacht Racing Association	1875
Cycling	Bicyclists' Union	1878
Skating	National Skating Association	1879
Rowing	Metropolitan Rowing Association	1879
Boxing	Amateur Boxing Association	1884
Hockey	Hockey Association	1886
Lawn tennis	Lawn Tennis Association	1888
Badminton	Badminton Association	1895
Fencing	Amateur Fencing Association	1898

Source: McIntosh (1963)

Conclusion

1. It is necessary for people to put more emphasis on the "do your best" principle of sports than on the "nothing but victory matters" principle. When organisations follow the latter principle, international understanding is hard to achieve.
2. Competitiveness and play elements contained in sports themselves are easy to make use for other purposes. Therefore it is necessary to assess constantly the direction and content of the abuses of sport.
3. The content of increasingly diversified sports greatly influences people's consciousness. It is necessary to create characteristics of sport which encourage mutual understanding.
4. It is necessary for sports organisations to retain independence and freedom. The present situation of our society makes it very difficult for sports organisations to act independently of politics and economics, as we recently saw in the Olympic Games and in other sports meetings. Therefore, it is very important for these organisations to exercise wisdom, thought and economic power that they might judge and act independently in critical cases.

These four problems are probably very difficult, and the last one extremely so. But it is most important today to achieve international understanding; thus people from all countries of the world should discuss these problems and act wisely and cohesively to achieve their solution.

References

McIntosh PC (1963) Sport in society. Watts, London, p 63 Niwa T, Muramatsu H (1983) The cultural characteristics of sports as determined by examining the attitudes of sports club members of universities. The Japanese Committee on Sport Sociology (ed) Sociological Journal of Physical Education and Sport, vol. 2. Dowa-Shoin Pub., Tokyo, pp 1–23

Niwa T (1982) (ed) Sport and human life. Asakura-Shoten, Tokyo, pp 72–74

The Economic Planning Agency (ed) (1980) The white paper of national life. The Printing Bureau of Finance Ministry, Tokyo, p 53

The Information Unit of the Prime Minister's Secretariat (ed) (1972) The survey of public opinion on sport. The Printing Bureau of Finance Ministry, Tokyo, p 14

The Prime Minister's Office (ed) (1965/1979) The survey of public opinion on sport. The Printing Bureau of Finance Ministry, Tokyo

The Statistical Bureau of the Prime Minister's Office (ed) (1981) Statistics of Japan. The Printing Bureau of Finance Ministry, Tokyo, p 305

The Statistical Office of the United Nations (1977) Statistical yearbook: twenty-eighth issue. United Nations, New York (Japanese edition)

The Tax Administration Agency (ed) (1976) Statistical yearbook. The Printing Bureau of Finance Ministry, Tokyo

III

The Extent and Content of International Co-operation in Sport

1. Competitive and Top-Level Sport

On the History of International Sporting Co-operation: Some Trends

A. Hietanen

Introduction

"Without trying to understand the past, it is impossible to understand the present or to predict the future." This common aphorism serves as a point of departure for this brief analysis of the general trends in international sporting co-operation. Various approaches can be used in the analysis of historical evolution. This paper aims at synthesising some of the main approaches in order to clarify the historical trends of international sports.

The internationalisation of sports was a comparatively slow process before it was accelerated by social evolution and technological revolution during the second half of the nineteenth century. Intranational sporting activities, the necessary prerequisite of international co-operation, led gradually to the formation of national sports associations. In England, the first national associations had already been formed in the eighteenth century (e. g. McIntosh 1963; Wildt 1972). Elsewhere the organisation of sport first took place in the nineteenth century.

The Internationalisation of Sports

The spread of sporting activities inside nations was due to many factors. In some countries university sport was a significant factor in the promotion of sports. Often the university sporting contests antedated the formation of national associations, as is shown in the case of England in Table 1. It can also be seen from Table 1 that there is usually a clear time-lag between the formation of national associations and the formation of international federations. Likewise, the internationalisation process seems to advance in different stages, usually from one continent to another.

In the case of the Olympic Games, the diffusion process (i. e. internationalisation) involved several stages. In the beginning, there were 13 countries (Australia, Bulgaria, Chile, Austria, Denmark, France, Germany, Great Britain, Greece, Hungary Sweden, Switzerland and the United States) from three continents with 310 sportsmen (Krotee 1981). After this characteristically Eurocentric phase, the actual intercontinental diffusion started. In the first stage of this diffusion, many Latin American countries were integrated into the Olympic movement. By 1936, 14 South American and Central American countries were participating in the Games. It can be argued on good grounds that the Olympic system was by no means a global entity before the Second World War. Therefore the Olympic Games in 1948 and 1952 represented a fundamental leap to the second phase, which involved the participation of several Asian countries (a total

Table 1. The dates of the first Oxford versus Cambridge sports contests and of the formation of British national associations and international federations (Palmer 1977)

Sport	Date of first contest	Date of formation of national association	Date of formation of international federation
Cricket	1827	1788	1909
Rowing	1826	1882	1892
Shooting	1863	1860	1907
Athletics	1864	1880	1912
Football	1874	1863	1904
Bicycling	1874	1878	1900
Tennis	1881	1888	1912
Hockey	1890	1886	1924
Swimming	1892	1869	1908
Fencing	1897	1902	1913
Ice hockey	1900	1908	1908
Table tennis	1923	1927	1926
Judo	1930	1948	1951
Basketball	1931	1936	1932

of 14 in the 1952 Olympic Games (Kieren et al 1977). In addition, there were some signs of the entry of black Africa into international sport. The African countries taking part in the 1952 Olympic Games were Egypt, Gold Coast, Nigeria and South Africs (Jokl 1956).

The 1952 Helsinki Games were meaningful also in the sense that the socialist countries made their first large-scale appearance in the Olympic Games. Some socialist countries had participated in the 1948 Olympics, but the Soviet Union took part for the first time in 1952. Before the Second World War the Soviet Union had preferred to co-operate with the workers' sports federations in Eastern and Western Europe, but shortly after the war this policy was changed (e. g. Espy 1979). Already during the years 1946–1948 Soviet sports associations affiliated to 11 international federations (see Table 2).

Table 2 also shows how rapidly the international contacts of the German Democratic Republic increased in the 1950s. Her entry into international sport took place simultaneously with the affiliation of new African countries to international federations. Kenya, Liberia, Ethiopia and Uganda part in the 1956 Olympic Games and in the late 1950s Nigeria, Ghana and Uganda affiliated to the International Federation of Association Football (FIFA) (National associations of FIFA 1978). In practice the African connection emerged in international sport in the 1960s, although in some sports the rate of African participation is still low or nil; for example, there are very few African member associations in the International Gymnastics Federation.

The diffusion process seen in respect of the Olympic Games apparently applies to other sports as well. In the case of FIFA, the diffusion pattern was repeated: The Euro-centric phase was followed by the affiliation of 15 South and Central American countries in the 1920s and 1930s. In a similar manner, the Asian countries became members after the Second World War, Especially in the years 1947–1954.

Table 2. The affiliation of the sports associations of the USSR and the GDR to international federations, 1946–1967 (Riordan 1977; Hietanen and Varis 1982)

USSR	Year	GDR
Basketball, soccer, skiing, weight-lifting	1946	
Athletics, chess, speed and ice skating, swimming (incl. diving and water polo), wrestling	1947	
Gymnastics, volleyball	1948	
Boxing	1949	
Soviet Olympic Committee affiliated to the IOC	1951	Skiing, table tennis, volleyball
Cycling, canoeing, equestrianism, fencing, ice hockey, modern pentathlon and biathlon, shooting, rowing, yachting	1952	Archery, basketball, boxing, canoening, soccer, swimming, wrestling, yachting
	1953	Bowling, skating
Table tennis	1954	Ice hockey, judo
Bandy	1955	Cycling, rowing, weight-lifting, GDR Olympic Committee affiliated to the IOC
Draughts, tennis, motorcycle racing, motor racing	1956	Athletics, fencing, handball, hockey, rugby
	1957	Angling, bob-sleighing, tobogganing, motorcycle and motor racing, motor boat sport, gymnastics
Gliding, handball	1958	Badminton, billiards, modern pentathlon and biathlon
	1960	Aeronautics, shooting
	1961	Orienteering
Judo, radio sport	1962	
	1964	Tennis
Sub-aqua sport	1965	Equestrianism, water-skiing
Model boatcraft sport	1966	
Archery, mountaineering, orienteering	1967	Amateur cycling

The Dynamics of Change

The trend towards internationisation in sports can be analysed as a process between feudality and entropy interaction systems. In the feudal system there are three main rules: interaction between centre and periphery is vertical, interaction between periphery and periphery is missing and the multilateral interaction of these three is missing. In addition, the centre monopolises interaction with the outside world (Galtung 1971). As to the entropy model, it suggests that a high entropy system consists of relatively equal actors involved in a symmetric and horizontal interaction network (e. g. Galtung 1968). In the historical development of sport, there seem to be characteristics of both systems. For quite a long time the interaction between the centres (Europe and North America) and peripheries (Africa, Asia and Latin America) remained vertical (Coubertin 1961). As to the interaction between the peripheries in international sport, the interaction pattern has not traditionally existed, with the exception of the last three decades. However, the third rule of the multilateral interaction does not hold true in the case of sports. On the contrary, the bulk of sporting co-operation is organised multilaterally. Sport differs from many other fields of activity in the sense that there are no interational governmental organisations (so-called IGOs) in sport. Instead, there are a large number - approximately 130 - of international non-governmental organisations (INGOs) (e. g. Hoefnagels 1981). Probably this lack of governmental involvement at the international level is due to the activities of the International Olympic Committee. In recent years this lack of inter-governmental sporting co-operation has in part been compensated by the European Sports Conferences and the Intergovernmental Committee of Physical Education and Sport in UNESCO. On the whole the present structure of international sport is closer to the model of high entropy than to the feudal model.

The structural development of international sport has had quite unique phases. The multilateral interaction has not totally concealed the feudel rules of sports interaction. The feudal system was dominant during the early part of this century, but both the gradual globalisation and the regionalisation of sporting interaction brought changes. Thus the only sign of the existence of some kinds of feudal rules is the lack in inter-regional, i. e. inter-periphery, interaction. The only bi-regional links within the periphery consist of Arab regional organisations, e. g. the Arab Table Tennis Federation, the Arab Weight-lifting Association and the African and Near East Billiards Confederation (Hart et al. 1974). At present no other region-to-region or periphery-to-periphery relations exist, although the regionalisation trend in general has been strong in international sporting relations. Nevertheless, there are regional organisations, which provide a useful link between the periphery and the centre. For example, in the Mediterranean area there are several such organisations.

Notes on the Conflictology of International Sporting Relations

As was noted above, the general structure of international sport as such is not a barrier to the promotion of international understanding through sport. Yet there is a kind of in-built conflict potential in the international sports system. This is due to the fact that the so-called Olympic ideal and the practice of the Olympic Games developed separately in the nineteenth century. Nationalism was not left outside the Olympic practice, and thus there have been more or less violent and more or less political conflicts, as Table 3 reminds us.

Table 3. Some political disputes in the Olympic Games, 1896–1980 (Seurin 1980; Kieran et al. 1977)

1896: Dispute between France and Germany
1908: Confrontation between USA and Great Britain
1912: Flag dispute between Finland and Russia
1920: The defeated of the First World War excluded
1936: The Jewish issue and the Peru–Austria–Germany dispute
1948: The defeated of the Second World War excluded
1952: The China issue and dispute between USA and USSR
1956: Hungary issue: Egypt, Lebanon, Iraq, Spain, the Netherlands and Switzerland boycotted
1960: The Taiwan and South Africa issues
1964: The GANEFO dispute: Indonesia and North Korea excluded
1968: The South African issue
1972: The Middle East issue and terrorism
1976: Boycott by the African countries
1980: The Moscow boycott

Conclusions

The structural development of the international sports system has, in recent years, started to follow the model of high entropy, which as such is necessary prerequisite to the peace mission of sport. The traditional feudal structure has still not been wholly superseded, and in the near future this issue may cause disputes. However, far more problematic are the issues related to the political disputes, which have not remained outside the stadia. Sport cannot be practised in a political vacuum; owing to its dialectical contents, sport can have an influence on politics, including international politics.

References

Coubertin P (1961) Colonization of sport. Bull CIO 76:31-32
Espy R (1979) The politics of the Olympic Games. University of California Press, Berkeley, pp 25-28
Galtung J (1968) Entropy and the general theory of peace. In: Proceedings of International Peace Research Association Second Conference, vol 1. Assen, pp 3-37
Galtung J (1971) A structural theory of imperialism. Peace Res 8:81-117
Harf JE, Coate RA, Marsh HS (1974) Trans-societal sport associations: A descriptive analysis of structures and linkages. QUEST Monogr 22:52-62
Hietanen A, Varis T (1982) Kansainvälisen urheiluyhteistyön rakenne ja kehityslinjat. Polit 24:208-233
Hoefnagels M (1981) Growth of international organizations since 1945: Interpretations of quantitative and qualitative evidence. In: Jütte R, Grosse-Jütte A (eds) The future of international organization. London, pp 14-36
Jokl E (ed) (1956) Sports in the cultural pattern of the world. A study of the Olympic Games at Helsinki. Institute of Occupational Health, Helsinki
McIntosh P (1963) Sport in society. Watts, London
Kieran J, Daley A, Jordan P (1977) The story of the Olympic Games. 776 B.C. to 1976. Lippincott, New York
Krotee ML (1981) Sociological perspectives of the Olympic Games. In: Segrave J, Chu D (eds) Olympism. Stipes, Champaign, pp 207-226
National Associations of FIFA: Zurich, 1978.
Palmer RW (1977) The development of university sport in Britain from the early Oxford v Cambridge contests up to the present day. Mimeo
Riordan J (1977) Sport in Soviet society: Development of sport and physical education in Russia and the USSR. Cambridge University Press, London, p 365
Seurin P (1980) The future of the Olympic Games and tomorrow's sport. FIEP Bull 50:7-16, 2
Wildt KC (1972) Daten zur Sportgeschichte, part 2. Hofmann, Schorndorf

Sport and International Understanding: A Survey of the Structure and Trends of International Sporting Co-operation

A. Hietanen and T. Varis

Introduction

The history of international sporting co-operation goes back some 100 years. Throughout this era there has been some discussion on the relation between sport, peace on earth and the mutual understanding between peoples. This relation was analysed by Baron de Coubertin and in recent decades it has been discussed at several conferences. In contrast to the widely shared general interest in this theme, very few scientific studies have been carried out on the overall development of international sport. This can be said to be true of both the theoretical and the empirical approach to the subject. The backwardness of the political science of sport may partly explain this state of affairs (Güldenpfennig and Schulke 1980). This article includes a review of the structure of international sport and summarises the results of the study carried out by the Tampere Peace Research Institute.

Sport, Peace and International Understanding

The relations between sport and international understanding have not been discussed very frequently since the Coubertinian era, obviously because the issue has been considered rather unproblematic. Some conceptual analyses have, however, been published in recent decades. The approaches to the relation between sport, international understanding and the promotion of peace vary in several aspects and stress different factors. Firstly, some authors (e.g. Milshtein and Molchanov 1976; Noel-Baker 1962) have considered the positive influence of sport to be self-evident: "sport due to its nature" is "the best weapon in the struggle for peace on earth". Secondly, some analyses mention state-level factors as those preventing sport from making its contribution to international understanding. For example, Jones (1960) mentions such factors as aggressive nationalism, political interference and the spectacular character of sports. Heinilä (1971) also stresses the negative impact of the totalisation process of sport on the peaceful potential of sport. Thirdly, several authors emphasise the importance of sociocultural factors in evaluating the impact of sport on international understanding (e.g. chapter in this volume by Stolyarov and Sanadze; Kyröläinen and Varis 1981). The main argument is that the practice of sport does not take place in a social or political vacuum. Of these sociocultural factors, mass media and communication have often been evaluated as the most important, e.g. in the studies by Heinilä

(1971) and McIntosh (this volume). The principle of fair play in sport has also been emphasised quite frequently, although there does not seem to be unanimity on the actual contents of fair play (Heinilä 1982; McIntosh 1974, 1979).

Also with regard to international understanding, there has been much controversy on the functions and disfunctions of sport. On the one hand, there have been views emphasising the integrative and peaceful influence of international sport. One example of this is to be found in the International Charter on Physical Education and Sport, which was approved at the 20th General Conference of UNESCO in 1976:

> Through co-operation and the pursuit of mutual interests in the universal language of physical education and sport, all peoples will contribute to the preservation of lasting peace, mutual respect and friendship and will thus create a propitious climate for solving international problems.

This ideal was also the basis of Coubertinian ideology, and it has been accepted to a surprising extent both in the West and in the East. On the other hand, there have been more sceptical appraisals of the role of sport in international relations. George Orwell's comment on competitive sport: "It is bound up with hatred, jealousy, boastfulness, disregard for all rules and sadistic pleasure in witnessing violence - in other words, it is war minus the shooting" is a case in point (New York Times 1959).

Some authors (e.g. Natan 1969) have accused sport of being an instrument of chauvinism and nationalism. It is quite clear that sport has disfunctions, too - linked in particular to commercialism, professionalism, doping and nationalism. The last-mentioned factor has, however, two faces: it consists of nationalistic feelings and nation-building, and it is worth noting that nationalism has been one of the prerequisites of international sport. As regards the negative impact of sport on society, Huxley (1937) argued in the 1930s that sport is a substitute for war, since it is used to prepare men for the militia and to score points in political propaganda. Huxley also analysed the global role of sport: "In a world that has no common religion or philosophy of life, but where every national group practices its own private idolatry, international football matches and athletic contests can do almost nothing but harm". From a historical viewpoint, it is quite true that sport has often been subordinated to militarism, e.g. in nineteenth century Germany and in several countries in our century (Wagner 1959; Rittner 1976).

The definition of sport as war-minus-shooting or war-without-weapons has also resulted in positive appraisals of the role of international sport. These analyses have viewed sport as an alternative to war. For example, Bertrand Russell argued in his Reith lectures in 1948 that sport might provide an outlet for the the savage inside all of us (McIntosh 1963). His view was that there is some kind of a competitive instinct in human beings and that this instinct could be satisfied trough sport, instead of war. In a similar manner, George Santayana (1954) pointed out that a means of preventing wars could be found in sport: "The arduous and competitive element in sports is not harmful, if the discipline involved brings no loss of faculty or of right sensitiveness, and the rilvalry no rancour. In wars states wish to be efficient in order to conquer, but in sport men wish to prove their excellency because they wish to have it."

The most popular and widespread example of the emphasis on the positive potential of sport is the theory put forward by Konrad Lorenz (1963) that sport is a safety valve for aggressive behaviour. In the 1970s Lorenz admitted that his safety valve thinking was too optimistic and that he had "strong doubts whether watching aggressive behaviour even in the guise of sport has any cathartic effect at all" (Psychology Today 1976). The idea of cathartic function of sport is as such quite persuasive and it can be effectively used in the legitimation of sport. It was also used as a theoretical basis in a book by Goodhart and Chataway (1968) on the history of international sport. However, in aggression research the safety valve model of aggression has been abandoned and therefore it is misleading to discuss sport only in terms of aggression and catharsis, because sport has other more important characteristics.

It is here worth quoting Paul Weiss, a sport philosopher, who argues that "sport is not aggression controlled and harmless. It is constructive activity in which aggression plays a role together with dedication, co-operation, restraint, self-denial, and a respect for the rights and dignity of others" (Weiss 1969).

As regards the nature of sport, it ought to be borne in mind that sport is not a zero-sum game, but in sport competition is complemented by association, i.e. both sides respond to a mutual system or to mutual interests without expecting to get a prize as a compensation. This kind of "antagonistic co-operation" is an essential part of the raison d'être of sport. It can be said that in sport the association aspect is dominant and the conflict aspect is only secondary (Lüschen 1970). Nevertheless, in the mass media this view of sport is often distorted. To quote W. Phillips Davison (1974): "Sports reporting is unintentionally dishonest in that the focus on the contest obscures the enormous amount of co-operation between the contestants: the acceptance of the referees' authority and the often complicated infrastructure of rules, prior arrangements, and sponsorship." We argue that too little attention has been paid to the associational and constructive structures of sport, especially at the international level, and to the institutionalised mechanisms of conflict resolution within sport as an alternative to war.

The dialectics of international sport means that sport can be both a means of power politics and an instrument for improved international understanding. As to the difference between ideals and reality, it is useful to recall the results of a study by Hans Lenk (1964). In his analysis Lenk points out that the only element of the Olympic values which had not been fulfilled was religious affiliation, including the truce (*ekecheiria*) and the peace mission. Lenk presents nationalism and chauvinism as the explanatory factors preventing the realisation of those values. However, the non-realisation of the truce and the peace mission can also be explained by the fact that the Olympic Games and Olympic ideals have developed separately. The modern Olympic Games are not a revival of the Ancient Games, but a modified version of the Scottish Caledonian Games, the British Olympic Festivals held in Liverpool and the Greek Olympic Games of the nineteenth century. The Olympic ideal had its roots elsewhere: in aesthetics, humanism and Hellenism combined with the ideals of English sport (Lucas 1981).

Baron de Coubertin (1931) also referred in his memoirs to the role of sport as a world religion uniting the peoples of the world. On the whole it seems that the failure of the peace mission of the Olympic movement and the international sports organisations in general may in part be explained by this contrast between the old ideals and the actual contents and reality of the Olympic Games and international contests.

There are conflicting views on the role of cultural exchange in international relations as well as on the conditions under which such exchange contributes to the promotion of international understanding. It can be said that cultural exchange, including sport, has a great potential for the strengthening of peace, particularly in times of international tension when such exchange may function as a stabilising factor. The impact of sport on international understanding can be defined as a complex, multifactor issue. Firstly, it is influenced by the structure of international sport and the contents of sporting exchanges. Secondly, the peace potential of international sport depends on the development aid and co-operation in sport and on the social context of sport on a natiomal level. Thirdly, the mass media and communication have an important role in the relationship between sport and international understanding. International sporting co-operation does not automatically or self-evidently promote mutual understanding among peoples; rather most often the impact of sporting relations is indirect.

As regards the role of sport in uniting peoples, it has been estimated that during the 1972 Olympic Games in Munich only some 10% of the West German spectators came into direct contact with foreign spectators (Hackforth 1975). For the mass media audience the contact with foreigners is always indirect and filtered. Consequently, the impact of international sporting contacts on mutual understanding among peoples should not be overestimated, although there is no reason for underestimation either.

The Structure of International Sport

The development of the structure of international sport has been comparatively random. The evolutionary phase of structural development took place in the second half of the nineteenth century. The institutionalisation of international sport started in the 1870s with the rugby and yachting clubs having members from both England and abroad. Thus the first element of the structure of international sport emerged. The second element was constituted in 1894 when the International Olympic Committee was established in Paris after an 8-day conference. In the same year the first national Olympic committees were formed. Thereby the four main elements of the international sports system existed by the beginning of this century. The main actors in international sports are the International Olympic Committee (IOC), international sports federations, national Olympic committees and national sports organisations.

For decades the structure was quite heterogeneous and there were no formal linkages between these actors, with the exception of the eight Olympic Congresses between the years 1897 and 1930, in which there were participants from the IOC, the international federations of the Olympic sports and the national Olympic committees. The organisational disorder is demonstrated by the fact that it was not until 1920 that the IOC delegated to various sports federations the responsibility for conducting competitions in their respective sports at the Olympic Games (Glader 1978). The structure became increasingly complex as the number of international federations multiplied in the transnationalisation process. The transnationalisation of sport took place rather late, the great leap forwards not occurring until the 1920s and then again after the Second World War.

During the last two decades the general structure has become more complex. There has been a trend towards *homogenisation* and increased *co-operation* both among the international federations and among the national Olympic committees. Thus far, the results of this trend have been the General Assembly of International

Sports Federations (GAISF) and the Assembly of National Olympic Committees (ANOC). The GAISF was established in 1967 with the purposes of expanding the co-operation between the federations and of dividing the television revenues. The motives behind the establishment of the GAISF were mainly financial, but dissatisfaction with the IOC also gave momentum to the plan (Espy 1979).

The superfederation of the national Olympic committees had a rather similar background. The Permanent General Assembly of National Olympic Committees (GANOC) was established in Mexico in 1968. Besides the issue of independence, one issue of controversy between the IOC and the national committees was the development aid in sport. Gradually the IOC adapted to the situation and new kinds of plans for development aid and inter-organisation co-operation were presented (Espy 1979; Jacobsen 1981). At the 1973 Olympic Congress, the motto of which was "Sport for a World of Peace", a new Tripartite Commission was founded consisting of members from the IOC, international federations and national Olympic committees.

The integration of the co-operation between these organisations has not been the only structural change in recent decades. A notable trend has been the *regionalisation* which has occurred everywhere in the international sports system. Firstly, regionalisation has taken place within the Olympic system. For example as a result of the idea of Pan-Americanism, The Pan American Sports Organization was founded in 1940 and in 1951 the first Pan-American Games were held.

The trend towards regionalisation in the international federations started as a substitute for the lack of global co-operation within the federations. This took place much earlier than in the Olympic system: the first South American regional sports organisations were established as early as the 1910s.

In Africa, the African Football Confederation was established at the end of the colonial era in 1956 and in the 1960s confederations for basketball, tennis and judo were formed. In Asia the regional efforts started in 1952 when the table tennis federation was established. In Europe, regionalisation started before the Second World War, when, for example, the European Swimming League was founded. In the Australian and Oceanic region, regionalisation started in the 1950s, when the Fencing Confederation of Oceanic Zone and the Oceania Judo Union were founded.

As a complementary phenomenon to regionalisation, *interregionalisation* has also taken place. Most interregional federations have been organised between the Americas. Outside the framework of The Pan American Sports Organization, there exist several federations. As a linkage between Europe and Africa there are Mediterranean Games and the International Mediterranean organisations, such as the International Committee for the Mediterranean Committee of Table Tennis. Interregional co-operation is also organised between Africa and Asia. The Arab Table Tennis Federation was established in 1956 and the Arab countries also have other co-operation organisations.

The third trend in regional co-operation has been *subregionalisation*. The subregionalisation trend started in the Far East when sports associations from China, Japan and the Philippines organised a total of ten Far Eastern Championship Games between 1913 and 1934, but the conflict between Japan and China put an end to these games (von der Laage 1977). In a similar manner, subregional co-operation in sports was organised in the Nordic countries as early as the first decades of the twentieth century. The co-operation between the national sports organisations of Denmark,

Finland, Iceland, Norway and Sweden was institutionalised in the Faelles Committee, and Nordic federations were established in almost all sports, from gymnastics and weight-lifting to rowing, orienteering and judo. Only some regions can match this vast amount of subregional co-operation in sport. The Balkan region has some similarities, since there are several subregional organisations in the co-operation between Bulgaria, Greece, Rumania, Turkey and Yugoslavia. This co-operation, which ranges from athletics, gymnastics and handball to judo and table tennis, would be worth a closer study, for in that region the structures of the bloc politics of the post-war era have been broken in a unique way. Another area with long traditions in subregional sports co-operation is the Caribbean region, where the first Central American and Caribbean Championships were held in 1926.

As regards the impact of sport on international understanding, one interesting issue is the relation of sports integration to political and economic integration. In the integration studies, the main hypothesis usually declares that the deeper the bloc conflict, the more intense the integration within the blocs. The socialist integration in the field of sport consists of several elements: the socialist countries have a standing committee dealing with the co-ordination of their sports policies. In addition to this committee, which was established in 1974, there is an annual conference of the sports administration of the socialist countries. The armies and security organs have a separate organisation, the Sports Committee of the Friendly Armies (SKDA), which was established in the 1950s. The socialist countries also have championship games in several sports. As to the so-called Western bloc, sporting co-operation takes place within the framework of the Council of Europe, including the conferences of the West European sports ministers and the Committee for the Development of Sport. Thus, the bloc conflict has not deeply penetrated the structures of international sport. On the contrary, there are many more organisations linking the socialist and capitalist countries than there are separating these countries. It seems that the political and economic integration within the blocs is much more severe than the sports integration. This study of integration supports our view of the relative autonomy of sport in international relations.

The Commonwealth Games Federation is a relatively independent element in the international sports system. The first practical steps to organise the British Empire Games were taken in 1928 and the first Games were held in 1930. Ever since, the Federation has arranged Empire and Commonwealth Games every 4 years, with the exception of the Second World War period. Although quite imperial in the beginning, the Federation has been able to adapt to the changes in the external environment, which is reflected in the changes in its title – from the British Empire to the British Commonwealth and finally to merely the Commonwealth Games Federation. At present, 54 national associations are affiliated to the federation and over 40 of them represent developing countries, which are former colonies.

A relatively recent element in international sporting co-operation is the intergovernmental co-operation in sport and physical education. To develop further the détente power of international sports, UNESCO activated its sports profile in the mid-1970s. In 1976 UNESCO arranged an international conference of ministers and senior officials responsible for physical education and sport in the education of youth and in the following year the Interim Intergovernmental Committee for Physical Education and Sport held its first session. After the 20th General Conference of UNESCO this committee became permanent. In addition, UNESCO has, with the help of the International Fund for the Development of Physical Education and Sport, (established in 1978), shown new efforts to develop sport and physical education, especially in its poorest member countries.

Another new form of intergovernmental co-operation in the field of sport was started in the 1970s, when the first European Sports Conference was held in Vienna in 1973. The biannual conference has turned out to be a useful forum of co-operation, although - or because - there have not been very complex or wide-ranging issues on the conference agenda. In addition to the European Sports Conference, the Council of Europe has also organised intergovernmental co-operation in sport. The Council has a Committee for the Development of Sport and it has thus far organised three Conferences of European ministers responsible for sport. It is worth noting that the conference of sports ministers has dealt with such issues as the deficiencies in the structure of international sports, the role of nationalism, the costs of international sporting events and the role of development aid in sport.

As regards the intergovernmental co-operation, we have to take into account the work in the United Nations, which has dealt with the prohibition of apartheid in sport. Thus far, the work has resulted in a declaration adopted by the General Assembly of the United Nations in 1977, the International Declaration against Apartheid in Sports. An a hoc committee is still working in the United Nations on drafting an international convention against apartheid in sport. Furthermore, we need to mention the active role in regional intergovernmental co-operation of the Nordic Council, which took up the issue of sports co-operation in the mid-1970s. On the whole the 1970s was a decade of increased governmental activities in international sporting relations. Before the 1970s the international sporting relations had in fact been a strange exception in the group of intergovernmental organisations, since no intergovernmental sports organisations had existed.

Relations Between East, West and South

Although the present tendency seems to be towards homogenisation of international sport, there have been quite different trends in international sporting co-operation during this century. Prior to the Second World War, international sporting co-operation during this century. Prior to the Second World War, international sport meant in practice sporting relations between indutrialised Western countries, which had received the Olympic Games and started the activities of most international sports federations. In addition, the working class movement gave rise to the workers' sport internationals in the 1910s and 1920s. The internationals, the Socialist Workers' Sport International (SASI, originally the Lucerne Sport International) and the Red Sport International, both counted well over two million members by 1928. The latter played an important role in establishing links with sportsmen of the newly born and internationally isolated Soviet Union. In the 1937 Workers' Olympics, these two internationals showed their total strength in a protest against Hitler's Olympics of 1936 (Steinberg 1978).

The diffusion process of international sport started at the beginning of this century. In the first phase of internationalisation, Latin America was integrated to international and intercontinental sport. This integration culminated in the first World Championships in football in 1930. The championships were held in Uruguay, the host country playing Argentina in the final. In a sense this indicated the end of the Eurocentric phase of sport. Before the Second World War,, three continents - Europe, the Americas and Australia - participated actively in international sports. The second phase of the internationalisation process in sport came after the war, in the late 1940s and early 1950s. Within the Olympic framework, this phase started with the participation of several Asian countries in the Olympic Games: as many as 14 competed in the 1952 Summer Games in Helsinki. Of perhaps greater importance was the entry of socialist countries and countries of Black Africa into international sport: seven socialist countries and two Black African countries (Nigeria and Gold Coast) participated in the 1952 Summer Games. The entrance of newly independent Third World countries progressed with the pace of the decolonisation process, and this third phase of the internationalisation of sport is still continuing.

After the Second World War, a major change took place in the international sport policy of the Soviet Union. The new Soviet sports policy was mainly formulated by Lavrenti Berija. During the leadership of Berija the Soviet Union affiliated to over 20 international sports federations. Another alternative would have been to join only the International Workers' Sport Committee (CSIT), but the Soviet Union preferred co-operation on a broader basis. Finally, in 1951 the Soviet Union was accepted on to the International Olympic Committee, which resulted in an expansion of international co-operation in the field of sport (Riordan 1977). The international sporting contacts of the German Democratic Republic expanded in a similar manner in the 1950s. It is worth noting that in 1958 the sports associations of the GDR were affiliated to a larger number of international federations than the associations of the USSR.

In the East-West dimension it is interesting to analyse the sporting co-operation between the Soviet Union and the United States. The sportsmen and sportswomen of these two countries met for the first time in 1952 in the Helsinki Olympic Games and after this the bilateral sports co-operation progressed. In 1955 the first contest was arranged in weight-lifting. The incidents of Suez and Hungary do not seem to have affected the U.S.-Soviet sporting contacts, since the United States did not join the Netherlands, Spain and Switzerland in the 1956 Olympic boycott. On the contrary, during the Melbourne Games the United States and the Soviet Union agreed upon the initiation of yearly competitions in athletics in 1958. The Soviet Union had met Great Britain in athletics as early as 1955. Without doubt the Geneva spirit of the mid-1950s had an impact on the progress in the sporting co-operation between the United States and the Soviet Union. The year 1958 was in many respects a culmination point in sporting relations between the two countries: meetings were organised in athletics, wrestling and basketball and, furthermore, the sporting relations were institutionalised in the Agreement between the USA and the USSR in the Cultural, Technical and Educational Fields USSR-USA Sports Encounters 1977).

Later, sporting relations were included in the structures of détente. During his visit to the United States in June 1973, president Brezhnev signed the General Agreement between the USSR and the USA on Contacts, Exchanges and Cooperation, in which Article XIII reads: "The Parties will encourage exchanges of athletes and athletic teams as well as visits of specialists in the field of physical education and sports under arrangements made between the appropriate sports organisations of the two countries". Sporting co-operation reached its peak in the mid-1970s, but sporting relations did not totally break up in the post-détente era. The Olympic boycott of 1980 naturally caused a rift in these relations, but, for example, the series of athletic meetings has continued until the present, the latest being held in the United States in the summer of 1982. On the whole, sporting relations between the USA and the Soviet Union have shown signs of the relative autonomy of sport from international relations. Yet this autonomy is not absolute, as was demonstrated by the 1980 Olympic boycott.

One of the greatest upheavals in international sport since the Second World War has been the increasing success of the socialist countries. Since 1956, with the exception of 1968, the Soviet Union has led in the harvest of medals. Furthermore, as some statistical studies show, the German Democratic Republic has been the most successful country in relative terms in the 1972, 1976 and 1980 Summer Olympic Games. The other upheaval, the strong entrance of the developing countries and especially of African countries had as its landmark the gold medal won by the Ethiopian Abebe Bikila in the marathon at the 1960 Olympic Games in Rome. The majority of developing countries belong to the Movement of the Non-Aligned Countries. During the 1970s this movement started to activate its policy in the field of sport and physical education. For instance, a separate committee for sport and physical education was established in the Movement of the Non-Aligned Countries. This committee has organised various sporting events and the 1979 Non-Alaigned Summit Conference approved a sports programme in which references were made in particular to the necessity of democratising the decision-making structure of international sport and to the abolition of all racial, political and religious discrimination in sport. In recent years the non-aligned sports movement has also presented a demand for a new international sports order, which would balance the existing inequalities in the field of international sport. In 1981 this was the main demand of the Conference of the Movement of Non-Aligned Countries on Sport and Physical Education.

The role and representations of China in international sports organisations is a classic example of the interplay between international politics and sports. In the International Olympic Committee Taiwan represented China after 1952 and there was strong pressure to maintain Taiwan in the Olympic movement under the name Republic of China in 1959-1960. Even Today the China issue causes debate and boycotts in some international federations and international contests, and there are no Chinese representatives on the IOC (von der Laage 1977). Although China did not participate in the Moscow Olympic Games in 1980, it has had active sporting relations with other countries and Chinese sportsmen have participated in several international competitions. In 1976 China was a member of 13 international sports federations, and her affiliations have increased since.

The oil-rich OPEC countries have in recent years shown great interest in international sport. Especially Kuwait, Saudi Arabia and Iraq have perceived the role of sport in international relations in a new manner. Libya has also shown efforts to make progress in sport. Mention should also be made of the so-called pariah states, which include such countries as Israel, South Africa, Taiwan, sometimes the Republic of Korea and some other states (Harkavy 1981). For the pariah states, which are at least in part outside international co-operation or even in international isolation, sporting contacts may become a means of breaking the isolation. Therefore the pariah states often stress the meaning of sporting contacts. In the international community this kind of instrumental use of sport has been resisted by some measures. For example the United Nations Centre against Apartheid has in the last 2 years published a register of sporting contacts with South Africa (Un Centre Against Apartheid 1981, 1982).

On the whole, the world map of international sport is quite versatile and pluralistic. It includes the traditional great powers of sport in Europe and North America, the new strong groups such as the socialist countries and the non-aligned sport movement, countries taking their first steps in international sport and also some regional power centres. The latter include Nigeria and Kenya in Africa, Cuba in the Caribbean region, Argentina and Brazil in South America, and Japan and Iran (until recent years) in Asia.

Empirical Results

A total of 1364 research questionnaires were sent out in the autumn of 1980 to international sports federations, national associations and Olympic committees as well as to the governmental sports administrations in various countries in order to survey the present situation in sporting relations between states and organisations and to evaluate the role of sport in international relations.

Approximately one-third (32%) of the recipients returned the questionnaire with an uneven level of accuracy and geographical representation. The overall breakdown of returned questionnaires is a follows:

National associations	33% (364/1109)
Olympic committees	34% (46/135)
International federations	31% (26/70)
Ministers and central organisations	10% (5/50)
Total	32% (441/1364)

Of the national associations, the European ones tended to respond more often than those of other regions. The answers from the Olympic committees, however, represented a wide geographical distribution. Although many of the replies are far from satisfactory and the information provided is often only fragmentary, certain tentative conclusions can be drawn on the basis of this material.

The Extent of International Sporting Co-operation

The international federations create continuity in international sporting relations and increase the value of international competitions. There are dozens of international federations, with the number of member associations varying from a few to well over 100. Table 1 illustrates the size of some of the largest federations. Quite a few federations are actually global in their activities.

With the exception of the International Table Tennis Federation, all the federations listed in Table 1 are included in the Olympic Games. ITTF is recognised by the IOC. There are major sports federations outside the Olympic connections, too, such as the World Chess Federation (FIDE) with a membership of 92, and the International Federation of Body Builders (IFBB) with 94 members.

Table 1. Some major international sports federations

Name	Founded	Member associations
International Amateur Athletics Federation (IAAF)	1912	162
International Amateur Basketball Federation (FIBA)	1932	150
International Federation of Association Football (FIFA)	1904	150
International Amateur Boxing Association (AIBA)	1946	132
International Volleyball Federation (IVBF)	1947	129
International Cyclist Union (UCI)	1900	119
International Table Tennis Federation (ITTF)	1926	116
International Amateur Swimming Federation (FINA)	1908	112
International Weightlifting Federation (IWF)	1920	106
International Judo Federation (FIJ)	1951	104

Our survey confirms the view that the extent of international sporting co-operation has increased rapidly over recent decades. Table 2 illustrates the expansion and diffusion of international sporting relations. The globalisation trend has been most rapid in soccer, athletics and table tennis. Handball has also expanded rapidly throughout the world.

The rapid increase of membership in the international federations is largely due to the affiliation of the associations of developing countries, which has occurred in almost all major federations.

Table 2. The growth of membership in international federations

Year	Football	Handball	Badminton (1934/9)	Table tennis (1926/8)	Athletics (1912/17)	Boxing (1946/21)	Gymnastics	Rowing	Orienteering	Korfball (1933/2)
1960	90	27	41	72	103[a]		45	39	10[b]	3
1970	132	49	54	85	143		63	47	16	4
1980	150	80	64	116	162	132	79	53	26	11
Active members (million)	23	3.8			17					

[a] 1962 [b] 1961

The Flow of Sportsmen and Coaches

Many factors influence the international profile of different sports: these include socio-cultural factors, climate and geography. Different sports do not seem to have the same kinds of international consequences or portential. The traditional way to classify sports has been to draw a line between contact sports (e. g. boxing, wrestling, ice hockey and football) and non-contact sports (e. g. rowing, volleyball, weight-lifting). In a similar manner, a distinction could be made between team sports and individual sports. In analysing the conflict potential of sports this kind of classification is not useful, although empirically we could argue that contact sports and especially team contact sports results more easily in conflicts between the parties. However, it is necessary to emphasise that in modern society and especially in international relations practically all sports are connected to the mass communications and other sociocultural factors which in the final analysis determine the potential of various sports to contribute to international understanding. Instead, a distinction between high-performance sport emphasising the competitive aspect and non-competive sport for all might be more relevant, since the continuous emphasis on the competitive aspect has resulted in the totalisation of sport with all its co-phenomena, from doping to commercialism and professionalism. Originally sport has its roots in the Latin word *"desporto"* which had a meaning "to carry away from work". This word *desporto* has become disport and sport, but it seems that sport has lost almost all of its disport nature and has become far too serious a business (Glader 1978).

In our analysis we found that there were great differences in the international contacts and the flow of sportsmen and coaches in different sports. On the one hand, in some sports there turned out to be almost solely intraregional co-operation and exchange. In our material these sports included handball, orienteering, canoeing and skiing. On the other hand, some sports were characteristically intercontinental in their interaction patterns. Volleyball, rowing, football, basketball, fencing and table tennis belonged to this group. As regards the extent of East-West co-operation in sports, there were notable differences in various sports. In some, such as basketball, handball, gymnastics, ice hockey , weight-lifting and table tennis, there was active interaction between East and West, while in others, such as wrestling, yachting, tennis, golf and orienteering, there was little co-operation. In the case of tennis and golf, this can be partly explained by the professional rules. In the co-operation between industrialised countries and developing countries, the exchange of sportsmen seemed to be most extensive in volleyball, fencing, table tennis, gymnastics and basketball. All these sports are quite suitbale for co-operation with the developing countries, since they do not require a large infrastucture or material facilities, unlike, for example, yachting, motor sports, cycle racing or golf. As regards the flow of coaches, only general conclusions could be drawn from our material. In ice hockey the flow of coaches was from Northern America to Western Europe; in football, weight-lifting, volleyball and gymnastics, from Eastern Europe to Western Europe.

Political Commitments and Financial Support

The respondents in our survey were asked if the international activities of their organisations reflect any political commitment. The results indicate that the sports organisations perceive their role and profile as non-political. In other words, the sports organisations believe that the *"Freiraumthese"* of unpolitical sport also holds true in practice and that sport is outside all politics, in a vacuum. Only some 20 national associations out of 364 answered that they had some kinds of political commitment in their activities. The political commitments were reflected in their attitudes towards apartheid in the Republic of South Africa and towards racism in general. As any as 15 of the 20 replies dealt with apartheid. Twelve of the answers came from sports organisations which were either un*willing* or un*able* to compete with South Africa. Two South African organisations answered that they were against apartheid policy and one of them was therefore under suspension. The replies from members of federations in which South Africa still has membership did not mention apartheid or racism in their answers, with two exceptions. In contrast to this, members of federations in which South Africa is not a member reacted to the apartheid policy. South Africa still has membership in 37 international federations (Hunter 1980).

As to the other kinds of political commitments, three associations referred to "global principles, UN principles and non-grata countries". In two cases Taiwan was mentioned together with South Africa. One Japanese association admitted that the non-participation in the Moscow Olympics constituted an exception to their non-political profile. Four references were made to government financing and its political implications. Associations from Australia and New Zealand announced that they could not use government money for competitions with South Africa. In addition, one French sports organisation argued that the dependence on government financing means, in practice, a political commitment. However, most sports associations have not found this issue problematic, although almost all of them receive government support. Of course, money can be used as a means of persuasion or blackmail, as was shown in the 1980 Olympic boycott. Still, it is necessary to separate financial support and direct political involvement in the study of governmental involvement in sport.

Table 3 shows the percentage of governmental financial involvement in national sports organisations. The statistics show that the differences in the financial support provided by the governments are notable. On the one hand, a group of countries with great dpendence on governmental financing can be discerned. These include many Latin American countries such as Mexico, Chile, Brazil and Argentina and Nordic countries such as Norway and Finland. In addition to the socialist countries, France, Canada and the traditionally independent sports country Great Britain belong to this group, together with Turkey and South Africa. On the other hand, there are countries with low rates of governmental financing, including Switzerland, Japan, the United States, Australia and New Zealand. Naturally, the rate varies from one sport to another, as can be seen from the Table 3. Between these two extremes there are many countries where governments provide moderate financial support. These include the Federal Republic of Germany, Spain, Italy, the Netherlands, Ireland and Austria.

Much of the obscurity in the discussion of sport, politics and financial dependence is caused by loose definition of the concept "politics". Instead of studying the relationship between "sport" and "politics", it would be analytically interesting to study the phenomenon "politics in and politics against sport". Thus far, the political analysis of sporting relations has been an almost unexplored field in sports sciences, despite the fact that sport has been increasingly integrated into its social environment (Güldenpfennig 1981).

Table 3. The percentage of governmental financing in national sports associations (1980)

Australia	
Skating	50
Gymnastics	30
Cycling, athletics	20
Orienteering	14
Icehockey	10
Brazil	
Table tennis, basketball	100
Football	80
Canada	
Table tennis, weight-lifting	90
Fencing, handball, skating	
Basketball, cycling, wrestling	85
Football	40
Icehockey	20
England	
Boxing, fencing, volleyball	75
Water-skiing	70
Table tennis	61
Basketball	30
Federal Rep. of Germany	
Equestrianism	65
Fencing, handball	50
Volleyball	30
Yachting	25
Finland	
Cycling	60
Weight-lifting	48
Volleyball	45
Swimming	44
Football, orienteering	40
Ice hockey	7.5
France	
Fencing, gymnastics	90
Rowing, canoeing	80
Volleyball	70
Athletics	60
Handball	50
Japan	
Fencing	21
Skating	20
Volleyball	16
Cycling	3.5
Waterskiing, football	0
Mexico	
Handball, wrestling	100
Table tennis	80
New Zealand	
Wrestling	60
Fencing	30
Skiing	20
Equestrianism	15
Canoeing	10
Switzerland	
Wrestling	30
Golf	20
Skating	0
Turkey	
Judo, rowing, table tennis, yachting	100

The Role of Development Aid

Development aid is a relatively recent issue in international sport. The emergence of newly independent nations in the 1950s and the 1960s had an influence on the international sports movement. In the International Olympic Committee the development aid issue was discussed for the first time in 1961. On the initiative of the French Count de Beaumont and the Soviet Andreanov, the IOC appointed an International Olympic Aid Commission to "study ways of helping African and Asian nations to improve their sports programs" with de Beaumont as the chairman. However, owing to political considerations the work of the committee was suspended in 1963 (Espy 1979). The IOC returned to the development issue 5 years later, when a new Aid Committee was appointed at the Mexico meeting and Juan Samaranch, the present IOC president, was elected as chairman of the committee. No separate funds were given to the committee and thus its work was purely administrative. Some progress was made in 1972 when a new Olympic Solidarity programme was established under the auspices of the IOC, after long debate between the IOC and the national Olympic committees.

The multilateral development aid and co-operation in sports includes the IOC Olympic Solidarity programme, UNESCO's International Fund for the Development of Physical Education and Sport, and the aid programmes of the international federations. The UNESCO sports fund is financed by the UNESCO members in accordance with their willingness. The financing of the Olympic Solidarity programme is on a somewhat firmer basis, since it is being financed from the national Olympic committees's share of the Olympic television revenues. The television revenues are shared in the following way: the Organizing Committee of the Olympic Games takes two thirds, and the remaining third is divided between the IOC, the national Olympic committees and the international sports federations into three equal parts. The financing of the Olympic Solidarity Programme has been strongly critised because the funds are taken from the national Olympic committees's share and not from the share of the international federations. In practice, the poor developing countries, which from the majority in the national Olympic committees, are helping themselves through this Solidarity programme, i. e. poor developing countries, and the IOC and the international federations, are consuming the national committees' share of the television revenues. Nowadays, the television contracts and revenues are worth hundreds of millions of dollars; the conflict between the national Olympic committees and the international federations is therefore not merely about principles, as can be seen from Table 4.

Table 4. The overall television revenues of the summer Olympics (Hackforth 1975)

Rome 1960	$ 1.2 million
Tokyo 1964	$ 4.1 million
Mexico 1968	$ 4.5 million
Munich 1972	$ 12.0 million
Montreal 1976	$ 43.6 million
Moscow 1980	$ 85.0 million
Los Angeles 1984	$ 225.0 million

Sources: Hackforth J (1975) Sport im Fernsehen. Münster; McCollum R, McCollum D (1981)Analysis of ABC-TV coverage of the 21st Olympiad Games. In: Segrave J, Chu D (eds), Olympism. Champaign

In our survey the channelling of development aid was studied. Of the 364 national sports associations, 26 (7%) were giving some kind of development aid. The main channels of aid were financial support and the sending of coaches. Twelve associations announced that they gave financial aid to the poorer associations abroad. Fifteen organisations were sending coaches within their aid programmes. In addition, three associations had sent referees to hold courses in the developing countries. According to our data, only five associations were sending sports equipment and technical experts to the aid recipients.

The development aid of the international federations is more extensive and versatile than that of the national associations. According to the survey, 10 federations out of 26 have given some kind of development aid. In some sports, there are special funds or foundations for this purpose, e. g. the International Korfball Federation has an international propaganda foundation and the Badminton Federation has a coaching fund for countries where this sport is not well developed. On the whole, the aid takes various forms: reduced membership fees in international federations, seminars for developing countries, sending of books, film and equipment, the training of sports officials and referees, financial, technical and coaching aid and the construction of the infrastructure of sport in developing countries. The largest federations have special programmes of development aid and co-operation: the International Federation of Association Football has development projects with Coca Cola Inc., e. g. an International Football Academy, and its own programme of technical aid, grants and loans. The International Amateur Athletics Federation has a separate Development Programme Commission in co-operation with the Olympic Solidarity programme of the IOC.

Extensive development aid and co-operation in sport is without doubt an important factor in the promotion of international understanding. In addition, it is one way of making progress in the establishment of a new international sports order. However, development aid in sport involves several problems, including the relation of development aid in sport to the international physical culture in developing countries (Hietanen 1982). The crucial issue is whether development aid is merely a means of expanding European physical culture to developing countries or whether the cultural interaction perspective is emphasised. Thus far the cultural context of development aid in sport has been a neglected issue (Galtung 1980). Another problem related to development aid in sport is that the aid activities have mostly been left to the international federations, national Olympic committees and national sports associations - in addition to the IOC and UNESCO - and therefore international sports solidarity has not reached the grassroot level of local sports clubs and sports fans. However, in recent years there have been some encouraging trends, especially in the Nordic countries. In Denmark, Norway and Sweden measures have been taken to integrate local sports clubs into development co-operation in sport. These projects have been trying to avoid the third major problem of development co-operation in sport, namely that the sports projects have not been integrated adequately into governmental projects in development co-operation.

A more fundamental problem is that the developing countries are not likely to be interested only in receiving financial and material aid but also in the demand for equity in international sport. In the 1960s and 1970s the affiliation of several developing countries to international sports federations resulted in some protectionist measures by the industrialised world in order to prevent drastic changes in the policies of the federations. For example, weighted voting systems were introduced in several major federations. Furthermore, other kinds of organisational imbalances exist in the decision-making structure of international sports federations. However, some signs of change can be observed in this respect.

Conclusion

The rapid expansion of international sport has had several consequences. Of great importance is the fact that sport has become more social all over the world. The global social, economic and political realities are reflected in international sports relations.

The impact of sport on international understanding is to a large extent dependent on how the sports relations are adjusted to these realities. It seems possible that in a world of rapid change, instability and tension, international sport can function as a stabilising factor. Our study has indicated that sport has had relative autonomy even in the relations between the great powers and that the bloc-based integration is not strong in the field of sport.

In spite of the fact that sport has become more social and perhaps more political, most sports organisations perceive their role and activities as non-political. Nevertheless, governmental involvement is increasing both in national and international sport, especially in the form of financial support. As regards the order trends in international sports co-operation, there has been on the hand a tendency towards global homogenisation, and on the other hand a tendency towards regionalisation. In addition, the status of the developing countries in international sport has been a topical issue. Especially the Movement of Non-Aligned Countries has paid increased attention to sport activities, and development co-operation in the field of sport can be seen as a trend towards a new international sports order. However, today there do not seem to be great prospects for structural changes in international sporting relations.

References

de Coubertin P (1931) Mémoires Olympiques. IOC, Lausanne

Espy R (1979) The politics of the Olympic Games. University of California Press, Berkeley

Galtung J (1980) Cultural contact and technical assistance as factors in peaceful relations. In: Galtung J (ed) Peace and world structure. Essays in peace research, vol IV. Ejleres, Copenhagen, pp 482-511

Glader E(1978) Amateurism and athletics. Leisure West Point (1978)

Goodhart P, Chataway C (1968) War without weapons. Allen, London

Güldenpfennig S (1981) Internationale Sportbeziehungen zwischen Entspannung und Konfrontation. Der Testfall 1980. Pahl-Rugenstein, Cologne

Güldenpfennig S, Schulke H (1980) The need for politological research on sport and its relation to the sociology of sport. Int Rev Sport Soc 15:127-140

Hackforth J (1975) Sport im Fernsehen. Verlag Regensberg, Münster

Harkavy R (1981) Pariah states and nuclear proliferation. Int Org 35:135-163

Heinilä K (1971) Sport and international understanding. In: Mass media, sport and international understanding. Report of an International Seminar. ICSPE, Paris pp 15-18

Hietanen A (1982) Towards a new international sports order? Curr Res Peace Viol 5:159-175

Hunter MG (1980) The United Nations and the anti-apartheid in sport movement. Can J Hist Sport Phys Ed 11:19-35

Huxley A (1937) Ends and means. Chatto and Windus, London

McIntosh PC (1963) Sport in society. Watts, London

McIntosh PC (1974) Mass media: Friends or foes in sport. QUEST Monog XXII:33-44

McIntosh PC (1979) Fair play. Ethics in sport and education. Heinemann, London

Jacobsen TH (1981) Det internasjonale Olympiske system. En nasjonsbasert tilnaerming til utviklingen i det internasjonale olympiske system 1945-1978. Universitetet i Oslo, Oslo

Jones RW (1960) Sport and international understanding. In: Sport - Work - Culture. Helsinki, pp. 159-170

Kyröläinen H, Varis T (1981) Approaches to the study of sports in international relations. Curr Res Peace Viol 4:55-88

Laage von der R (1977) Sport in China - Eine Entwicklungsskizze und Bestandsaufnahme. Bartels and Wernitz, Berlin

Lenk H (1964) Werte - Ziele - Wirklichkeit der modernen Olympischen Spiele. Hofmann, Schorndorf

Lorenz K (1963) Das sogenannte Böse. Vienna

Lucas J (1981) The genesis of the modern Olympic Games. In: Sedgrave J, Chu D (eds) Olympism. Human kinetics. Stipes, Champaign, pp 7-21

Lüschen G (1970) Cooperation, association and contest. Confl Res 14:21–34
Milshtein OA, Molchanov SV (1976) The shaping of public opinion regarding sport by the mass media as a factor promoting international understanding. Int Rev Sport Sociol 11: 71–82
Natan A (1969) Sport and politics. In: Loy JW, Kenyon GS (eds) Sport, culture and society. McMillan, London, pp 203–210
Noel-Baker P (1962) Sport and international understanding. Int J Ad Youth Ed 14:962
Phillips Davison W (1974) Mass communication and conflict resolution. The role of the information media in the advancement of international understanding. Praeger, New York
Riordan J (1977) Sport in Soviet society: Development of sport and physical education in Russia and the USSR. Cambridge University Press, London
Rittner K (1976) Sport und Arbeitsteilung. Zur sozialen Funktion und Bedeutung des Sports. Limpert, Bad Homburg
Santayana G (1954) The life of reason: or the phases of human progress. New York
Steinberg DA (1978) The workers' sport internationals 1920–1928. Cont Hist 13:233–251
United Nations Centre Against Apartheid - Notes and Documents 18/1981 and 7/1982. Register of sports contacts with South Africa.
USSR-USA Sports Encounters (1977). Progress, Moscow
Wagner H (1959) Humanismus - Militarismus - Leibeserziehung. Barth, Munich
Weiss P (1969) Sport - A philosophic inquiry. Southern Illinois University Press, Carbondale and Edwardsville

Competitive Sport and International Understanding: Some Sociological Observations on the World University Games of 1983

P. A. Saram

Introduction

The city of Edmonton and the University of Alberta (both located in Alberta, Canada) will co-host the World University Games of July, 1983. Events such as the Games provide an opportunity to examine the assumption that competitive sport promotes international understanding. This paper contains a summary of the initial phase of sociological research on this topic.

Universiade '83, a corporation representing the city and the university, is responsible for organising the Games. Its theme, "Welcome the World", reflects three domains of activity associated with the Games. The primary activity will be the *international sporting* event for some 3500 athletes from 101 countries. A second component, the International Sports Congress, will be an *international scientific* gathering drawing scholars from 50 to 70 countries. Third, Kaleidoscope '83, the *international cultural* festival which includes a competitive component, is expected to attract some 500 participants from about 100 countries.

Purpose

The broader purpose of this sociological research is to ascertain the nature of the relationship between competitive sport and international understanding. With reference to the Games, three topics of inquiry are: plans intended to promote international understanding; plans intended to prevent or minimise international misunderstanding; and aspects of international understanding that are merely assumed and, therefore, not integral to the planning process.

Procedure

A sociological study of this nature involves three phases of research covering the planning, operational and follow-up stages of the Games. The present inquiry is based on the initial planning stage and therefore the information on which the analysis is made is both selective and inconclusive. The information has been obtained from officials associated with the Games, Universiade '83 information brochures, community relations publication of the University of Alberta, and news and information releases in the Edmonton mass media.

For the research, the conceptual status of several terms requires some initial explication. *Competitive conflict* is a concept basic to the study. That varieties of conflict are inherent to all social relations and stable social systems has been elaborated in the sociology of Georg Simmel. In contrast to antagonistic conflict, the conflict element in competitive conflict is only indirect and involves parallel efforts by the competing parties concerning the same prize which may not even be in the possession of any of them. Competitive *sport* is a typical example of competitive conflict in this sense. Competition in the field of *science* assumes a common aim from which all participants could benefit, although the competitive efforts are not required to be identical. In *artistic* competition, such efforts are almost presumed to be different. In all three kinds of competitive conflict however, the subjective motives of the competitors contribute to the realisation of some objective social values that are even independent of these motives (Simmel 1955, pp 13-17, 34-35, 57-85). Different assessment criteria as they pertain to truth and validity in science, philosophy and art have also been clarified by Mannheim (1952, 1953).

As a concept, *international understanding* is elusive. "Understanding" is the empathic appreciation of action attributable to a different perspective or set of circumstances and contains the potential for certain relations with the actor including those of co-operation in areas of mutual benefit. Understanding between nations in this sense involves perspectives and circumstances that are essentially political in nature. The potential for international relations, especially those reflecting conspicuous co-operation is determined according to the acceptability of politically relevant action on the part of respective nations.

The term international understanding is sometimes taken to mean awareness, appreciation and relations of goodwill that some individuals have in reference to other nations. Such understanding is neither a necessary nor sufficient condition, though it is perhaps a contributory one, for international relations.

Events are planned or unplanned happenings that affect the course of biography and social history. A *pageant* is a dramatised event reflective of a given order of things and reinforced in an audience by way of a spectacular socio-cultural experience. *Incidents* are unanticipated happenings that undermine the success of a planned event.

Results

Some observations based on the *initial planning* stage of the Games are that:

- Even at this stage, the World University Games seem to have been transformed into an international pageant of spectacular expectations.
- International understanding is a precondition for the staging of major events involving competitive conflict in such fields as sport, science and art. The international standing of the host country, the sponsoring organisations and the participating countries is significant in this regard.
- Through conspicuous co-operation, these events reflect and reinforce the nature of international understanding at a given time.
- Such events provide a "non-political" controlled setting for a "claim to equality" on the part of all competing nations and a "claim to superiority" on the part of those declared to be successful.

- The inclusion of science, and especially art and culture, provides foci that diffuse the otherwise conspicuous distinctions between clear winners and losers.
- In the minds of spectators, such events could re-affirm the ideological and cultural differences that prevail between nations and groups of nations.
- Events of this nature involve considerable planning although efforts designed to promote international understanding are unclear and perhaps only latent to the planning process.
- International understanding seems to be assumed with reference to the staging of such events, the preservation of the former and the success of the latter being considerably dependent on the absence of "incidents".
- Such events call for efforts designed to prevent or minimise "incidents" that are likely to provoke international misunderstanding.

Discussion

The above observations are admittedly tentative; some are necessarily hypothetical, requiring refinement and verification during subsequent stages of the Games. However, what is apparent is the preconditional fact of international relations in determining the very possibility of competitive conflict. On the one hand, events of this kind, especially those of pageant-like proportions, become occasions of conspicuous co-operation that reflect and reinforce a given nature of international understanding. On the other hand, given the potentially fragile nature of international relations, planners of such events must take effort to prevent or at least minimise incidents that could lead to international misunderstanding and thereby undermine the success of the event. From a planning point of view, the success of such an event lies not so much in tangible accomplishments of international understanding, but in the absence of incidents.

At present it has not been possible to detail specific planning efforts directed towards the preventin of international misunderstanding. This is due to such plans being unformulated as yet or to their inaccessibility to the public. Also, the role of competitors, spectators and organisers as potential agents of international understanding, and the role of the Games in the realisation of higher order social values cannot be ascertained. I hope to explore these questions in the light of more information available during the remaining phases of the research.

References

Edmonton Journal (1982) Edmonton, Canada
Folio (1982) University of Alberta Community Relations Publication, Edmonton, Canada
Mannheim K (1952) Essays on the sociology of knowledge. Routledge and Kegan Paul, London
Mannheim K (1953) Essays on sociology and social psychology. Routledge and Kegan Paul, London
Simmel G (1955) Conflict and the web of group affiliations. The Free Press, New York
Universiade '83 (1982) Information brochures. Edmonton, Canada

2. Sport for All

The Extent, Content and Organisation of International Co-operation in the Past, Present and Future in Respect of Sport for All

T. Wolańska

Introduction

International co-operation in the sphere of "sport for all" takes place both in an organised and in an informal way; it occurs on a global scale and also within various regions, continents and political blocs. It is co-ordinated by international organisations or by such bodies as UNESCO, the International Council for Sport and Physical Education, the Federation International d'Education Physique and the World Leisure Recreation Association. In addition, co-operation may be on a bilateral basis between various countries, national sports organisations and twin cities.

Side by side with the trend organised by international agencies, there is a lively exchange of experiences in an informal and spontaneous way as a result of international tourism and the influence of the mass media. Organised and purposeful as well as spontaneous activity brings in its wake the universalisation of patterns of sport for all, which finds its expression in very similar recreational models. K. Heinilä (1977) writes that lively cultural exchange on the international level adds international features to the culture of the individual countries. Active participation in competitive sport helps to accelerate the rate of internationalisation of physical culture and the disappearance of purely national features.

The International Development of Sport for All

The development of physical culture made it necessary to set apart the competitive trend from sport for all. Sport for all as a more large-scale social phenomenon made its appearance only in the 1950s and 1960s. In many countries in which there is a development of the trend called sport for all, "mass physical culture", "gymnastique volontaire", "trim", "trim and fitness" or "physical recreation" is gradually being set apart from the rest of physical culture. The consequence of the pluralistic conception of physical culture has begun to come to the fore in international organisations. They now concentrate more and more not only on sport and physical education, as was the case until the 1950s, but also on trends in physical culture which take into account the human being during his entire life, i.e. children, youth, families, the aged, handicapped people - i.e. on sport for all. New organisations are being set up and already existing organisations like the International Olympic Committee and FIEP are beginning to take into account sport for all.

New organisations for the co-ordination of exchange of experiences regarding sport and leisure include: ICSPE, the World Leisure Recreation Association (WLRA), the European Leisure and Recreation Association (ELRA), the "Trim and Fitness International", the International Council on Health Physical Education and Recreation (ICHPER), and the Comité Sportif International du Travail.

A special ICSPE Committee, "Sport and Leisure", was set up in 1964. This is a specialised organ of ICSPE for the co-ordination of international exchange of experiences regarding sport for all. It regularly organises international seminars every two years which try to find answers to the most urgent proplems of sport for all, such as the development of sport in residential districts, physical fitness norms and badges, organisation and administration, training of professional and voluntary personnel, and sport and the family. But not less appreciated are the results achieved by other international organisations and bodies that have developed activities supporting the exchange of experiences relating to sport for all, e.g. the FIEP congresses, seminars and vacation courses, the international seminars and congresses organised by WLRA, ELRA, the "Trim and Fitness International", the ICSPE and ICHPER congresses, organisations of women's sport, the Van Clé Foundation, the International Commission for Advancement of Leisure Leadership (INTERCALL) and finally many initiatives for the exchange of scientific findings from universities or of practical material collected by national sports organisations.

More lively international co-operation could be observed in the 1970s, when many international congresses and seminars were held to deal with the above-mentioned problems and when a number of important documents were adopted and declarations made, e. g. the Charter for Leisure (1970), the Sport Manifesto (1964) and the FIEP Manifesto on Physical Education (La FIEP 1974).

In 1972 ICSPE issued a document entitled "Sport for All" in which it laid down the principles for sports policy. This document stressed the necessity to attract people to practice physical activity regularly, to combine sport with culture and to make sport attractive for all age groups (Sport für Alle 1972).

A good example of exchange of international experience and of the idea of understanding was the international conference held in 1975 to celebrate the 700th anniversary of Amsterdam, entitled "City on the Move" ("Stad in Beweging"). Along with specialists on physical recreation, the mayors of many capitals of the world were invited. Beginning in 1975, UNESCO started to show more active interest in "sport for all", mainly through conferences of ministers of sport. G. Młodzikowski (1979) thinks that these conferences are an expression of new, higher forms of international sporting relations which permit unhampered exchange of opinions, interformation and experience on the role, function and significance of sport in various countries and on the international level. As a result of the first conference, an Intergovernmental Committee for Physical Education and Sport was set up, and in 1978 during the general UNESCO conference the International Charter of Physical Education and Sport was adopted. Article 1 of this Charter stresses that all human beings have the right to participation in physical education and sport, to the extent to which this is indispensable for the full development of the personality. To date this is the most important document on the international level related to physical education and sport. N. Moolenijzer (1980) indicates that this "Magna Carta" contains important implications for all those who deal with sport in terms of filling the large gap between the developed theory and philosophy connected with sport for all and its implementation.

P. McIntosh (1980) is quite correct in saying that the criterion for the analysis and evaluation of "sport for all" should be Article 1 of the UNESCO International Charter of Physical Education and Sport, which most thoroughly formulates the aims and tasks of "sport for all", though this actual term was not used.

Current Situation in International Sport for All

The many activities now being undertaken demonstrate the growing significance and the ever higher level of sport for all, which from a marginal position has in many countries already attained equal rights with other forms of sport, and even a leading position in relation to them. The content of international exchange reflects all the features of activity in the sphere of sport for all, i. e. programmes, organisation and administration, methods and means of popularisation, facilities, training of personnel, information and documentation, publications, exchange of students and finally international research. Examples of such exchange are the initiatives launched by UNESCO as well as by other internatioonal organisations, universities etc.

The mass media, above all television and publications, contribute markedly to international exchange and mutual understanding regarding sport for all. A special ICSPE document entitled *Mass Media and Mass Sport* (1979) is a good example.

In a report prepared for UNESCO and entitled *Sport for All – Program Throughout the World by ICSPE* (1980), the situation regarding "sport for all" in the world was presented in a comprehensive way on the basis of material collected from 14 countries as well as selected source material. The author stresses that so far neither information and documentation centres nor occasional reports by UNESCO have fulfiled their tasks satisfactorily, because ICSPE and UNESCO both need to consider the possibilities of still better and more effective exchange of international information. UNESCO should more intensively inspire and popularise seminars, conferences and discussions, should encourage people to embark on international research (above all on the problem of motivation for "sport for all"), and should encourage people to make more use of mass media and technical means. McIntosh suggests that UNESCO should encourage the members of its governmental and non-governmental sub-committees to draw up plans and programmes for the development of sport in individual countries.

The activity of many organisations so far reveals considerable achievements but also certain weaknesses. One of the weaknesses especially pointed out is insufficient help and commitment to the popularisation of sport in developing countries. E. Beyer (1980) points to the lack of co-operation and international planning as regards aid to the developing countries, and, thinks that priority should be given to the training of animators, teachers of physical education and coaches. McIntosh (1980), on the other hand, asks UNESCO to oblige its Intergovernmental Sub-committee to establish priorities in research related to "sport for all" for developing countries.

The spontaneity and diffusion of many valuable initiatives and material means are another weakness of the existing system of international co-operation in the area of "sport for all". There is insufficient access to countries and milieux which require aid and consultation. There are too many neglected aspects while at the same time there is an over-exploitation of certain subjects by various organisations almost simultaneously. It is not enough to conduct research into sport for all from the point of view of psychology, economy, law, ecology etc. Adjustments in the training programmes of specialised personnel to cater for the needs of sport for all have been too slow. There has also been insufficient co-ordination in planning conferences and congresses in terms of both dates and subject matter. Finally, there have been too few international research projects concerning sport for all.

The Future of International Sport for All

If P. Seurin's (1980) definition of sport for all as the sport of tomorrow is to be accepted, then reflections on the future of international co-operation will arouse hopes for change and progress. Growing interest in the problems is to be expected on the part of international organisations - not only sport organisations but others such as those related to health, education, culture, environmental protection, architecture and the family. With such a development, the need for better co-ordination of activities at the international level on the part of UNESCO and ICSPE will increase.

It is to be expected that new fields of activity and integration will appear. It is also to be expected that there will be more active co-operation with developing countries, and that their presence in international organisations as partners on an equal footing will enrich the forms and content of exchange and deepen mutual understanding.

The further development of international tourism will show progress, especially in relation to the search for healthy recreational regions in the context of the further degradation of the natural environment. The further increase in the number of trips to foreign countries for sport vacations will ensure better use of the world's regions suitable for sports and recreation (there are many possibilities with regard to skiing, sailing, mountaineering, hunting, angling, surfing and orienteering). This will bring in its wake a more frequent exchange of sport patterns between tourists from various countries and the local people. In addition, stronger informal contacts will be established in connection with the practice of sport for recreational purposes, i. e. on the beaches, on the ski lifts, on the tourist routes, at camping sites and in hotels (which will be supplied with ever better sports equipment). This is why there is an urgent need for closer co-operation between international sport and tourist agencies. The future will bring a further stepping up of bilateral co-operation between various countries, cities and sports organisations in the field of sport for all. The principal means of international co-operation in respect of sport for all will continue to be organised forms.

Recommendations for the Future Development of International Sport for All

On the basis of an analysis of the present state of affairs, certain recommendations may be made which will increase the effectiveness of the international system of sport for all:

- Better co-ordination of the still scattered initiatives and activities is needed, as, perhaps is a more clearly outlined profile of some of the international organisations.
- There should be better co-ordination in respect of the dates and subject matter of conferences and, more importantly, congresses.
- It is necessary to embark on international research on problems connected with sport for all, and co-ordinated research plans on certain subjects should be drawn up.

- Through the intermediary UNESCO, representatives from more countries should be persuaded to join sports organisations.
- It is necessary to identify neglected areas on the geographical map of sport and to draw up a list of problems to be dealt with by science and practice, making use of the best experience in the world.
- It is necessary to improve and to allow much broader access to the system of information and documentation regarding sport for all.

References

Beyer E (1980) Problemes de la promotion de l'éducation physique et du sport dans les pays du thiers-monde. Analyses dans l'optique d'un pays industrialisé. Bull FIEP 4:15–23

Charter for Leisure (1970). Genève

Heinilä K (1977) Social factors affecting sports and recreation. Sport and leisure. The Finnish Association of Architects, SAFA, Helsinki, pp 3–4

ICSPE (1979) Mass media and mass sport. Maison de L'UNESCO, Paris

La FIEP (1974) Cinquante années au service de l'éducation physique dans le monde. Bull FIEP (Suppl.) 4

McIntosh P (1980) Sport for all: Programmes throughout the world.

Młodzikowski (1979) Polityka i sport. Sport i Turystyka. (Politics and sport. Sport and Tourism). Warsaw, pp 145–160

Moolenijzer NJ (1980) Professional responsibilities for implementation of the International Charter of Physical Education and Sport. Bull FIEP 3/4:7–10

Seurin P (1980) The future of the olympic games and tomorrow's sport. Bull FIEP 2:7–16

Sport für Alle (1969) Doc ICSPE-CIEPS. Buc/69/12/ Rev 72.5.

European Health Tour 1984 – Promoting Health Through Sport and International Co-operation

N. Daly

Introduction

In the medium programme for the 7th General programme of Work 1984–1989 there was a call by the European Office of the World Health Organisation to consider health promotion in Europe. A document surmised that programmes of health promotion were far more developed in North America than in Europe, and they adopted the definition of health promotion employed by the American Office of Health Promotion: "Any combination of education in related organisational, political and economic intervention designed to facilitate behavioural and environmental adaptation that would improve or protect health."

The concept of health promotion requires an examination in qualitative terms of the life-style of the population under consideration. Crucial to the success of any health promotion initiatives would be an understanding of the limitations placed upon the community by their environment. The physical, social and psychological environment can in many instances be barriers to behaviour options which may be offered during health promotion programmes. The World Health Organisation European Regional Headquarters has as its responsibility mainland Europe and parts of North Africa, i. e. areas large numbers of differing life-styles and life expectations within distinct communities. In an attempt to provide a single unified template with which each individual country within the region could articulate, the European Office commissioned a feasibility study on a health promotion event to be held throughout Europe during 1984. On examination of the experience in Ireland, Scotland and the United States with regard to health promotion events, the feasibility study examined the possibility, management and funding of a major European cycling event entitled "The Euro Health Tour 1984". I would like to stress that the choice of an international cycling event by the health education organisations in Ireland and Scotland merely reflects the facility provided by stage cycle tours for interaction with large numbers of people within their own communities. The Irish example in 1980 and the Scottish example in 1981 demonstrated that over half a million people out of a total combined population of eight million became involved in associated health week activities because of the media interest generated by the international cycle race. Cycling was chosen by these countries after analyses of other sporting events and after tentative sports sponsorship initiatives using other sports. It was felt that cycling offered the best possible sport to allow a centralised health education to interact with as many grass root organisations as possible in the shortest space of time.

It would be important for the World Health Organisation to realise that although it may be seen to be promoting cycling in essence, the function of the cycling promotion is to help individual national organisations to come to terms with the currently accepted principles of health promotion which have been determined by "The Working Group on the Concepts and Principles of Health Promotion" in Copenhagen.

In terms of the potential for behaviour change resulting from a range of such initiatives, we have to look to the United States for an example. There, the rate of coronary heart disease has declined by approximately 23% over the last 20 years. This represents an enormous saving both in human misery and also in health service resources. This dramatic change in coronary heart disease is reflected across all racial groups and social classes in the United States with, in fact, a larger percentage decrease amongst the non-white community than amongst the white community. There are several dominant hypotheses which attempt to outline the causes of this reduction, but all include a component which ascribes an element of this success story to the change in life-style which American communities have experienced over the last 20 years. Among the reasons for these behaviour changes on such a vast scale are an increased awareness of the health risks assocciated with coronary heart disease and an increased awareness of the steps which can be taken to reduce these risks. It is crucial in the American experience that all parts of the community became involved in the prediction of risk and its consequent reduction. The initiation of health promotion/health education programmes within the medical services, at the work-place and in the home and the way in which health promotion became fashionable as the concept of possible health became a high priority on the national agenda were of significant importance.

In general terms, it would appear that the knowledge and expertise are available for the World Health Organization to effect in the first instance an attitudinal change on a Europe-wide basis. Further, the World Health Organization European Office, because of its significant political and diplomatic situation, can influence the priority given to health education and health promotion by individual governments if it can demonstrate that the existing movement for good health can be expanded and increased in terms of the numbers of individuals participating both intellectually and physically. The concept of the European health week in association with the sporting event is crucial to the aims of the World Health Organization regarding health promotion. The World Health Organization will never be in a better position to interact directly with distinct local communities throughout Europe.

As part of the feasibility study, consultations took place with organisations involved with health education and promotion in the following countries: Austria, Belgium, Denmark, France, Holland, Luxembourg, the USSR and West Germany.

Outline of the Event

Stage cycling offers the possibility of covering over 100 miles per day. Several different styles of cycling event were offered for consideration by countries participating in the feasibility study. In general terms there are three major options as regards the organisation of such an event:

1. *The star tour.* A single location would be chosen in mainland Europe and individual countries would be asked to mobilise their own populations with the aim of attract-

ing members of the public to cycle on a specific date over a specific route to the "Star" centre. The essence of this event is folk participation.
2. *The non-competitive tour.* This event closely resembles a stage cycling race, where fairly large distances are covered throughout Europe in a linear fashion. The participants in this event would not be top athletes but a combination of health, environmental and educational respresentatives, perhaps with some celebrities and political figures being recruited.
3. *The competitive health race.* This would be a full international amateur competitive cycling event. Each participating country would send their top national cycling team to participate in the event with the aim of demonstrating their expertise and fitness through cycling.

The merits and demerits of the options were discussed with the representatives of the countries visited. In general terms, the following is a summary of comments made regarding the three types of events:

The Star Tour

The star tour was seen as potentially the most difficult to organise. The focus of the event was seen very much to be the star centre, and it was suggested that in terms of media and potential subsidiary sponsorship there would be no unifying event for coverage and to attract finance. Further, each Health Education Authority in countries other than the host country for the star centre would be seen to be participating in an event which had its focus in another country. Because of the difficulty of split focus and low attractiveness for the media and sponsorship, this style of event was seen as possibly more costly and uneconomic than the other two. Further, it was suggested that politically a star centre would present problems in terms of participation from Eastern bloc countries.

To be truly successful, such an event would need to attract thousands of participants from each country, thus making the organisation in terms of policing, management, feeding, accommodation etc. a major problem. There would also be an imbalance in route planning in that non-competitive cyclists might require several weeks to reach the star centre from those countries furthest from it.

Although this event was seen philosophically to be most acceptable, it was recognised and suggested that in terms of the aims of the World Health Organisation in providing a unified strategy, this was perhaps the least suitable of the three options. Nevertheless, it was felt that such star tours on an individual national basis were worthy of consideration by the least several of the countries visited.

Non-competitive Tour

A non-competitive tour was seen as potentially the most appropriate style of event. But during discussion with representatives of the countries involved in the study, it became apparent that there would be difficulties in organising such an event internationally because of the lack of specific organisations already in existence that could undertake this task. It was felt that the mechanism for the election of participants would be dubious in some countries and totally inappropriate in others. The Health Education

Authorities were diverting their responsibilities away from the organisation of health weeks and more towards the health tour and its philosophy in providing a vehicle for the organisation of national health weeks. The commercial interests contacted with a view to providing outside sponsorship declared themselves relatively uninterested in this style of event because of the lack of an existing cohesive organisation to make preparations for it. The event was also suggested as being relatively unattractive to the media in Europe, given the enormous coverage of competitive sport.

The duration of a non-competitive tour was also problematic. Given that each individual country would control the selection of participants, the age and state of fitness to a large extent would act as a limiting factor in the distance which could be covered in each day's cycling. Consequently, choosing a specific distance which everyone could cover would be most difficult.

Competitive Cycle Race

Although several countries felt the philosophy of a competitive cycle race was not totally in accord with the aims of health education and health promotion, in terms of organisation this was seen as perhaps the easiest option. There already exists an international organisation for the organisation of such international events. This organisation removes from each individual national Health Education Department the need to be involved in the organisation of the tour per se, and allows them to devote the bulk of their energies to the organisation of the national health week which should be organised in conjunction with the cycle tour. The proposed event, were it to be a competitive cycle race would be virtually guaranteed to attract major media coverage. This media coverage in turn would allow national health education interests to involve non-health organisations, both statutory and voluntary, during the planning of the national health weeks, and thus would achieve one of the main aims of the health tour/health week matrix, i. e. to bring together environmental agencies to discuss with health agencies the role of the environment as a limiting factor in positive health. A competitive cycle tour was also seen as providing a focus for fringe events which would cover sub-groups within the community, e. g. the elderly, the handicapped and the young. In terms of raising finance to fund the Europe Event 1984, the competitive tour demands most commercial backing for health promotion and for the race itself. Further, the competitive cycle tour could involve countries other than those selected for the race route.

Euro Health Week 1984

Regardless of the style of event which is eventually chosen, the aim of the organisation of the Euro Health Tour is to set the scene and provide the stimulus and focus for the organisation of a European Health Week in 1984.

A major international sporting event can provide national health education authorities with the necessary vehicle for mobilising national, voluntary and statutory organisations to participate in the planning and organisation of associated events. One of the aims of such events is, in fact, this cross fertilisation and introduction of different governmental and non-governmental agencies with the sole aim of providing health

Table 1. Sample local health week module: organisations that could be involved in various health activities

Health	Activity	Organisation
Health and body	Active participation in sport, keep fit, covering all age groups Demonstrations of health, i. e. dance; participatory events	Sports councils/ recreation bodies Dance groups
Healthy mind	Relaxation Stress/anxiety/depression	Yoga organisation, self-help groups Trade unions, womens' groups, grass roots community groups
Health and nature	Health foods and diets Plant care Wildlife study Nature conservation Nature study Environment of the disabled	Dietitian/health food shops Botanic gardens, open exhibitions Disabled people's organisations

promotion initiative. According to the paradigm previously tried in the United States, Ireland and Scotland, participatory events would be organised to cover the entire week, culminating in the arrival of the European Health Tour in that particular location.

As it is the aim of the European Office of the WHO to provide a strategy into which each individual national identity can comfortably be fitted, it was not the function of the feasibility study to prescribe activities which could or may be organised. Nevertheless, a sample health week module was developed from the report (cf. Tables 1 and 2).

Conclusions

It would appear that with the exception of West Germany, all the countries visited during the course of the feasibility study were positively disposed towards the World Health Organization suggestion that a European Health Tour 1984 be organised. Several countries stressed the important nature of this new departure by WHO in terms of its health promotion activities.

In terms of choosing an option for the style of event, there seems to be a split between the non-competitive and the competitive health tour. Philosophically the non-competitive health tour seems to be the more attractive, but from an organisational point of view the competitive health tour, which would be organised by the International Cycling Federation, was seen as being the better option. The star tour was seen as impractical from a European viewpoint in that the star centre would be the focus of most of the interest. The distances that some countries would have to cover in order to participate were perhaps too large. The choice of options for the event were divided between the non-competitive and the competitive tour. In terms of feasibility, the competitive tour is preferable because of the possibility of raising the amounts of

Table 2. Sample local health week module: activities appropriate to distinct population groups

Participant	Activity	Venue
Families	Mini marathon	
	Jogging	
	Generation tennis	
	Fil rouge knockout	Local park
	Orienteering and picnic	Woods, forests
	Family volleyball	Recreation centre
	Fun run "Clean up the hedgegrows"	
Children (schools, youth and sports clubs)	Relay/obstacle races	Parks/playgrounds
	Trampolining	Recreation centre
	Round the table - Table tennis	
	Nature hunts	Wood/forest
	Treasure hunts	
	Invent a game	
	Sand castle competitions	Beach
	Outdoor art	
	Netball	
	Walt Disney cavalcades	Park
	Swimming gala	
	Cycling proficiency test	School
	Country dancing	Town hall
	Disco dancing	Town hall
	Roller disco	Town hall
	Clubs/brownies	Town hall
	Scouting/guiding	Town hall
Senior citizens	Bowling	Local
	Swimming	Local
	Golf	Local
	Fishing	Local
	Floral arrangements	Local town hall
	Flower/vegetable shows	Local town hall
Handicapped	Wheelchair races	
	Volleyball	
	Netball	
	Table tennis	
	Boat trips	
	Sports centres	
	Organised open days	
	Able-bodied and handicapped joint events	
Adults	Bowling	
	Cross-country running	
	Cricket	
	Canoeing	
	Gliding	
	Golf	
	Mountaineerting/rock climbing	
	Sailing	
	Parachuting	
	Cycling	

money required to fund such an event. The non-competitive tour is also potentially feasible with the caveat that the contributions required from participating countries would proportionally be much greater than for a competitive tour. This entire concept is obviously a new departure both in terms of philosophy and funding for the World Health Organization European Office and as such has received a much warmer reception from individual countries than most new initiatives have.

A meeting is being convened by the European Office of the World Health Organization in Copenhagen in September to discuss the findings of the feasibility study and to decide whether or not the European Health Tour in 1984 will in fact take place.

Marathon Peace March: A Demonstration of International Understanding

A. Laitinen

How can anyone be worthy of a prize for peace when we are so far from it? In the face of stupendous risks, public opinion is asleep.

Alva Myrdal
(Einstein Peace Prize, March 1980)

Introduction

In recent years, especially in Finland, the Peace Movement has used physical activity (walking, cycling, skiing, rowing etc.) as a political means in its efforts to maintain peace in Europe. By adopting physical activity as one form of peace work, the Peace Movement is trying firstly to make the political decision makers take notice of public opinion on the subject of peace, and secondly, to offer "ordinary" citizen a possibility of working together for peace.

The first international marathon march for peace was the idea of three Norwegian women. The peace March 1981 started from Copenhagen on 22 June 1981, the route passing through Denmark (7 days), Germany (17 days), the Netherlands (5 days), Belgium (7 days) and France (13 days) to Paris. The march ended on the 6th of August - the day the first atomic bomb was dropped on Hiroshima. The distance covered in a day varied from 20 to 45 km. Sundays were rest days.

By marching, the participants wanted to demonstrate their strong desire for a peace policy instead of a war policy and their despair at the global situation, at the arms race and at nuclear arms. This march was the first march for peace that demanded both mental and physical efforts.

The Subject of the Study and the Method Used

This is a case-study about the action of the peace movement. The idea of doing this research was aroused by the questions: "What meaning has physical activity among the marathon peace marchers [1] who walked through the European countries?, "What are the main characteristics of the international Peace March?" and "How does the Peace March demonstrate international understanding?" Being a teacher, I decided to carry out this research with a group of students in physical education, who helped me in planning the questionnaire. Thus one purpose of the study was that it should serve as a part of peace education; in addition it represents a personal contribution to peace.

The study was conducted from the phenomenological perspective, accepting that "being truly objective about people means trying to hear precisely what they are saying, letting them tell their story in their own words and opening ourselves to the

---

1 With one exception, the Finnish marchers achieved the marathon distance (42.2 km), and usually more. Ten women and two girls from Finland walked the entire way (1250 km) to Paris. Eight of these 12 answered the questionnaire.

reality they are trying to convey rather than applying our own categories." (Whitson 1976). Accordingly, this paper and its structure are based on the experiences of the marchers themselves.

In this study, I attempted to develop an empathic understanding with the peace marchers by gathering different kinds of research material for the study - written, verbal and visual. The mail questionnaire with a great number of open questions was sent first in March and again in April 1982, and was returned by 19 (68%) Finnish peace marchers. Other sources of data were in-depth interviews (four, all tape recorded, taking a total of 10 hours), cassette recordings (two), newspaper articles, a periodical and about 100 pictures from the march. The research data were explored thoroughly by reading all the questionnaires and other material and calculating the frequencies of various types of statement, as well as by listening to the tapes and looking at the pictures.

The Peace March as a Social Movement

According to Tournaire (1981), it is the very character of a new social movement, such as the Peace Movement, to unite the professionals, who speak in the name of knowledge, and those who want to stay on the sidelines or are forced to do so by a central apparatus. In this case, the professionals of the Peace Movement were a core group of Nordic women, from Norway, Denmark, Sweden and Finland.

The Finnish core group in the Peace March had the political support of all Finnish parties, although they did not all have official delegates walking the 1250 km from Copenhagen to Paris. There were official delegates from the Social Democrats, the Swedish National party and the Liberal National party. The rest were from different action groups and associations.

The other participants in this social movement, who represented the "ordinary" women/men from Finnish grass-root organisations, also had different political backgrounds. In general, this group committed itself more to the left-wing than to the central and right-wing parties. This is not surprising, because up till now (i. e. before the anti-nuclear movements) the left-wing has been more active in peace work. Many of the Finnish marchers belonged to some new social movement or at least had read about them and supported them in some way. According to Finguelievich (1981), it is typical of these kinds of urban movement that they unite different social forces (old ones like political parties and new ones like action groups, alternative groups and citizen committees) when handling concrete political issues - in this case creating a non-nuclear Scandinavia and Europe from Portugal to Poland.

If we look at the political background of the march accordung to an "interview" with a member of the core group, it seems that this new social movement of peace has succeeded in its efforts to unite the professionals who are active in peace work and the ordinary citizen. She reported as follows:

> I asked many...why are you here...I mean I don't mean the core group, but those who came for a few days or for a few weeks...most of them answered...I have not been in any Peace Movement, I don't belong to any political organisation, I am not at all interested in confidential activities, but I have felt so worried about the global situation and...I have felt that I would like to do something concrete that an ordinary citizen can do....

This kind of heterogeneous political reality has been one typical characteristic of new social movements and can be seen as a criticism of the established political set-up. According to Tournaire (1980), these kinds of action are new ways of influencing politics. Both people who are not very interested in politics and those who are involved in it form the new social forces which will influence the politics of futre society. These new social movements are an expression of the collective will and lie at the heart of social life. With their different kind of action, social movements inform the policy makers what the common citizens think and what public opinion is.

The Social and Physical Background of the Peace Marchers

The typical Finnish peace marcher is a woman aged between 30 and 49 years (range among the Finnish marathon marchers: 12–65) who has had a higher level of education than the population in general and whose work is physically light. The numbers of single, married and divorced women were similar; they had more children than in average Finnish families ($\bar{x} = 2.0 > \bar{x} = 1.7$) (Marin and Stolte-Heiskanen 1980).

If we compare the participants of this peace movement with those of another Finnish social movement, the environmental movement of Koijärvi (Järvikoski 1981), we notice that there are some differences in terms of background: In the environmental movement the participants are young people coming mostly from middle-class families, while participants in the Peace March were from many age groups (but were mainly middle-aged) and the social background of their childhood families was bi-curved. In other words, some were from families of common labourers, lower administrative workers (clerical employees) and independent farmers/workers whereas others were from the highest class of society. Middle-class background was not represented at all among the peace marchers.

Before the Finnish core group (10) joined the other Nordic core groups in Copenhagen, they prepared themselves for the march both mentally and physically. One marcher reported that when she was asked to be an official delegate of her party, the following thoughts came into her mind:

> When I heard about the theme of anti-nuclear Scandinavia, anti-nuclear Europe, it was clear to me that I could accept it, but the practical question...shall I be able to stand it? I'm not a sportswoman, I don't do any physical exercise except that I don't have a car and I usually make all trips by bicycle and walking. But I'm not an active person...I was scared of this kind of practical thing. Although I have travelled and have had experiences, the situation was new and I had delusions about how people would take it on the way through Europe and that...that the core group of Nordic Women would walk alone over there on the roads in Europe. I could never have imagined that it would attract so many people...it is one of those things that carries one along right away.

The training profile of the marathon walkers (two of whom made part of the journey by bicycle) differed from the Finlandia marathon runners (Kannas et al. 1980), who trained intensively almost every day. Only two of the walkers took physical exercise continually. Thus they generally had little physical preparation for the march; for instance, one participant who completed the entire walk, described her training as follows: "Before the March I walked 20 kilometres two or three times to test myself." Another, who walked about 80 km in 2 days, asserted "This question does not concern me!" Most of the walkers prepared for the march by walking and cycling, but five participants did not train at all. Those who classified themselves as joggers (four) were the most active in training. In spite of this lack of physical training as compared with marathon runners, the marathon walkers, and especially those who had trained at least twice a week over 3 months, considered their training to have been sufficient.

Peace Work at Different Levels

At the local level the aim of the march was to bring the professional peace workers into contact with the citizens of European countries. The march succeeded in creating international relationships, especially at the local and personal level. According to this peace group, one of their most important achievements was that they managed to make people wake up to the importance of peace and to make them active in peace efforts. Hence comments were made like "it developed the Peace Movement in Europe", "we made people wake up" and "people have noticed that peace work is for all".

During the march the number of walkers varied between 300 and 700 persons. At the most (just before Paris), there were ten thousand people walking. About 110 people walked the entire way from Copenhagen to Paris.

The most impressive experience during the march was to see the friendly smiles of the ordinary citizens when the march passed by. The organised help and care on a group level was also remarkable; e. g. the help provided by the Women for Peace and other women's organisations and by the Church was unforgettable. One beautiful memory was the ringing of church bells when the marchers entered a town or village – this happened all the way through the Netherlands.

At the global and national level the Peace March tried to connect the professional policy makers and the grass-root organisations by sending telegrams both to the superpowers and to the leaders of the countries through which the march passed. This interaction was successful with the Soviet Union. Brezhnev was the only leader who sent a return telegram to the peace marchers. UNESCO also acknowledged the march and inivited about 500 peace marchers to a party in Paris.

The Peaceful Demonstration

The Peace March had some degree of organisation and some rule regarding how to reach the destination (Paris) and the goal (peace). At the same time the organisation was open, free and flexible. Anybody who wanted to join in could do so and could stay as long as they wanted. The very character of the march was, according to a participant, "like the camp of gypsies on their way to heaven".

The Peace March was like a small community with a life of its own. The marchers received and sent letters. They held meetings in their community, which had political, personal and practical problems of its own.

The core group stated that the most important aim was to keep the Peace March peaceful. There existed political and strategic disagreements at the beginning and at the end of the march, but the core group succeeded in keeping the demonstration peaceful after consulting in long, overnight meetings.

The atomosphere of the march was described by one member of the core group as follows:

> Our march was so peaceful and quiet. We never shouted any slogans...and nothing like 'we want peace, we want peace'; in a way it would have been beautiful, but still noise. We sang only folk-songs and peace songs, the soft ones, and we waved our hands and smiled... usually demonstrations are noisy and violent, but this on e was not. Also the policemen in Germany noticed that the masses can move and be without violence...so femininely soft even though 50% of the marchers were men.

Thus, the march always adhered to its principles of being politically neutral and reacting non-violently in the face of obstacles like the strategy of civil defence. The whole march demonstrated, put into practice and developed a positive conception of peace (Galtung 1970).

The Meaning of Physical Activity Among the Peace Marchers

The peace marchers gained their strength to continue more from the other walkers, from singing and from the common aim - peace - than from their own physical condition. The continuing movement and the social life of the march was one main source of strength. The Buddhist monks played an important role in this feeling of continuity by calling the peace marchers with their drums every morning to start moving on their way to Paris. Thus the march itself gave people power to carry out the plan. The participants reported how once a person had joined the march, the march itself carried him or her forward towards the common goal.

Marching has a very important social meaning for peace work and international understanding in many respects. Firstly, everybody can walk and can express her/his opinion regarding peace policy without political knowledge and political discussions. Most of the marchers reported that they had come along to express their anti-nuclear opinion by walking for peace. Secondly, while walking it is possible to walk to other peace workers and to create contacts with people from different countries. Thus marchers said "I wanted to get to know personally other peace workers in different countries" and "I wanted to feel myself a part of the Eurpean Peace Movement". Moving from Copenhagen to Paris made them feel that they had done something concrete for peace: "I have been in the Women for Peace Movement since 1980. We have talked and discussed a lot. I wanted to do something concrete for peace, I wanted to make a self-sacrifice." An old peace-work activist felt that for the first time in her life she had really achieved something, despite the fact that she had talked and listended to speeches at international level, e. g. at UN conferences and meetings of different states.

Almost everybody's best experience was the mutual interaction and feeling of solidarity. The Peace March gave strength to the participants and reduced their feeling of powerlessness. According to Tournaire (1981), one of the attributes of new social movements is that they give the participants the same feeling of togetherness that used to be present in earlier communities with face-to-face relationships. Thus through the march the Peace Movement offered people in mass society a chance to experience social reality with a common goal. The Peace March made the participants feel that they can still make their own history instead of leaving it to the professional policy makers.

The Finnish Peace Marchers were critical of organised sport. They felt, for instance, that the Olympic Games may even have a negative influence because they arouse ultranationalism and develop national values and ethnocentrism rather than international goodwill. Some did not understand how competitive sport could promote co-operation and international understanding because it is based on the attitude that one competitor must be better than the other, which is analogous to the situation in the arms race, when the superpowers think: "One must be more powerful than the other".

Thus the Peace Marchers agree with Heinilä's criticisms (1971), believing that while sport promotes goodwill and international understanding among athletes, it may simultaneously have latent negative effects in establishing negative attitudes towards other nations. The most active members of this peace group in terms of physical exercise had the most positive attitudes towards sport, seeing it mainly as promoting international understanding.

Conclusion

This case-study on the Peace March 1981 supported Tournaire's (1981) conception about a new social movement being *a heterogeneous political reality*. Further, the movement brought together *the professionals* of knowledge (in peace and politics) and people who were not active in these matters - *the "ordinary" people*. The main characteristic of the Peace March was that it was *a peaceful demonstration for peace*. Physical exercise and sport did not play a big role in the participants' everyday life and they did not train for the march (according to the criteria of sportswomen/men). Their physical activity predominantly takes place during the summertime and consists of taking a walk, riding a bicycle or wandering in the countryside. Nevertheless, it was the physical activity of walking which enabled the participants to meet and converse with others; and even when there was no common language, *walking* together side by side was in itself *a common language* symbolising peace, the marchers' common goal. Similarly, walking made the abstract concept of peace something real and concrete.

The most imortant aspect of the physical activity of marching in relation to "the peace process" was the way it involved not just the mind but the whole body and the feelings as well. Thus one marcher reported:

> Before the peace march I had ambivalent feelings towards peace work. It was the most important thing to me in the world, yet at the same time the fear of nuclear war and the feeling that there were no possibilities, nothing for me to do, depressed me greatly. The main effect of the Peace March was that this desperate depression disappeared. I was very surprised by this change. During the march I did not do any other peace work except walking. The discussions were rare and did not concern world policy at all. Berit Ås thought that the change was caused by the fact that I participated in peace work with my whole being, the whole of my body, my muscles, my will power etc. and...the most important thing is that the perfomance demanded all my energy - I had to put all my effort into the perfomance of the task...

This statement reflects the fact that physical activity has a very important role in the peace process, because it works even without words and conversation. This presupposes that the idea for which one is working is clear and accepted. According to the research data, physical exercise is probably one way to change entrenched attitudes.

All of the marchers became more active in peace work; in the words of one marcher: "Participants became peace activists for the rest of their lives." By walking together in this transpolitical and transnational march, the feeling of powerlessness turned into a feeling of strength. The march led to a deeper level of understanding, sympathetic understanding, and thus promoted an attitude of patience in mutual interaction.

Thus, finally, we can reply to Alva Myrdal's statement, quoted at the start of this paper: According to this case-study, public opinion is no longer asleep. This conclusion is supported by the many local peace marches that took place in the autums of 11981 (World Students News 1982).

References

Brock-Utne B (1981) The role of women, as mothers and members of society, in the education of young people for peace. Paper presented at the Expert Meeting on the Role of Women in Education for Peace, Mutual Understanding and Respect for Human Rights. United Nations Educational, Scientific and Cultural Organization, New Dehli, India, 7-11 Nov 1981

Finguelievich S (1981) Urban social movements and the production of urban space. Acta Sociologia 24/4:239-249

Galtung J (1970) Rauhanomaisen poulustuksen strategia. (The strategy of peaceful defence.) Kirjapaino Jaarli, Hämeenlinna

Galtung J (1975) Peace: Research - education - action. Copenhagen

Heinilä K (1971) Notes on inter-group conflicts in international sport. In: Dunning E (ed) The sociology of sport. Cass, London, pp 343-350

Heinilä K (1975) Kilpaurheilun säätelyjärjestelmä. (The regulation system of competitive sports.) Jyväskylän yliopiston Liikuntasuunnittelun laitos. Tutkimuksia 9:1

Järvikoski T (1981) Alternative movements in Finland: The case study of Koijärvi. Research Note. Acta Sociologica 24/4:313-320

Jensen J, Simonsen K (1981) The local state, planning and social movements. Acta Sociologica 24/4: 279-291

Kannas L (1981) The life-style of active joggers: A study of Finlandia marathon-runners. A paper presented at the first ICHPER Europe Congress: Social aspects of physical education and sport. Wingate, Israel, 28 Dec 1980 - 2 Jan 1981

Marin M, Stolte-Heiskanen V (1981) Suomalainen perhe eristyy, yksityistyy, yhteiskunnallistuu. (Finnish families are getting more isolated, private, communal.) Tiede 2000 2:5-10

Pietilä H (1981) Women for peace. Development Forum 11

Touraine A (1981) The voice and the eye. An anlysis of social movements. Cambridge University Press, Cambridge

Whitson DJ (1976) Method in sport sociology: The potential of a phenomenological contribution. Int Rev Sport Soc 4 (11):53-70

World Student News 36/1:18-21, 24

Ways of Promoting Voluntary Physical Activity in Present-Day Society

L. Heinilä

Introduction

Background

Addressing himself to the important question "Why coluntary gymnastics?", Pierre Seurin (1968), President of the F. I. E. P., stated in a paper presented at an international congress in Madrid in 1966: "Greater health means greater happiness, less expense on *(sic)* the family level and greater social output." The world 'health' here (as in all studies of physical activity) refers not only to the absence of illness but also to the ability of the body to defend itself against and to tolerate these and other 'attacks' made upon it by the social environment, as well as to the ability to face current and future events in a favourable, creative, confident and optimistic way (Langlade 1980). Hilma Jalkanen (1961), who instigated the development of women's gymnastics in Finland, put it concisely as follows: "Physical activity should engender 'vigour' in the individual, i. e. a strong taste for life, a readiness to lead a diverse and rich life."

Discussing the problem of the development of voluntary physical activity Pierre Seurin (1968) laid special emphasis on the significance of practice: "Our aim is to determine... the best means to put into practice hygienic and recreational physical exercises for adults." How well has this aim been achieved in recent decades, what are the problems for the practice of voluntary physical activity in the next decade, and how should it be promoted? It is obvious that there are indeed problems and a need for development, as only one in three people participate in some type of physical activity (and of those who do, only a third are women).

Aims

It is my aim in this short article to discuss the methods through which voluntary physical activity could be promoted in the context of the physical culture in present-day society, and the ideology of 'sport for everyone', i. e. equality, implemented more effectively. I will consider the question mainly with regard to sociology and psychology, and I will attempt to set up a model which includes them both.

The European Sport-for-All Charter defines sport-for-all as a comprehensive concept, embracing sport in many different forms, in which all people have the right to participate, of whatever sex or age and at whatever level of skill or commitment (The greater involvement of women in sport 1980).

Physical Activity and Equality

Human needs, such as physical exercise, are the motivating force of man's physical activity. However, they are by no means the only factor determining such activity. In the individual, physical culture appears in the form of his participation in various sporting activities - the term referring to actual physical exercises as well as to the sum total of the needs, aims, motives and interests related to and influencing those exercises (Ojala 1980).

From the viewpoint of the individual, physical exercises are more than just an attempt to maximise physical performance; they are a means of maintaining and improving the basis for physical, mental and social activity, of expanding one's frame of reference in life. Physical exercises provide the opportunity to enjoy an active leisure time, relaxation and recuperation.

The individual, however, is a member of society even when engaging in physical activities. In contemporary, competitive society, the social status of the individual is determined by his or her achievements. The content and form of these may vary a great deal between the sexes and age groups, for instance. *Equality is not the same as similarity. In a cultural setting, equality can be looked at from the viewpoint of the distribution of power. 'Power' here denotes an extensive set of concepts which includes an individual's right to express himself or herself, to satisfy his or her needs, and to participate in societal decision making - including that on issues related to physical activities.* It is this level of decision making that has assumed a considerable importance during the past decade. Therefore, those who engage in voluntary physical activities should recognise the influence of this factor on 'happiness'.

Environment of Physical Activities as a Cultural Unit

In the present context, the term 'physical culture' refers to the sum total of the physical activities practised in a given society, determined as this is by the values, norms and beliefs prevalent in that society, and by the hierarchy of these, i. e. the cultural ethos. One can thus differentiate between the physical cultures of various nations, e. g. between "Swededucation", "Finneducation" etc. These man-made settings are, of course, based on the natural environment, on climate, terrain and the characteristic of the people. In Scandinavian countries, for instance, the seasons are one factor regulating and directing physical activities.

Within the realm of physical culture, too, equality can be looked at with respect to the use of power. Power is maintained both by internal and external actions. The internal ones inhere in the sports setting itself, and consist of the values, ideologies and myths used in order to maintain the prevailing distribution of power. These values ideologies and myths are acquired during the time one is growing up, through the physical education environment. They include such factors as the time, facilities and resources available for a given physical education purpose. By the external uses of power, the means of suppression, are here understood various external forces brought to bear on sports, i. e. social factors such as laws and norms. These internal and external uses of power determine the make-up of our physical education environment by producing conditions either favourable or unfavourable to specific individuals and groups of individuals engaging in physical activities (Fig. 1).

Value / Physical culture		External use of power	
		Favourable	Unfavourable
Internal uses of power	Unfavourable	+ −	− −
	Favourable	+ +	− +

Fig. 1. Environment of physical activities as a culatural unit
(+, promoting voluntary activity; −, militating against voluntary activity)

Physical Culture Today

Changing Environment of Physical Activities

The development of physical culture and its contemporary manifestations have been greatly influenced by the social changes of the past decades. The most important of these include production-related and technical progress, motorization, automation and urbanisation, as well as changes that have affected the whole of the societal system, e. g. democratisation and bureaucratisation. The decrease in the opportunities for what might be called natural physical activity has been accompanied by an increase in the need for organised physical activities.

Sports organisations of considerable magnitude have been established lately, and a great deal of money is being spent on building facilities for various physical activities. An increasing number of physical activity services are being offered, e. g. the facilities and services provided for the members of society by various physical education organisations at purely nominal rates.

Within the world of physical culture, and also in the field of physical education, there has been an *increase in the conformity to norms.* Physical education policy has become significant, as has research into physical education, financially supported by the Finnish Government. Finland was the first Scandinavian country to bring into force in 1980 a law and a corresponding statute concerning physical education. They define the methods for implementing decisions related to physical education policy. The law provides a description of the general principles of physical education administration and of the system of financial support from the Government, and sets down the regulations concerning Government support of both voluntary physical activities and those organised by local authorities.

As financial contributors to these physical education services, i. e. as taxpayers, we all are in a fairly equal position. But what is our position with respect to the use of these services? On whose terms do we actually engage in physical activities, today and tomorrow?

It is reasonable to ask whether 'humanity' is on the verge of disappearing. To take one example, the sex test carried out before any major international sporting event reveals a lot about the values prevailing in one subarea of physical culture, in competitive sports: strength, aggressiveness, a fighting spirit, endurance, ambition. Also, materialistic and commercial values have entered the picture, and professionalism has become more widespread. Is the world of physical activities a "man's world"? Are the ideologies of 'Sport-for-All' and amateurism adequately realised in it? When physical education services are offered, is there a bias towards materialistic values - does the individual become a production unit, a part of a machine? Sports should not be abused. Obviously, we cannot hope to do more today than to try to stop the world from destroying itself, to quote freely from Albert Camus, winner of the Nobel Prize for literature.

Values Guide Our Physical Activities!

Research (Kenyon 1968) has indicated that attitudes towards physical activities are related to the instrumental value of a given activity. The most distinct of these attitudes are:

1. Physical activity as a social experience: provides a medium for social intercourse, i. e. to meet new people and perpetuate existing relationships
2. Physical activity for health and fitness: desire to improve one's physical performance, strength and endurance
3. Physical activity as the pursuit of vertigo: desire to experience thrill, speed, danger and novel feelings
4. Physical activity as an aesthetic experience: desire to enjoy a beautiful, polished performance and the atmosphere, to feel the rhythm and to express it and/or oneself in physical movement
5. Physical activity as catharsis: desire for relaxation through physical activity, for going at one's own pace
6. Physical activity as an ascetic experience: desire to become an athlete, to engage in long-term training, to work hard to achieve a certain end
7. Physical activity as chance: desire to experience change and unexpected situations, to refresh oneself

In the international study mentioned above, it was shown that attitudes were related to sex. Women's (girls') attitudes were more favourable towards physical activities which incorporated social-, health- and fitness-related and aesthetic experiences. On the other hand, boys' attitudes were more favourable towards activities which contained elements of thrill, ascetic experiences and chance. People in older age groups were more inclined towards appreciation of activities with ascetic and cathartic experiences. Attitudes towards physical activity are also related, to some extent, to other behavioural preferences, to understanding and appreciation of one's own body, to a need for attention from others and to one's relationship with one's parents.

The Kenyon scale has been used in Finland as well, with similar results (Telama et al. 1981; Laakso 1967). The most important motive was health and fitness, the second most important, recreation. It must be noted, however, that the concept of health turned out to be very broad in this study. As obstacles to participation in physical activities, the following factors were mentioned: laziness and desire for comfort, other interests, lack of time and homework.

The familiy also influences the extent to which individuals participate in physical activities (Engström 1975; Fasting 1980; Vuolle et al. 1981). What is more, such participation has been shown to be related to social class membership (Fasting 1980). For instance, Norwegians in the upper social class have been shown to be physically more active than Norwegians in the lower social classes - which is the reverse of the situation prevailing in France (Fasting 1980).

Research evidence suggests that women's participation in sport has increased. However, their share in the decision making in sport is rahter modest, as was noted by Monique Berlioux (1980), President of the Olympic Committee, in a Council of Europe seminar on the promotion of women's participation in sport. Moreover, research findings (Ferris 1981; Wilmore 1979) show that there is little difference between the level of physical performance in men and women who participate in sports on an active basis. By means of physical activity, a women can maintain, from age 10 throughout her life, the same level of endurance, for instance, as a man of equivalent age. As to the differences in the values espoused by the sexes, witness the fact that women's interest in gymnastics is limited hardly at all by factors such as the seasons or age. Rather, women remain faithful to the sport.

Towards Humanity and Equality in Physical Culture

In both research and the increasing physical education planning based on it, the deficiencies of voluntary physical activities have been clearly recognised, and action is underway to eliminate them. For instance, in 1981 the sports committee of the Council of Europe published a set of directives and recommendations intended to promote women's participation in sport (The greater involvement of women in sport 1980).

In Finland and in other Scandinavian countries, physical education planning teams have been active, emphasising the need for the sports policy of the twentieth century to develop physical education services suitable to all, as well as different kinds of physical activiy. To give an example, Juppi (1980) has advanced the following three points:

1. Given the increasing differentiation of human life, and the attendant emphasis on specialisation, stress should be laid in physical education not only on specialisation but also on *natural, holistic physical activities.*
2. As alternatives to specialisation, links should be established between physical activities, on the one hand, and *activities of the spiritual culture such as art,* and *social interaction,* on the other.
3. The monotonous and extremely *serious* type of fitness exercise of today should be replaced by *more relaxing and joyful physical exercise.*

In order to achieve these goals, it is necessary to study not only the content of teaching but also its methods, in other words the way in which the interaction between individuals is carried out during the teaching event (Heinilä 1977).

Finally, I am glad to be able to say that physical education planners, who control decision making in sports at the various levels, have increasingly come to appreciate natural physical activity, including, for instance, the ideology and methods of women's gymnastics, as was noted above. Also, the need for co-operation between the generations has been recognised, as has the relevance of the family unit to the level of physical activity.

In an attempt to promote physical culture, we should strive to influence it by employing both internal and external means of using power. We should try to make an impact on the formation of the structure and the value hierarchy of physical culture as well as on the environment in which it takes place so as to enable it to express on an even higher level the ideology of 'sport for everyone' - humanity. *It is important that we recognise what we are doing, but even more so* how *and* why *we do it.*

References

Berlioux M (1981) Women in the promotion and administration of sport. The greater involvement of women in sport. Seminar report. Council of Europe, 1980, pp 75-81. FIEP Bull 51/2:22-27

Engström L-M (1975) Fysisk Aktivitet under Ungdomsåren. (Physical activity during adolescence.) Pedagogiska Institutionen, Lärarhögskolan i Stockholm

Fasting K (1980) Et litteraturstudium og en ampirisk undersøkelse on hvilke faktorer som er av betydning for utøvelse av fysisk aktivitetet i fritiden. (A review of literature and an empirical study of the significant factors related to physical activity in leisure.) Norges Idrottshøgskole

Ferris E (1981) The physiological make-up of women and its effect on their participation in sport. The greater involvement of women in sport. Seminar report. Council of Europe, 1980, pp 53-55. FIEP Bull 51/2:7-12

Heinilä L (1977) Analysing systems in the evaluation of the teacher-pupil interaction in physical education classes. In: Tammivuori T (ed) Evaluation in the development of physical education. Congress report. The Finnish Society for Research in Sport and Physical Education 64:37-58. FIEP Bull 47/1:20-34

Jalkanen H (1961) Voimistelu voi antaa arvokasta lisäsisältöä elämälle. Kisakenttä 50/1:8-10

Juppi J (1980) Liikuntakulttuurin yleiset kehitysnäkymät 1980-luvulla. (The development of physical culture in the 1980s.) In: Lagus P (ed) liikuntasuunnittelu. Liikuntatieteellisen Seuran julkaisu 77:42

Kenyon G (1970) Attitude toward sport and physical activity among adolescents from four English speaking countries. In: Lüschen G (ed) Cross-cultural analysis of sport and games. Stipes, Champaign, pp 138-155

Laakso L (1979) Evaluation of lifelong sport interest. In: Tammivuori T (ed) Evaluation in the development of physical education. Congress report. The Finnish Society for Research in Sport and Physical Education 64:176-182

Langlade A (1981) La santécomme objectif de la Science des Activités physiques. Conférence présentée âla "Gimnasiado Americana de Santo Domingo", October, 1980. FIEP Bull 51/2:13-20

Ojala R (1981) Liikuntasuunnittelun käsitejärjestelmä. (The conceptual structure of planning of physical culture.) In: Lagus P (ed) Liikuntasuunnittelu. Liikuntatieteellisen Seuran julkaisu 77:11-14

Seurin P (1968) How to develop adults physical education (voluntary keep-fit gymnastics). FIEP Bull 38/3-4:39-47

Telama R, Vuolle P, Laakso L (1981) Health and physical fitness as motives for physical activity among Finnish urban adults. Int J Phys Ed 18/1:11-16

The greater involvement of women in sport. Seminar report (1980). Council of Europe

Vuolle P, Laakso L, Telama R (1981) Physical and sport activities and their prerequisites: differences between married Finnish men and women. Paper presented at the IX International Seminar. "Sport Leisure and the family", Brussels, 9-13 Sept 1981. In: Reports of Physical Culture and Health 34. Research Institute of Physical Culture and Health, Yearbook. Jyväskylä, Finland, pp 57-67

Wilmore JH (1979) The application of science to sport: physiological profiles of male and female athletes. Can J Appl Sport Sci 4:103-115

3. Sport for Special Groups

The Extent, Content and Organisation of International Sport for the Disabled in the Past, Present and Future

K.-A. Jochheim

Analysing international involvement in sporting competition about 30 years ago, E. Jokl (1956) used the XVth Olympic Games in Helsinki to carry out an international study which was introduced with the following preface:

> The sport movement has become a part of modern civilization. The Olympic Games bring representatives of nations all round the world to meet each other and compete in accordance with a set of rules accepted by all contestants. Participation and advancement at the Olympic Games reflect, within certain limits, the extent to which each nation shows interest in competitive athletics. Changes in the contribution of different nations to the games and in the general level of results may reveal interesting and important trends.

A fairly similar position my be taken towards the international sporting activities of disabled citizens insofar as they constitute a quite accurate yardstick of the relationship between rehabilitation in general and special methods promoting health education as well as community-based long-term rehabilitation programmes.

The Development of International Sport for the Disabled

It is interesting to realise that those disability groups which receive quite early support in society, namely the deaf, the blind and physically disabled war victims, achieved a world-wide sports organisation almost 20 years ago (Guttmann 1979). On the initiative of the World Veterans' Federation, a working group was set up in 1960 on Sport for the Disabled. However, because of insurmountable differences of opinion this group had to be dissolved in 1964. Finally under the patronage of the World Veterans' Federation the International Sports Organisation for the Disabled was founded and became an independent body in 1967. Apart from this international movement, Sir Ludwig Guttmann had introduced sport into his paraplegic centre in Stoke Mandeville and held a small competition between paraplegics and war and accident victims, most of whom were unable to survive until the change from passive treatment to active involvement had been made. In 1960, with the first competition of wheelchair-bound athletes in Rome, the International Stoke-Mandeville Games Committee was founded; after that the celebrated Para-Olympic Games were held with growing success in Tokyo in 1964, Jerusalem in 1968 and Heidelberg in 1972.

Competition between organisations frequently led to a unification of activities, and finally the International Sports Organisation for the Disabled and the International Stoke Mandeville Games Committee unified to hold joint competitions. The first of these was held in 1974 in the Stoke Mandeville sports stadium. Since that time the Para-Olympic Games of 1976 in Canada and 1980 in Arnheim have been powerful demonstrations of a unified international sports organisation, supported more or less substantially by a national sport orgnaisation for the disabled. Governments, social services and private donators have been helpful in organising not only the regular national activities but also the international competitions and the medical provision. In addition, the physical educators have been involved in safeguarding adherence to rules and regulations and the proper classification of the disability groups. However, in these competitions the classic disability groups - the blind, the amputees and now the paraplegics, with their well-defined programme of wheelchair sport - have been the main competitors. These groups could be considered healthy despite their disability and therefore have not suffered from medical restrictions as far as the competition itself is concerned. This remark does not, however, cover every discipline, and there are certainly some physical activities which cannot be performed without considerable risk of accident. Such hazards as bicycle riding for the blind or sprinting for above-knee amputees should certainly be excluded by rules and regulations in connection with the classification. In the meantime rehabilitation procedures have been applied to many other disabilities and handicaps resulting from congenital deficiencies, accidents and acute and chronic diseases, some of which were fatal at an earlier stage of medical development. These disability groups, e. g. those whith coronary heart disease, frequently need a much higher level of medical supervision and a higher level of skill as far as coaching is concerned, because the area of treatment and the area of sport come together much more closely, sometimes overlapping considerably. Hence close co-operation between doctors and coaches is necessary.

The WHO Classification as a Basis for Research into the Present and Future Development of Sport for the Disabled

Two volumes collected by Jochheim and van der Schoot (1981) demonstrate in which areas of research much has still to be done nationally and internationally in order to evaluate world-wide model activities and to guide those activities through accompanying research towards local, national and international comparison. The tools for such evaluation have been published recently by the World Health Organisation (1980) in a volume entitled *International Classification of Impairments, Disabilities and Handicaps.* Many of the health deficiencies result in a loss or anormality of psychological, physiological or anatomical structure or function - this is termed *"impairment". "Disability",* on the other hand, is defined as any restriction on or lack (resulting from an impairment) of ability to perform an activity in the manner or within the range considered normal for a human being. Finally, *"handicap"* describes the disadvantage for a given individual resulting from an impairment or a disability that limits or prevents the fulfilment of a role that is normal (depending on age, sex, and social and cultural factors) for that individual.

Sport for the disabled therefore aims, within the context of rehabilitation, to prevent an impairment if possible, increasing function by means of exercises and technical aids, and removing the disadvantages of handicaps by fostering social integration in an adapted environment. Research has to envisage these different targets in order to produce convincing results.

Table 1. Classification of disabilities needing a long-term programme of physical activity

Classification of disabilities	Clinic	School	Vocational training	Leisure time
1. Physical disabilities				
Heart and vascular diseases	+	-	(+)	+
Hypertension, peripheral vascular disease	+	-	(+)	+
Coronary disease	+	-	(+)	+
Congenital and acquired heart failure	-	-	-	-
Pacemaker clients	(+)	-	-	-
Impairment of lung function (i.e. athma)	+	-	+	+
Impairment of liver function	(+)	-	-	-
Impairment of renal function	(+)	-	-	(+)
Impairment of metabolism (diabetes, adipositas)	+	(+)	-	+
Haematological diseases	+	-	-	-
Dysfunction of the autonomous nervous system	+	-	(+)	(+)
Tumours	+	-	-	(+)
Motor system disabilities				
Amputations	+	-	+	+
Congenital limb impairments	+	(+)	+	+
Joint impairments and rheumatism	+	(+)	+	+
Congenital muscular dystrophy	-	(+)	-	(+)
Disabilities following imlpairment of central and peripheral nervous system				
Cerebral palsy	(+)	+	-	+
Brain damage in adulthood	(+)	+	-	+
Epilepsy	+	(+)	(+)	(+)
Spinal cord lesion in childhood	(+)	+	-	(+)
Spinal cord lesion in adulthood	+	+	+	+
2. Disability involving sensory organs and communication				
Blindness	(+)	(+)	+	+
Visual impairment	-	(+)	+	+
Deafness	-	(+)	-	+
Hard of hearing	-	(+)	-	+
Deafness and dumbness	-	+	+	+
Deafness and blindness	-	-	-	-
Voice and speech impairment	-	-	-	-
3. Learning disabilities				
Moderate mental retardation	-	+	-	+
Severe mental retardation	-	+	(+)	+
4. Behavioural disabilities				
Psychosis	(+)	-	-	-
Neurotic behaviour	(+)	(+)	-	+
Drug abuse	(+)	-	-	+
Alcoholism	(+)	-	-	+
Social deviation	(+)	(+)	-	(+)
5. Multiple disabilities				
Including geriatrics	+	(+)	-	+
6. Other disabilities e.g.				
Oncological and dermatological disorders	(+)	-	-	-

[a] + Scientific reports available
(+) A few incomplete descriptions of sporting activities in the field are available
\- No activities or no scientific evaluation

WHO policy on disability prevention and rehabilitation has also stressed the need for community-based activities to avoid or at least shorten the institutional care of disabled persons. Sport for the disabled, however, has to be introduced in institutions in order to foster skills and the motivation to continue on a community level. The need for a long-term continuation of physical activity goes closely in hand with the need for cheaper and more effective domestic programmes for disabled persons. Community-based sport programmes with sufficient variety for the different disability groups may provide one of the answers, since resources become more restrained and the disabled proportion of the population increases with greater longevity and the improvement of medical services. The recent research results are presented in Table 1. These results need to be translated into an active programme for the coming years. Basic criteria were developed during the international year for disabled persons, but there is a common understanding that the implementation of such programmes on regional, national and international levels will require at least a decade to achieve tangible results. The United Nations are presently discussing the feasibility of a long-term programme, and we should urge our governments to support such planning for a decade, hoping that the international disabled sports movement would benefit from such a co-ordinated effort.

Priorities for a Long-Term Programme

The working panel on sports in the German National Commission for the International Year of Disabled Persons (1981) stated that insufficient use is still being made of the opportunities for sport therapy in connection with in-patient treatment and for out-patient sport for the disabled. Certain groups of disabled persons, such as emotionally disturbed persons, are not given an opportunity to take part in sports for the disabled. Sport for the disabled, whether in the out-patient sphere or with a more specific target in out-patient rehabilitation, must be intensified by better staffing and equipment.

Sports should also be available for the emotionally disturbed and (on a wider scale than hitherto) the mentally handicapped, and the requisite instructors must be trained. Where suitable sports methods are lacking, they should be developed. Furthermore, the sheltered workshops should provide more sport for the disabled than in the past.

Ordinary sports clubs provide few facilities for either leisure-time sports for the disabled or vocational rehabilitation.

Therefore a long-term programme should have the following priorities:

The sports clubs should establish sports groups for the disabled and in particular for handicapped children and adolescents. The institutions for vocational rehabilitation should incorporate a wide range of leisure-time sport for the disabled within their programme.

The current scientific studies on sport for the disabled have produced some significant and detailed findings, for example on the mentally handicapped and on persons exhibiting disturbed behavior. As a whole, the research results to date do not suffice for most groups of handicapped persons as a basis for responsible planning. Improvements should be made in introducing and financing research projects on sport for the disabled and on evaluating their findings. The results ought to be made available to all interested organisations. Appropriate subjects for research projects would be:

- The opportunities and limits of sport for the disabled with regard to various types of handicap
- The range and nature of sports facilities
- The question of altering attitudes by means of sport for the disabled
- Social re-integration via sport for the disabled
- Programme of training and further education

Since the sports movement is playing an increasing role in modern civilisation, the integration of disabled persons into society has to utilise sport for the disabled as a means to increase and improve physical activities, leisure-time planning and social acceptance for those members of our population who suffeer from diseases or accidents, with more or less permanent impairment.

References

Guttman, Sir Ludwig (1979) Sport für Körperbehinderte. Urban & Schwarzenberg, Munich

Internationaler Arbeitskreis Sport- und Freizeiteinrichtungen e.V. Köln (1981) Behindertengerechte Sport-und Freizeitanlagen

Jokl E, Karvonen M J, Kihlberg J, Koskela A, Noro L (1956) Sports in the cultural pattern of the world. Kirpe Mono Oy, Helsinke

Jochheim K-A, van der Schoot P (1981 a) Behindertensport und Rehabilitation, Teil I (Schriftenreihe des Bundesinstituts für Sportwissenschaft, vol 37). Hofmann, Schorndorf

Jochheim K-A, van der Schoot P (1981 b) Behindertensport und Rehabilitation, Teil II (Schriftenreihe des Bundesinstituts für Sportwissenschaft, vol 38). Hofmann, Schorndorf

International Year of Disabled Persons (1981) Report Nr. 9: Sports for the Disabled. In: Report and recommendations presented by the National Commision of the FRG. Federal Minister of Labour and Social Affairs, Cologne

WHO (1980) International classification of impairments, disabilities, and handicaps. World Health Organization, Geneva

The Improvement of International Co-operation and Exchange of Information in Relation to Sports for the Disabled and Other Special Groups

M. Jääskeläinen, E. Heikkinen, K. Koivumäki, U. Lahtinen and V. Puputti

Background

By order of the Finnish Ministry of Education, a plan for the improvement of sports for the disabled and other special groups was completed at the end of 1981. In this plan, handicapped, chronically ill and elderly persons were considered as special groups. The plan was drawn up by a committee of experts set up for this purpose (Opetusministeriö 1981).

When preparing the Finnish national plan, the committee made comparative analyses of corresponding systems in four other countries: Sweden, Norway, the German Democratic Republic and the Federal Republic of Germany. In the comparisons emphasis was laid on the organisation of the sports and physical education offered to the special groups. The information was obtained via official ministry channels, orientation trips and literature from the countries to be compared. In addition, the knowledge gained through the international connections of Finnish organisations of sport for the disabled was used. The information collected concentrated on the sports facilities (teachers, transportation etc.) for the special groups and ways of organising and improving sporting activities. The comparative study demonstrates that the problems in these different countries are basically the same, whereas organisational aspects vary greatly.

In the past, international exchange of information on sports and physical education for special groups has been rare. International contacts in sports for the disabled do, however, have a more established basis than co-operation in sport for the other special groups, which is still at an initial stage.

In the four compared countries, the essential feature of the arrangement of sporting activitiy is the co-operation between one large federal sport organisation for the handicapped and the official administration. In the countries in question the national sports organisations sport for the disabled were established during the 1950s or 1960s. The state and communities support these organisations in all four countries. All the countries have tried to specify the groups that should be included in the activities of the sports organisation for the handicapped.

The division of labour between the sports administration and social and public health care aroused some discussion among the officials in Finland. The reason for this is the significance of sport for the disabled in terms of rehabilitation and the fact that rehabilitation is an important function of the social and public health care organisation.

In several countries the sports organisations for the disabled arrange instructor training, but in Norway, for example, the department for sport and youth affairs participates in carrying out the training and in preparing the training material.

This paper, based on the material collected by the committee, will point out some aspects of the international connections in sports for special groups, as well as the ways of utilising the experiences of different countries to improve sport for special groups in Finland.

International Co-operation

During recent decades, active and fairly broad international co-operation has developed in sports for the disabled. In 1948 Sir Ludwig Guttman initiated the Stoke Mandeville Games for the disabled, which developed into an international event in 1952 and has been called, since 1960, the Special Olympics. Participation in the summer games of these Olympics has been constantly increasing; in 1980 in Arnheim the number of competitors exceeded 2000. Participation in the winter games, which were started in Sweden in 1975, is also constantly increasing. In addition to those disabled by motor and spinal malfunctions, people with a visual or hearing handicap or cerebral palsy participate in these Special Olympics. The mentally retarded have also had their own international competitions.

Several international organisations have been founded to promote international sporting activities for the disabled, the first significant organisation being the International Stoke Mandeville Games Federation (ISMGF). The International Sport Organization for the Multidisabled (ISOD) was established in 1964, and other organisations (CP-ISRA etc.) work in the same field. In addition to these specific sports organisations, some international physical culture organisations have dealt with sports for the disabled and other special groups in past years. UNESCO and the European Council have studied the question and made recommendations to governments and to ministries concerned with sport in the member countries. The Committee for Development of Sports of the European Council has initiated procedures for improving the sporting activity of the elderly. International symposia and seminars were organised in connection with the Year of the Handicapped in 1981. In addition, UNESCO organised an international symposium on sports for the disabled in the USA in the autumn of 1982. An important aim in the future should be to faciliate co-operation between different countries in questions of sports for special groups.

Suggestions for Developing Physical Education and Sports for Special Groups in Finland Based on the Comparative Study

The following findings of the comparative analysis were utilised in the plan to develop sport for special groups in Finland:

In Sweden transportation arrangements are, according to the Committee, well organised for severely disabled persons. Furthermore, the Committee was especially interested in the Swedish project to involve disabled children and recently disabled persons in sport, which has produced interesting results.

In both Sweden and Norway, important experience has been gained in relation to consultation arrangements at a national level regarding sport for the disabled.

From Norwegian experiences, useful conclusions were drawn concerning winter sport and recreation for the disabled and the instructor training appropriate for special groups. The Committee also considered the arrangement of annual national conferences on education and planning of sports for special groups in idea worthy of consideration. Sports education from the viewpoint of the special groups, as already practised in Norway and the Federal Republic of Germany, was also mentioned by the Committee in its report.

The report of the Committee outlines the rehabilitation law passed in 1974 in the Federal Republic of Germany and especially stresses the significance of this law for rehabilitation and the financial support of sport for special groups.

The good scientific and practical results obtained from motion analysis in sports for special groups in the Federal Republic of Germany and the German Democratic Republic were taken into account by the Committee. Furthermore, the German Democratic Republic's experiences in relation to co-operation with medical expertise and the medical control of special groups are presented in the report.

Of course, these examples are neither exhaustive nor necessarily the most representative from these countries. Furthermore, there were informative experiences to be drawn from other countries, too. However, in order to give some concrete illustrations of the significance of the exchange of international information, these examples were selected. The adaption of an operative system, or a part of it, used in another country requires complete knowledge of the details as well as flexibility and consideration of the circumstances in the adapting country. A comparison can, however, be significant in improving a national system.

Suggestions at an International Level

As a result of the national plan for developing sport for special groups, Finland has proposed to UNESCO the following three objectives for international organisations concerned with physical culture:

1. Improving the physical culture for special groups as a whole (attitudinal education, distribution of information, recommendations for realisation of the "Sports for All" ideal).
2. Promotion of co-operation between neighbouring countries, e.g. in co-ordinating the production of educational and informational material.
3. Concrete recommendations to render the sports facilities more suitable for the disabled.

Encouraging the sporting activities of the disabled and other special groups influences positively the entire physical culture. It emphasises the health-restoring influence of sport. The international Olympic movement might learn something from the International Sport for the Disabled movement. It is our sincere hope that in the future, international co-operation in physical culture will be fostered and thus help create better conditions for the participation of the disabled and chronically ill in physical activities. To achieve this goal, international organisations must strive to improve the collection and distribution of results of research into sports for special groups.

Reference

Opetusministeriö (1981) Erityisryhmien Liikuntatoimikunnan mietintö. Kom. miet 44. Helsinki (Ministry of Education. Report of the Committee of Physical Education and Sports for Special Groups)

Volunteers in Sport for the Disabled: A Case Study

J. Drowatzky and H. Marcal

Introduction

In September 1980 I (J. D.) was contacted to see if I would be willing to serve as a volunteer professional for 2 weeks in the state of Parana, Brazil. The goal of this volunteer project was to assist in the development of physical education and rehabilitation programmes for the mentally retarded and to establish an exchange between Toledo, Ohio and the Brazilian cities of Curitiba and Londrina. This project involving physical education and sport for the handicapped is a part of the Partners of the Americas programme, which links a United States state with a counterpart state, region or nation in Central or South America to share skills and work towards achieving greater international co-operation and understanding among the peoples of the Western Hemispheres. This case study presents the preparation, project execution and post-project phases involved in such a project.

Preparation Phase

In my opinion, the pre-trip preparations are the key to a successful project. The process that appears to be most successful is similar to the process that must be followed when developing any new curricula. The steps that appeared to be most helpful are listed in Table 1, a pre-trip check-list.

Table 1. Preparation Check-List

Background reading	*Preparation of material*
History of region	Verbal
Governmental form	Written
Control of schools - local or central	Audio-visual
Financial support of education	Other (catalogues etc.)
Geography of region	
Climate of region	*Others*
	Travel arrangements
Develop questionnaire	Passports etc.
Goals of community	Housing, meals
Resources	Transportation on site
Facilities	Clothing
Equipment	
Training of staff	
Present programme (curriculum)	

One of the important sources of information in preparation for this trip to the state of Parana, Brazil was the background material obtained through reading a variety of books on the area. A knowledge of the history of Brazil was important in understanding the development of the region and specific problems that might need to be addressed. Other particularly pertinent information useful in planning the programme concerned the form of government and the nature of financial support for education. Knowledge of the form of government and financial support assisted in understanding the type of control that was exerted over education. Such knowledge helped me to understand at what level any educational changes should be suggested.

Two other types of information were also of practical significance. These were a knowledge of the geography of the region and of the climate of the region. Such information was useful in determining the type of sports and physical activities that would be useful in the region and in forming recommendations about facilities and equipment. Once this general knowledge was collected, the next step was to gather more specific information about the area.

The primary tool used to collect more specific information about the region was a questionnaire. This questionnaire was administered to several people: educators, physicians and the co-ordinators of my trip. Some responses were obtained verbally and others in writing. The topics that I requested more specific information about included the following: goals of the co-ordinators; goals of the community; community and educational resources available; sports facilities and equipment; training or background of the staff; and the present sports curriculum of programmes being used.

The topics that needed particular emphasis emerged from the information-gathering process. They were: the use of behavioural objectives in programme development and evaluation; activities, in addition to sports, that should be included in programmes for the disabled; types of fitness and skills tests available; the development of fundamental psychomotor skills; and equipment and facilities developed for the disabled. Once this step was completed, it was possible to prepare materials that were used on the trip.

The materials that proved to be particularly beneficial for this trip were the verbal presentations, written material for the participants, audio-visual materials and miscellaneous articles such as catalogues and samples of material. All seminars were accompanied by two written copies of an outline, one in English and the other in Portuguese, enabling the participants to follow the presentation in the language of their choice. Likewise, drawings and instructions for the construction of special equipment were provided. Slides of activities, facilities, equipment and written material to accompany the verbal presentations were also prepared. Of particular interest was the material showing the problems encountered during the development of facilities and equipment for the retarded and how they were resolved. (See Table 2 for seminar topics.)

Table 2. Seminar Topics

Definition and causes of mental retardation
Objectives of education for the mentally retarded
Physical education activities for the mentally retarded
Evaluation of programmes for the mentally retarded
Development of psychomotor skills in the mentally retarded
Methods of teaching physical education to the mentally retarded
Current trends in the United States

Travel Phase

The time spent in Brazil to work on this project relating to physical education and rehabilitation programmes for the mentally retarded was 16 days. The project consisted of 1 week of seminars in each of the two major cities of Parana, question and answer sessions with teachers and other professionals, visits to schools, conversations with government officials and interviews with members of the news media. Follow-up plans were made to continue my services as a resource person after my return to the United States.

Based on my experiences during the trip, I believe the following would improve this phase of service as a volunteer professional. First, the seminars were planned to last approximately 3 hours. Our experience was that any planned presentation should not exceed 2 hours; the remaining time should be used as a question and answer period. The most appropriate method of handling the questions was a requirement that any questions be submitted in written form. This allowed us to group questions by topic and issue and enabled all people to hear the question when it was read over the microphone. The other recommendations regarding these sessions would be that there should be an earlier meeting with the interpreter to go over any technical vocabulary, and provision of an extra outline so that interpreter understands what is transpiring. This was doubly important in the situation where simultaneous translation was not possible and participants could follow in both languages. In my opinion, a summary of the purpose of the trip, topics discussed and the professional's area of expertise should be provided to those persons planning interviews and courtesy visits. This prior information could facilitate the planning of these meetings and enable a focus on pertinent topics. Site visits were important, particularly early in the trip, because of their value in providing an understanding of local conditions and needs. Finally, the written material that was prepared before the trip proved invaluable; it served to anchor the seminar presentations and provided for a permanent source of information that remains after the professional has departed.

Trips such as this often involve attendance of official banquets and visits which, I feel, often serve to isolate the professional from the student participants in the seminar. Informal times scheduled to permit the students to interact with the professional can do much to improve international understanding as well as facilitate their ability to learn. These informal concats can be as valuable as the seminar sessions to some of the participants. Such events should be as much a part of the planning as the seminar sessions.

Post-Trip Phases

A part of the partners programme is that the volunteer professional become a contact person to form a link between the needs of the state of Parana and the resources of the state of Ohio. To this end, the following projects were initiated and are still in progress. Textbooks were solicited from professionals and book companies and sent to the Brazilian Universities; these books primarily dealt with physical education, sport and handicapped persons. A programme was established at the University of Toledo to enable Brazilians to come for specialised courses of study in addition to degrees. Specifications necessary to construct facilities and equipment were sent to Brazilian agencies and governmental offices. Duplicate sets of slides and visual materials were made and sent to Brazilian educators and officials. Student, faculty a physician exchanges have been co-ordinated. Finally, I have served as a resource person for volunteer professionals in other fields who are travelling to the same area on other projects.

Evaluation

Post-visit questionnaires indicated that the Brazilian organisers of the trip felt that the project was highly successful. The strong points reported by the evaluations were the breadth and depth of the material presented in the seminars, appropriateness of the presentation, extensive use of slides, preparation of written material and provision for continuing consultations. Examples of the more concrete results obtained from this project include the development of parks and recreation facilities accessible to all persons, removal of architectural barriers, development of physical education programmes for the handicapped based on scientific foundations, and travel by Brazilian professionals for study in the United States. Inquiries have also been made by Brazilian professionals about the feasibility of a second trip to develop further the original materials.

Summary

In addition to the items listed above, many intangible aspects of international understanding are associated with this type of project. The friendships that were made are continued through correspondence. Handicapped students and their families were most happy with the knowledge that a foreign professional communicated and worked with them; they develop a more positive attitude towards education. Teachers, coaches and the public become aware that sport and physical activity should be for all people, not just the most talented. I believe that these results depend upon two principles; first, pre-planning the trip to meet these objectives and second, that the professional is not isolated but has an opportunity to meet the public as well as the professionals. International understanding can be anhanced through all aspects of sport for all types of people.

IV

Measures Related to International Co-operation in Sport

1. Mass Media and International Understanding

International Communication, Sport and International Understanding

P. C. McIntosh

Introduction

To begin with an anecdote: The London Marathon of 1981 attracted 6500 entries. After 16 miles two of the runners, Dick Beardsley from the United States and Inge Simenson from Norway, broke away from the rest of the field and for the next 10 miles neither of them was able to establish a lead over the other. About 800 metres from the finish some communication took place between them, they clasped hands and crossed the finishing line together as joint winners. The interviewer for BBC television then asked Beardsley whether this sharing of victory as deliberate. He said it was and that there were other occasions for "duking it out at the finish". He also suggested that in the Olympic Games he would not have done it. This was without doubt a manifestation of international understanding but whether the behaviour of Beardsley and Simenson in giving up the competition before the end of the race was compatible with the Olympic motto "citius, altius, fortius", or even with the fundamental and principle aim of competitive sport, that is to determine a winner, is a matter of argument. Are competitive sport and international understanding incompatible or merely strange bedfellows? Millions of viewers vicariously shared the joint victory of the London Marathon through television. What was the effect upon them and upon their attitudes? We do not know because these are the kinds of question which very few researchers have asked and even fewer have tried to answer.

Lack of Research

When, in 1979, The International Council for Sport and Physical Education commissioned Dr. Halloran, Director of the Centre for Mass Communication Research at the University of Leicester, to review the literature and research on mass media sport and international understanding, he could find only one item in 263 bibliographical references which in its title directly addressed the subject of the review (Halloran 1981, Milshtein and Molchanov 1976, p2). UNESCO, which is dedicated to the promotion of international understanding, asked ICSPE in 1971 to organise a seminar on mass media, sport and international understanding. A report of the seminar was published but was no longer available in 1979. However, a committee of ICSPE has met annually since 1971 to follow up this concern. UNESCO, itself, however, in its recommendation concerning education for international understanding, co-operation and peace adopted at the General Assembly in 1974, specifically commended the use of the visual arts and music for this end but omitted all mention of sport (UNESCO 1974). Not until 1978 did UNESCO proclaim, in its International Charter on Physical Education and

Sport, the need for sport deliberately to promote mutual respect and understanding between peoples and individuals, and call upon the mass media to exert a positive influence (UNESCO 1978 Preamble and Article 8). There is a considerable body of research on sport and international relations, on mass media and international relations, and on mass media or mass communication and sport, but the complex relationship between all three items has been little researched. An examination of the problem and a partial analysis may suggest a way forward.

News vs. Entertainment

There are certain immediate difficulties. Sport does not fit into categories used to classify television or radio programmes. Katz, for instance, suggested among his proposals for research three headings - first news, information and current affairs: programming reality; secondly entertainment: programming pleasure and thirdly social differentiation: programming identity, but sport is all three of these (Katz 1978, pp 90–95). The media tend to present sport as entertainment but the result is always news and the entertainment includes a wealth of information about the players and the sport which spectators, viewers and readers expect to be given.

It may be that the classification is deficient for research purpose but the structure of broadcasting organisations and of the press also sharply separate news and comment from entertainment and often put sport in a house on its own. Cohen and Young were therefore able to produce a revised edition of their book in 1981 under the title *The Manufacture of News* containing 35 chapters on, among other topics, crime, accidents, scandals, strikes, women, alcoholism, racial conflict, photography, mugging and "the left", but they included no chapter on sport (Cohen and Young 1981). We need to examine the presentation of sports without adherence to existing classifications of news, comment and entertainment.

A second difficulty is that the newsworthiness of sport does not conform with concepts of newsworthiness which have been used by researchers. Many years ago, Galtung named eight factors which determine what will strike our attention and four more which influence the transition from events to news. The last of these was "reference to something negative", i. e. what most people refer to when they say "there is so little to be happy about in the news" (Galtung and Ruge 1965), but news about sports events always makes some people happy, namely the winners and their supporters, including those who have won money on the result. Sports news is always good news for someone. We cannot therefore transfer without qualification general theories about newsworthiness to the newsworthiness of sport. We must do our own research.

What Is International Understanding?

When we come to examine international understanding we meet a difficulty not peculiar to sport - the meaning of the term. Without attempting to define what may be indefinable I am suggesting that the term in the English language is commonly to embrace knowledge about people from other nations, co-operation with them and goodwill towards them. It is self evident that these three elements are not necessarily dependent upon each other. It is possible to have greater ill will towards a person or group the more you know about them it is possible to co-operate for purpose of sports competition with minimum knowledge of your opponents and without strong feelings of either goodwill or hostility. The suggestion by the International Olympic Committee in its Charter that a better understanding will, or even can, arise through sport and "thereby help to build a more peaceful world" (IOC 1979) and the firm statement by Milshtein and Molchanov that "sport, due to its nature is a factor promoting peace, friendship and mutual understanding" (Milshtein and Molchanov 1976 p 71) are not self-evident and cannot be accepted without supporting evidence. We need first, however, to examine the usage of the term "international understanding" to see whether it is capable of definition. Heinilä's study of varying interpretations of the term "fair play" by footballers in Finland, Sweden and England in 1974 provides a model which could well be used again for researching international understanding in sporting contexts before we look for causal relationships with vehicles of mass communication (Heinilä 1974).

Violence

There is some evidence that the admixture of news, information and entertainment in the presentation of sport determines its own peculiar pattern. Comisky and his associates found that viewers were easily convinced by the announcer they were watching a fiercely competitive game of ice hockey whereas the game, visually, was devoid of exciting play (Comisky et al. 1977). Givant reached the same conclusion in his investigation of American football (Givant 1978). There is one feature of sport and the presentation of sport which deserves special attention because of its relevance to international understanding, and that is violence. A recent study of terrorism and the Western news media in Holland established that according to Western news values, war is better television than peace and violence better television than non-violence (Shmid and deGraaf 1981). Consequently a British or American child in the course of 3 hours television will see about 20 violent incidents and the order of frequency of crimes in US television has murder first and burglary sixth, while in real life burglary is first and murder is seventh. Both the quantity and the nature of violence in the world is distorted. It would not be surprising, therefore, to find that violence in sport is similarly distorted. No sophisticated research is needed to support the assertion that most sport is non-violent. Throughout the alphabet of sport from archery to yachting, many sports are totally non-violent and even in contact sports, which are the only ones to provide opportunities for violence, there is very little violence in terms of time and crime. In 1972 Gabler recorded on videotape all the fouls which occurred in water polo matches played by the West German team during the Olympic Games in 1972. Following a classification of aggressive and non-aggressive actions he found that of 596 fouls which were penalised, not more than 15% could be regarded as aggressive (Gabler 1976). This is often not the picture presented by the media. A US film of the Winter Olympic Games at Lake Placid entitled, significantly, *The Spirit of the Olympics*, which was shown to the Olympic Congress in Baden Baden in 1981, devoted a disproportionate amount of film to violence and fighting in the final game of the ice hockey competition.

Even the supporters of extreme theories of catharsis would have difficulty in covincing anyone else that this film made a positive contribution to international goodwill. The effect of such distortion is insidious. More content analysis along the lines of Milshtein and Molchanov could reveal the extent of the distortion, but the question that would still remain is how media portrayal of sport could contribute to international understanding unless these values are changed.

It is not to be assumed that distortion is only a capitalist and Western vice. The television cameras at the opening ceremony of the Olympic Games in Moscow in 1980 showed the flags of only those teams which chose to march behind their national flag. The olympic flags which some countries chose in preference to their own were not shown. I am drawing attention to the fact of distortion not to its purpose nor to its effects. There is a natural tendency, confirmed by the Glasgow University Media Group, to regard our own national news as fair and impartial but other nations' views as biased (Glasgow University 1976 p 2). We know too from research in Finland that the kind of violence portrayed on television in the United States is different from that portrayed in the USSR (Pietilä 1976). In the former country violence against individuals and against property predominates and in the latter, violence against society and the environment. We need similar cross-cultural comparisons in the distortions of sport.

Attitudes to Other Countries

I have postulated that the concept of international understanding includes both knowledge and goodwill. Which comes first, the knowledge or the attitude? In a cross-national study on the development in children of concepts and attitudes about their own and other nations in 1966, it was concluded that in at least one of the countries, children learn which foreign countries are "bad" or "good" before they learn practically anything else about them (Tajfel and Jahoda 1966, p 23). At the age of 9–11 almost all preferences were highly polarised. It would be idle to pretend that American and Soviet children, Arab and Israeli children, Southern Irish catholic and Northern Irish protestant children are all developing attitudes of goodwill towards each other at an early age. However, the part that sport and media coverage of sport play in forming children's attitudes, or might play in improving them if deliberately used to that end, is difficult to determine. Halloran, in reporting on a contemporary study of children's attitudes to other countries in Canada, the Federal Republic of Germany, Hungary and Great Britain found that sport or media references to sport did not figure at all prominently in children's responses (Halloran 1981, p 51). However, as he himself says, "If you do not ask questions about sport you are unlikely to hear answers about sport". Johnson's study of English 8- to 10-year-old children's concept of Germany in 1972 also found that by far the most frequent information given in response to an open question was classified as Simple War information (Sport did not appear at all), and also that children acquire most information about nations they like and least about those towards which they feel neutral (Johnson 1973).

Two other points are worth making about children's attitudes: First, children are immature in self-identification and are less able than adults to distinguish fantasy from reality. It is even more difficult for children than for the rest of us to decide whether sport is fantasy or real life and many of them do use what they see on television as a guide to what is appropriate and justifiable in real life. Sport is unlikely to be an exception to this generalisation. Secondly, Halloran reports that "it was the media related family discussion which at least had the potential for having the most deep and enduring impact on reactions to other countries" (Halloran 1981, p 48).

Other research has shown that major determinants of socialisation are not sudden events but habitual events that form familiar and constant aspects of a child's environment over a long time (Howe 1977, p 36). In their investigations of racial conflict Hartmann and Husband concluded that short-term effects from the mass media were unlikely but that the media did define for people what the issues were and in what terms they were to be discussed (Hartman and Husband 1971). Attempts to find a causal link between watching violent television programmes and subsequent aggressive behaviour in sport and elsewhere have been inconclusive (Lefkowitz et al. 1973; Moriarty et al. 1979; Bandura and Walters 1963). Recently in some countries programmes of education in "Olympism" have been started with or without the help of the media. In due course we may be able to monitor the results and judge their effectiveness.

Sports Heroes Are Media Heroes

No research is needed to establish that sports heroes and heroines have for more than a century been made by the press and since World War I by radio too and since World War II by television. Because sport has become international, so have the heroes. Jim Thorpe, addressed by the King of Sweden in 1912 as "the most wonderful athlete in the world", was made into a hero and then unmade with the help of the press. 'Jesse' Owens, Abebe Bikela, Roger Bannister, Pele, Olga Korbut - everybody's daughter as one commentator called her - are just a few of those who have transcended their nationality and excited the administration and affection of people from all nations. The media can, of course, make heroes out of villains and this danger has recently been apparent in football, ice hockey and lawn tennis, but it is the international character of the star which is important. It was therefore possible for a poll, sponsored by Tass, to choose the American swimmer Debbie Myers as sportswoman of 1967, that is during the Vietnam war. Christopher Chataway comments "It is hard to imagine Tass publishing a poll which declared General Westmoreland as soldier of 1967; indeed, it is hard to imagine any other field in which Tass would have awarded such a distinction to an American" (Goodhart and Chataway 1968, p 153).

Internationalism of Sport

The supranational as distinct from international characteristic of sport merits further examination with especial reference to the media. Journalists and commentators are partial. The notion of cultural neutrality is never achieved. James Michenor is honest with himself when he writes "I am in favour of local partisanship, and to enforce a bland neutrality seems wrong. If I were a sports writer or broadcaster I would certainly be for my home teams .... I would also hope to be a just critic of their failures" (Michenor 1976, p 333). Many journalists are also subject to great external pressure and the best are no better than Montaigne: "I speak the truth", he said, "not as much as I would but as much as I dare, and I dare a little more as I grow older". (Montaigne 1580). Governments too are partial and use media coverage of sport for their own political ends. This was why Zaire and Malaysia staged major world boxing championships. King, the promotor of fights by Ali, was "shrewd enough to realise that championship bouts featuring Ali were the kind of promotion that developing nations like to stage" and he "courted heads of state in Cairo, Tehran, Lusaka and Kuala Lumpur" (Time, 30th June 1975, pp 55–56).

The international understanding of developing countries by the developed world has been increased by the media coverage of such major sporting events but is that all that has happened? It is possible to argue that an ideology and a system of values peculiar to international sport, different from and even in conflict with other political and cultural ideologies, has begun to evolve. It was therefore possible in 1980 for a non-governmental organisation, the International Olympic Committee, to oppose and to defy some of the most powerful governments of the world in the cause of Olypism and of international sport. The conflict was carried on before a world audience and in February 1980 the IOC decided by a unanimous vote to go ahead with the Olympic Games in Moscow despite the opposition of the government of the United States.

The nature of this internationalism and its system of values is still obscure. The nation state is an institution which originated in Europe in the fifteenth century. It still forms the basis of our international system, including governments which regard themselves as autonomous and sovereign in their relations with each other and governmental organisations such as the United Nations and its agencies. It also includes non-governmental organisations such as the IOC and the international federations of sport whose members or delegates are "national". National boundaries, however, are man made and may bear little relevance to cultural, ethnic, religious or political realities. Indeed, some of the bitterest conflicts today are not between nations but within nations, between religious, political or racial groups in, for instance, Iran, Ireland or South Africa. Understanding between these groups raises even more intractable problems. However that may be, supranational organisations based on common interests such as the European Economic Community, the Roman Catholic Church and International Communism exist across national boundaries, and so does international sport. Furthermore, while threats and diplomatic exchanges between nations make news, integration is also exemplified in such exercises as the geophysical year and communication satellites. Such moves may even be steps towards supranational unification.

International "Fair Play"

When international sport is viewed from this angle there are two factors which complicate and also distinguish it. The first is the concept of "fair play" and the second is the dependence of international sport upon mass communication. The term "fair play" has proved so difficult to translate that even the Paris-based Comite International de Fair Play uses the English words. The concept, however, has an international universality which is closely related to that of justice. There are, of course, arguments about what is and what is not fair. There are disputes between officials whose function is to decide what is fair and competitors who are required to accept the decisions. There are those who resort to deception and illegal practices to achieve success so that the cynics deny the existence of fair play, but sporting competition of any kind is possible only if reference can be made to an ultimate standard of fairness. This ultimate standard may be manifested not only in rules, regulations and sanctions, but in unwritten norms of behaviour which nevertheless have general acceptance. It is not possible or necessary in this short paper to enter into a philosophical discussion of fairness and justice. It is, however, both possible and necessary to assert first that fair play is the underlying condition of all sport, however abused it may be in practice, and secondly that it overrides national interests and gives to international sport a system of value of its own.

Responsibility and Partiality

The dependence of international sport upon mass communications has increased greatly since the Olympic Games were first televised in 1936. Within 10 years the International Olympic Committee has changed from debtor to creditor and draws its considerable income almost entirely from payments for television rights.

Even the rules and organisation of games, notably lawn tennis and golf, have been modified to satisfy the supposed wishes of the absent viewers. A feature of mass communications at the present time is their domination by a very few large news services. More than 100 countries lease services from the United States-dominated INTELSTAT. Associated Press and United Press International in the USA are the most important collectors and distributors of news all over the world. When Agence France Press in France and Reuters, based in the United Kingdom, are added with a smaller contribution from TASS in the USSR, news packaging is almost totally accounted for. The existing internatioinal communication system is characterised by uneven flows of information both between East and West and between North and South. This basic fact is bound to affect the international presentation of sport but not perhaps as much as some social scientists have suggested. Schiller, using the evidence of international boxing, and quoting Evelina Dagnino on Latin America, has claimed that national cultures have been deliberately submitted by governments "to a form of homogenization that is required for the maintenance of an international system" (Schiller 1976, pp 16-17; Dagnino 1973). However, the great North American sports of baseball and their own brand of football do not appear to command the world-wide interest that might be expected if domination of communications was exactly reflected in sport. Nevertheless, the clash of national cultures and international sport is surely possible. Even the MacBride Report to UNESCO, which sees no insoluble conflict between freedom of the press and its obligation to improve mankind, recognises that "distortions and imbalances reflect in some way the dominant interests of the societies from which they emanate" (MacBride et al. 1980, p 37). Shishigin claims that sports writers in the Soviet Union are given goals for sport set by the state which include love of one's country, devotion to its flag and friendship for the sportsmen and people of other countries (Shishigin 1975). Robert Helmick, speaking on behalf of the international federations of sport at the Olympic Congress in Baden-Baden in 1981, accused the press of heightening nationalism by overemphasising mistakes and "national scores" at the Olympic Games and challenged the press to find alternatives that would attract readers' and viewers' interest without having a negative effect (Helmick 1981). We do not know how the reconciliation between national and supranational presentation demanded by Shishigin and Helmick can be achieved or even whether it can be achieved.

The Need for Multidisciplinary Research

I return once more to a plea for research, but research of a special kind. There have already been strenuous efforts to investigate problems of international conflict and diplomacy by empirical methods. There have also been strenuous efforts by social scientists to keep abreast of the technological developments of mass communication, but the question "how is international sport related to these technological developments and to international conflict?" has yet to be answered. Moreover, because the conceptual frameworks which have been used in these related fields have not taken account of the peculiar features of sport, severe limitations are placed upon the inferences and extrapolations which we can make from the findings of this research. First then we need theoretical insights to identify the problems which international communication, sport and international understanding present to us. Thereafter we need field studies of a complex kind. Many years ago Kelman concluded that a key characteristic of behavioural study of international relations was that it could not be linked to a single discipline (Kelman 1965). His arguments apply with even greater force to the tripartite topic of this paper. This is not to deny the value of comparative and simple content analyses of the media coverage of sport, but even this will lack direction and relevance unless there is collaboration between a number of disciplines. Philosophy, history, political science, psychology, sociology, economics, law and other disciplines, too have contributions to make. As sports scientists we must excite the interest and enlist the help of colleagues so that they include sport in their conceptual frameworks and we, in our turn, must make use of their expertise in formulating and solving our problems.

In conclusion I confess to a fellow feeling with a certain character drawn by Lewis Carroll for that great English poem, *The Hunting of the Snark*. The leader of the hunt

> ... had brought a large map representing the sea
> With not the least vestige of land,
> The crew were much pleased when they found it to be
> A map they could all understand.
> Other maps are such shapes with your islands and capes
> But we've got our brave captain to thank,
> So the crew would protest, He has brought us the best,
> A perfect and absolute blank.

I very much hope that the crew at this congress will not be pleased with such a map but will try to fill in, by appropriate research, some landmarks and seamarks.

References

Bandura A, Walters R (1963) Social learning and personality development. New York
Carroll L (1876) The hunting of the snark. Macmillan, London
Cohen S, Young J (eds) (1981) The manufacture of news. Constable, London and Sage, Beverly Hills

Comisky P, Bryant J, Zillman D (1977) Commentary as a substitute for action. Communication 27: 150-153
Dagnino E (1973) Cultural and ideological dependence: Building a theoretical framework. In: Bonilla F, Girling R (eds) Struggles of dependency. Stanford
Gabler H (1976) Aggression and violence in sport. In: Schilling G (ed) FIEP Bull 46:4
Galtung J, Ruge M (1965) The structure of foreign news. J Int Peace Res 1:64-90
Givant M (1978) Pro football and the mass media. Rev Sport Leisure 3, 2:69-72
Glasgow University Media Group (1976) Bad news. Routledge and Kegan Paul, London
Golding P, Elliott P (1979) Making the news. Longman, London
Goodhart P, Chataway C (1968) War without weapons. Allen, London
Halloran JD (1981) Mass media sport and international understanding: A summary of a review of literature and research. ICSPE, London, p 2
Hartman P, Husband C (1981) The mass media and racial conflict. In: Cohen S, Young J (eds) The manufacture of news. Constable, London and Sage, Beverley Hills
Heinilä K (1974) Ethics of sport. Junior football players as cross national interpreters of the moral concepts of sport. Department of Sociology and Planning for Physical Culture, Jyväskylä
Helmick R (1981) Speech to 11th Olympic Congress, Baden-Baden, September
Howe MJA (1977) Television and children. New University Education, London
International Olympic Committee, Olympic Charter, Lausanne, 1979
Johnson N (1973) Development of English children's concept of Germany. J Social Psychol 90:259-267
Katz E (1978) Looking for trouble. J Communication 28/2:90-95
Kelman HC (ed) (1965) International behaviour. Holt, New York
Lefkowitz MM, Eron LD, Walder LO, Huesmann LR (1973) Preference for televised contact sports as related to sex differences in aggression. Dev Psychol 9/3:417-420
MacBride S et al. (1980) Many voices one world. UNESCO
Michenor JA (1976) Michenor on sport. Secker and Warburg, London
Milshtein OA, Molchanov SV (1976) The shaping of public opinion regarding sport by the mass media as a factor in promoting international understanding. Int Rev Sport Sociol 3 (ii):71-85
Montaigne ME de (1580) In: Tribaudet M, Rat M (eds) Complete works. Paris 1791, printed Bruges 1962
Moriarty R, McCabe A, Holman/Prpich M (1979) Studies on TV and youth sports. In: Avedon EM, Le Lierre M, Stewart TO (eds) Contemporary leisure research. Ontario Research Council
Pietilä V (1976) Notes on violence in the mass media. In: Instant research on peace and violence 4, Tampere Peace Research Institute, Tampere, pp 195-197
Schiller HI (1976) Communication and cultural domination. IASP, New York
Schmid AP, De Graaf J (1981) Terrorism and the Western news media in Holland. In: Halloran JD. Mass media sport and international understanding. ICSPE, London, pp 21-22
Shishigin MV (1975) Propaganda Fizicheskoi Kultury i Sporta, Moscow. (Publicity of physical culture and sport, Moscow.) Reviewed by Riordan J (1977) In: Sport Sociol Bull 6 (i)
Tajfel H, Jahoda G (1966) Development in children of concepts and attitudes about their own and other nations: a cross-national study. In: Cross-cultural studies in personality development. XVIII International Congress of Psychology, Moscow
UNESCO (1974) Recommendation concerning education for international understanding, co-operation and peace and education relating to human rights and fundamental freedoms. UNESCO General Conference, Paris, 19th November 1974
UNESCO (1978) International Charter of Physical Education and Sport, UNESCO, Paris

Sport in the Mass Media and International Understanding

A. Kirsch and W. Preising

Definition of the Problem

It is a widely held opinion that sport is an area of social reality where the idea of international understanding could meet with particular success. Therefore, within the framework of their sports commentaries the mass media are expected not only to report on the results of certain sporting events but also to convey the idealistic values of sport to the reader, listener or viewer.

It is, howeve, a characteristic feature of ideas that they formulate a certain claim and do not correspond to reality from the outset. This discrepancy is the reason why it is widely believed that sports reporting in the mass media prevents international understanding instead of promoting it. Those who make such a claim point out that both the language and the content of the reporting are governed by nationalistic or even chauvinistic criteria. Fundamental critics even doubt – with reference to the political abuse which occurs particularly during great sporting events like the Olympic Games or world championships – whether sport is at all capable of contributing to and promoting international understanding (Lüschen 1972). We will not analyse this question, but we would like to point out that the abuse of an idea does not reduce or jeopardise its worth, and that the promotion of international understanding is a value which is characteristic of sport and which should be supported despite all obstacles. Unfortunately, as yet there have not been any comprehensive theoretical or empirical investigations which have tried to establish to what extent the mass media contribute to the promotion of this value.

By referring to the results of individual research projects, we will now attempt to formulate some fundamental problems and questions for empirical investigation. We will proceed in three steps: firstly, we will analyse the relationship between sport and international understanding; secondly, we will discuss the influence of the mass media with regard to the effect of sport on international understanding; and finally, we will outline resultant scientific tasks.

The Relationship Between Sport and International Understanding

Lenk (1979, p 124) reported: "Many authors regarded the 'Olympic Idea' as a, or even the basic value for achieving friendly international relationships". The official *Olympic Rules and Regulations* (1974) themselves declare:

> The aims of the Olympic movement are to promote the development of those fine physical and moral qualities which are the basis of amateur sport and to bring together the athletes of the world in a

great quadrennial festival of sports *thereby creating international respect and goodwill and thus helping to construct a better and more peaceful world ...*

In these quotations, international understanding is understood as an idea with potentially worldwide educational consequences which can be realised if every nation regards sporting performance as a means of gaining international respect. Only if the personal performance of the individual athlete is, at the same time, seen and understood with reference to the nation he represents can such international respect flourish. It is held that this international respect can contribute to a better and more peaceful world.

If we think out this claim, it becomes obvious that:

- The prerequisite of the idea of international understanding is the recognition of national peculiarities
- Sporting performance is a field where each nation - if it sticks to the rules - can attain international recognition and respect
- Each individual performance of an athlete also has, or at least is considered to have, the function of representing the national performance capacity
- Sport is not the only means of protecting peace. By promoting international respect, however, it can make a contribution to peace

In addition, we would like to add a personal thought: at the very time and place where peace is in danger, where international understanding no longer seems possible, it is necessary to use sport as a reminder of the value of such understanding.

Today, this sense of international understanding, which was defined by taking the Olympic Games as an example, applies to all sporting events where the performances of different nations are compared. At the same time, it is identical with the term used in political sociology.

As Earl Zeigler (1977, p 71) has written:

In the English language the word 'nation' is generally used synonymously with country or state ... These individuals, members of a political community, are usually considered to possess a certain 'nationality' ... The word 'nationalism' itself might apply to a feeling, attitude or consciousness that persons might have as citizens of a nation. Nationalism might be defined as a political philosophy in which the good of the nation is supreme. The word is often used incorrectly as a synonym for chauvinism.

We think it is necessary to keep in mind that nationalism is not the same as chauvinism. Nationalism is an idea through which people can build up a group identity and, by feeling different from other people, can develop a concept of their own. While nationalism is associated with respect for others, chauvinism is just the opposite: it is associated with contempt for other nations. As an investigation supported by UNESCO and published in 1967 by Lambert and Klineberg has shown, children, as they grow older, show - to a degree which varies all over the world - increased prejudice towards other nations.

Regardless of how these stereotypes develop, we have to say that a realistic approach to handling this problem would be education aimed at the recognition of distinct nationalities and not at their abolition. It seems to us that sport, with its rules and values, can become a field of international respect, this respect being based on recognition of the achievements of other nations without the national identities of defeated nations being surrendered. A prerequisite of this, however, is that the competition rules are accepted and observed. Sporting competitions are characterised by their repetition at intervals, and any one performance is basically unique: a victory does not imply that the indivudual athlete or the nation he or she represents is raised once and for all above the group of losers, and conversely the same applies to the evaluation of a defeat. In addition, the ritual of the competition, which becomes particularly obvious in the festivities of the Olympic Games, unites all participating athletes and nations in one large community.

Thus the possibility of improving international understanding by means of sport lies not only in the various opportunities for holding competitions but also in the fulfilment of the sporting ideal that losers are also to be accepted because a victory is something transient. Of course, in practice it is just this ideal that is threatened again and again; it does not, however, lose its validity. To quote Aldous Huxley in his *Ends and Means*: "Like every other instrument that man has invented, sport can be used either for good or for bad purposes".

Influence of the Mass Media with Regard to the Effect of Sport on International Understanding

When analysing the role the mass media play in advancing the idea of internatiional understanding, the statements primarily refer to TV. Naturally, a thorough discussion must also consider newspapers, weeklies, radio and films. It must be said, however, that particularly TV has brought a new dimension into the broadcasting of events, including sporting events. The broadcasts are far more spontaneous than is possible in newspapers, the information being less preselected by the reporter and therefore of a different quality. Owing to the visual simultaneity of event and reporting on TV, not only the limited number of spectators sitting in the stadium but also those sitting in front of the TV set have the chance of seeing their own nation in contest with others and how the athletes of different nations fare in competition with each other. Statistics show how the size of audiences has thus been increased. The first TV broadcast where the reportage for the spectator and the actual event took place almost simultaneously (a delay of about 9 s) was during the XIth Summer Olympic Games in 1936 in Berlin (Hackforth 1975, p 15). In about 25 public TV rooms approximately 150,000 people watched the first live TV broadcasts (Hackforth 1978). Only 36 years passed until the Olympic Games in Munich in 1972; these years were characterised by great scientific progress and the triumphant advance of TV all over the world. It has been estimated that about one-third of the world's population watched these Games (Winkler 1973, p 40). Other estimates claim that approximately 1,5 billion people (Ruhland 1982, p 22) watched the TV broadcasts of the 1982 Soccer World Championship. Owing to the possibility of broadcasting matches via satellite, the simultaneity of broadcast and event is assured almost all over the world (McCollum and McCollum 1980). We can say that TV is able to create one single world society and that sporting competitions are probably the events where this potential is most often used. Expensive technical equipment made it possible during the Olympic Games in Munich to broadcast the competitions in more than 100 nations (cf. OC of the Olympic Games Munich 1972). Expenditure and broadcasting increased still further in Montreal and Moscow.

Given this expenditure and the increase of costs attaching thereto, the question arises whether this increase of international communication also helps to improve international understanding. Since we have little information on the effects of TV broadcasts in this field, we must, for the present, concentrate on the question of to what extent the sporting ideal is conveyed in the broadcasts, and since we do not have any reliable content analyses, we must give an indirect answer.

It is true that TV always broadcasts the opening and closing ceremonies - especially on the occasion of great competitions like the Olympic Games - so that the integration of the competitions into the fetivities becomes obvious. Afterwards the reporting primarily relates to the competitions, to their results, and to sport-specific analyses. This was shown by an investigation carried out on behalf of the Council of Europe, which revealed that the TV stations united in the EBU restrict their main sports programmes to news and competitions (Deutscher Sportbund 1977). The fact that TV considers the rituals of the festivities to a lesser degree is demonstrated by a statement made by the commentator of a German TV station (ZDF) after the opening ceremony of the Soccer World Championship in Spain. He introduced the first match after the ceremony with the words: "After all, we are approaching now what all of you have probably been waiting for all along." Such a statement depreciates that part of big sporting events which could particularly enhance international understanding (cf. ICSPE 1973) and lends support to criticisms that there are too few programmes directly related to the idea of international understanding. That the evaluation and the programming of sporting events are more directed towards their commercial and entertainment value than towards their idealistic value is proved by an analysis of newspaper reporting and interviews with the journalists concerned (Binnewies 1975). According to this study, sport is "one of the most attractive and vivid products of the modern entertainment industry" (p 173) and 77% of all sports journalists interviewed attached no importance to the political views of their paper (p 175). On a different page, Binnewies declares: "Apart from a few exceptions sports reporting is restricted to the reproduction of events taken place" (Binnewies 1973). That this is also true of TV reporting in the Federal Republic of Germany has been proved by H. Seifart (1976).

Also of interest is the method applied by national broadcasting stations when taking over multilateral programmes of the broadcasting station in the organising country or when producing their own unilaterial programmes. Hoyseater reports thatt during the Olympic Games in Montreal some of the stations added unilateral broadcasts to the joint programme in order to come up to the expectations of their viewers. He declares: "Roughly speaking, the situation appears to be the same in most countries: too many events were transmitted for which there was no great national interest." He continues: "When planning programmes, it may be a debatable point how much attention should be paid to this reaction, which has somewhat chauvinistic undertones" (Hoysaeter 1977, p 93).

Apart from *what* the media report on sports, it is also important *how* they report it. We have scant information on this question, but it is certain that the individual national TV stations choose very different productions of the various sporting events. While some investigations in the field of advertising psychology have analysedthe effects of certain images, their division, and their combination in sequences, no similar analyses have been made with respect of sports broadcasts. It is conceivable that the selection of a certain TV picture also contains a particular message. Whether riots among the spectators are broadcast or not, whether all rule violations by athletes are shown, whether such violations are emphasised in a particular way by repeating them or by stopping the film at that point - each of these, especially during international sporting events, could influence the way in which the viewer evaluates the event. We have, however, no reliable data to prove this.

A further problem concerns the language used in reports. On TV the importance of the picture considerably reduces the information content of the commentator's language (Bausinger and Stocker 1972), whereas on radio and in newspapers language is the most important purveyor of information and the only way of conveying meanings, including those of sporting events. In these media the often very loud language exaggerates the importance of certain aspects of sporting events (Becker 1983; Dankert 1969). Schmidt (1965) tried to show national tendencies in sports reporting. To what extent, however, the use of national stereotypes in reporting can prevet international understanding could only be shown in an exact effect analysis referring to viewers and listeners or newspaper readers. Evidence would also have to be gathered in order to assess the hypothesis that these national stereotypes are necessary in order to produce those identity patterns in the recipient which make it possible for him to understand other nations (as yet there have been no investigations in this field).

Up to this point we have asked only whether and how mass media convey the values inherent in sport. We have assumed that these values are actually realised in sport and are then conveyed by the mass media. However, we must also consider how the mass media, on the basis of their dramaturgy, which has its own special rules, might also change the message of sport. A primary possibility for this lies in the important role TV plays in the financing of great sporting events and the demands it can thus make concerning the course of these events. The latest example of this was the arrangement of the qualifying competitions during the Soccer World Championships in Spain, where the two decisive matches in one group were held at different times to that both could be broadcast live on TV. When the preceding results of three of the teams concerned were taken into account the spectator could have gained the impression that the result of the later match was manipulated in such a way that a team involved in the earlier match was handicapped. In this case, the dramaturgy of TV resulted in the violation of the principle of equal opportunities. At the same time, it may happen that the behaviour of a team can result in prejudice against the represented nation. Therefore, an exact scientific investigation should analyse whether and how the mass media change those rules of sporting competitions which make it possible for the recognition of a nation to be achieved through a sporting performance. That success is not the only criterion for such recognition can be seen from a German investigation in which only 48% of the interviewees felt that the medals won during the Olympic Games produce an effect on the way a particular nation is regarded by others. The other interviewees did not share this opinion or expressed no opinion at all. In his analysis of the Munich Olympic Games in 1972, Lenk expressed the fear that the exclusive orientation of the Games towards the entertainment function of TV might also support nationalistic prejudices (Lenk 1976, p 199).

In assessing the effect of the mass media on international understanding scientifically, we must bear in mind that in addition to particular productions of the media, international political situations are also influential. Despite those who are of a different opinion, we must conclude that in times of international conflict TV is influenced by political considerations. The Olympic Games in Moscow were an example of this: Most TV stations from countries which supported the boycott of the Games also considerably reduced their reporting. It would be interesting to examine whether in times of international conflict the mass media are no longer able to use sport to create a platform for mutual understanding.

Scientific Tasks for the Future

If we now consider what has so far been pointed out, we must say that, in a scientific sense, we have defined almost exclusively open questions. On the other hand, it is abvious that sport is becoming more and more dependent on presentation and dissemination by the mass media. Therefore the tasks formulated during a conference which UNESCO and ICSPE organised in London in 1973 still remain. We think it appropriate to repeat these tasks in our own words:

- Discussion of the idea of international understanding should be continued in a philosophical and empirical way.
- Sport must continue to examine the ways in which it can further international understanding. In particular, this applies to the rituals and ceremonies of great sporting events.
- As in the field of research into the influence of TV on aggression carried out by advertising psychologists, an effect analysis should be carried out to complement the merely descriptive analyses of viewing habits. This should be done by investigating the significance of the "language" of TV pictures.
- There should be continuous analysis of the influence the mass media have on the ideals and organisation of sport.

All this research, however, will not be very successful unless it is accompanied by international contacts between those who are responsible for sport and its representation. It is these contacts which will decide to what extent the findings of research can be put into practice.

References

Adefope HEO (1973) The role of sport in the creation of national identity and its contribution to the search for understanding between different communities and cultures. In: Grupe O, Kurz D, Teipel JM (eds) Sport in the modern world - chances and problems. Springer, Berlin Heidelberg New York, pp 580-582

Bausinger H, Stocker K (1972) Sprache und Umwelt. II. Reportagen. Ein Kapitel deutscher Sportsprache. Schulfernsehen 8:798-809

Becker H (1974a) Der olympische Aufstieg der DDR. Deutschland-Archiv 7:157-165

Becker H (1974b) Sozialisation durch Massenmedien im Sport. In: ADL (ed) Sozialisation im Sport. Hofmann, Schorndorf

Becker H (1983) Sozialisation durch Massenkommunikation im Sport-Sozialisationsfaktor Sportsprache. Unpublished manuscript, 4 pp

Binnewies H (1973) Das Bild des Sports in der deutschen Tagespresse. In: Gutsche KJ (ed) Sportwissenschaft in der Entwicklung. FU, Berlin

Binnewies H (1975) Sport und Sportberichterstattung. Czwalina, Ahrensburg

Dankert H (1969) Sportsprache und Kommunikation. Mohr, Tübingen
Deutscher Sportbund (ed) The role of television in promoting the practice of sport. Frankfurt
Hackforth J (1975) Sport im Fernsehen. Regensberg, Münster
Hackforth J (1978) Sport und Fernsehen. In: Hackforth J, Weischenberg S (eds) Sport und Massenmedien. Limpert, Homburg v.d.H., pp 29-37
Hoysaeter J (1977) The Games must go on - But with what kind of radio and television coverage? Olymp Rev 112:84-91
ICSPE (ed) (1973) Mass media, sport and international understanding. ICSPE, Paris
Lambert WE, Klineberg O (1967) Children's view of foreign peoples. Meredith, New York
Lenk H (1976) The 1972 Munich Olympic Games - a dilemma? In: Graham PJ, Uberhorst H (eds) The modern Olympic. Leisure, Cornwall, pp 193-203
Lenk H (1979) Social philosophy of athletics. Stipes, Champaign
Lüschen G (1972) Zur Soziologie des Sports. In: Baitsch H et al. (eds) The scientific view of sport. Springer, Berlin Heidelberg New York
McCollum RH, McCollum DF (1980) Analysis of ABC TV coverage of the 21st Olympic Games, Montreal. J Sport Soc Issues 4:25-33
OC of the Olympic Games (ed) (1972) Olympia und Technik. Munich
Ruhland W (1982) Freundschaftsspiele. Anmerkungen zu Sport - Kommerz - Fernsehen im Vorfeld der Fußballweltmeisterschaft. Medium 6:22-24
Schmidt HD (1965) Versuch einer Inhaltsanalyse nationaler Tendenzen in Sportreportagen. Psych Rundsch 16:43-51
Seifart H (1976) Berufssport am Beispiel des Fußballs und ein Vergleich zu den Professionalisierungstendenzen der Amateure aus der Sicht der elektronischen Medien. In: Paschen K (ed) Berufssport am Beispiel Fußball. Czwalina, Ahrensberg
Winkler HJ (1973) Sport und politische Bildung. Leske, Opladen
Zeigler EF (1977) Physical education and sport philosophy. Prentice Hall, Englewood Cliffs, NY

Mass Media, Sport and International Understanding

W. Gitter

Introduction

In its international activities the German Sports and Gymnastics Union (DTSB) of the German Democratic Republic bases its considerations on the fact that physical culture and sport can and must make an indispensable contribution to international understanding between nations, to a policy of détente and co-operation and thus to the preservation of peace throughout the world.

The development of sport at international level during this century, its worldwide dissemination, the widely ramified competition network and the proud development of the Olympic Games as a festival of friendship between peoples and of peace sufficiently demonstrate the above thesis. Athletes from all continents and states and with different social backgrounds meet to engage in fair competition, to get to know each other, to exchange their opinions and views, to become acquainted with other peoples' cultures, habits and customs, and, at the same time, to form a picture of their own homeland. Hereby, mutual respect is based on fairness and equality, thus promoting comprehension for common efforts towards understanding and peace.

As a result of the attention which they attract, international athletic competitions are capable of realising the humanistic goals of sport: Understanding directly materialises between athletes and, when reflecting upon their performances, among spectators in the stadium as well as among many television viewers, radio listeners and readers, the number of whom is continually growing in participating and other countries. In addition, however, co-operation between sports organisations at bi- and multilateral level, as well as work carried out by international sporting bodies and the sports scientific community, should also increasingly be directed at promoting the message of sport, namely international understanding.

One should not underestimate the part played by the mass media (press, television, radio, film), in the formation of public opinion by way of their coverage of and comments on international sport. It is astonishing that many sports sociologists do just this. They include in their research educational fields of any kind (parents, teachers, fellow sportsmen, lessons, self-interest etc.) as factors influencing sport, but the influence of the mass media on the ideology of sport is often neglected, and – in the extreme case – it is even asserted that the connection between the mass media, sport and international understanding is "apparently not a searchable concept" (UNESCO 1980).

In accordance with the International Charter of Physical Education and Sport of UNESCO (1978), the German Sports and Gymnastics Union of the GDR is strongly convinced that "... the mass media should exert a positive influence on physical education and sport". To this end, close relations between the governing bodies in sport and the mass media are recommended in the Charter; such co-operation will ensure objective and soundly based information.

Means of Co-operation Between Sport and the Mass Media

The DTSB of the GDR co-operates closely with both the mass media of the GDR itself and that of other countries. Within the last few years fruitful methods of co-operation have been developed which in the GDR are based on the fact that the mass media are governed by humanistic objectives and are also understood as a collective co-organiser of social life, including sport.

The following forms of co-operation have proved worthwhile:

- The DTSB holds regular press conferences at which up-to-date information is provided and views and experiences are exchanged with representatives of the mass media for mutual benefit. In this way, ideas and projects are discussed on a common basis, thus facilitating a streamlined promotion of physical culture and sport.
- The mass media launch their own initiatives both in popularising and in organising mass sporting competitions. The Association of GDR Sports Journalists, for instance, established a "mile committee" which in close co-operation with the bodies of sport helped the running movement immensely, in terms of both publicity and organisation. There are big relay races for children, a "table tennis tournament of the thousands", and many other events administered by large dailies and other media.
- Leading representatives of the mass media work as elected officials in the governing bodies of sports and lend their experience, opinions and methods to the work of these bodies to develop physical culture and sport. Such bodies are the National Executive of the German Sports and Gymnastics Union and the presidiums of national sports federations and organisations of sports science.
- Sports officials and sports scientists are included among the permanent staff of lecturers who provide training for sports journalists in the GDR. In this way sports journalists are enabled to work on a well-informed and factually correct basis.

The co-operation, only briefly outlined here, between our country's socialist sports organisation and the mass media proceeds from the principle reiterated in 1981 by the governing bodies of European sport at the 5th European Sports Conference in the final conference document (Abschlußdokument der V. Europäischen Sportkonferenz in Warschau, 1982): It was stressed unanimously that international sporting exchanges have become a firm and active element in the relations between people of different nationalities and help to further peace and friendship. They have a great influence on the education of young people, which is why in the present international situation more attention should be focused on the educational function of sport. In order to achieve this it is necessary "to exert influence on the mass media to the effect that they pay more attention to the realisation of the educational task of sport and develop their work considering this main objective".

The Committee for Mass Media, Sport and International Understanding

Knowing and considering all the relevant problems, we may assert today that during the 1970s a whole system of principles was created that encourage and enable the mass media to promote sport as a means of international understanding and of strengthening peace all over the world.

Some 10 years ago at the International Council of Sport and Physical Education (ICSPE), a committee entitled "Mass Media, Sport and International Understanding" and consisting of members from 11 countries was formed. This committee defined its aims as (ICSPE 1981):

- To promote the contribution of the mass media in the field of sport and of sports journalism to the furtherance of peace and international understanding and to the struggle against racism, apartheid and incitement to war or conflict
- To encourage the mass media to play an important part in educating young people in the spirit of peace, justice, freedom, mutual respect and understanding, with a view to promoting human rights and equality among people, nations and cultures in their social progress
- To promote - both at national and international level - co-operation between governmental and non-governmental organisations in the field of physical education and sport and the mass media in order to protect and implement the high ideals of sport

The foundations of the work of this committee, which includes among its members the president of the International Association of Sports Journalists (AIPS), are relevant UNESCO documents (*International Charter of Physical Education and Sport; Declaration on Fundamental Principles Concerning the Contribution of the Mass Media to Strengthening Peace and International Understanding, to the Promotion of Human Rights and to Countering Racialism, Apartheid and Incitement to War* - i.e., the *1978 Mass Media Declaration of UNESCO*) and suggestions arising from international conferences such as the Olympic Congress and the European Sports Conferences as well as from experience gained by the AIPS.

In December 1973 the first ideas for promoting the humanistic concern of this committee were set forth in a booklet entitled *Mass Media, Sport and International Understanding,* which was followed by another booklet *How Sports Journalists Can Contribute to International Understanding?* in March 1979 (ICSPE 1979). Studying the situation the committee focused on the following fundamental questions:

- The ethical and moral responsibility of the media for educating athletes and spectators and for promoting sport as a "bridge of understanding, comradeship and goodwill among nations without distinction as to race, colour, nationality and religion"
- The contribution of the mass media to the development of mass sports
- The professional qualifications of sports journalists
- Projects and subjects of research

Obstacles to the Flow of Information

What are the obstacles to the implementation of the high ideals and humanistic objectives outlined above? In our opinion, the barriers to the realisation of the humanistic task of sports journalists are inseparably connected with the commercialisation of sport and the mass media, which is increasing in many countries. This commercialisation militates against objective information, dissemination and responsible journalistic work in various ways.

The report to UNESCO mentioned at the beginning of this chapter (UNESCO 1980) drew attention, among other things, to the concentration of news information. A big American news agency, for example, supplies more than 1350 editors' offices in over 100 countries with information, while another agency has 2000 clients in 62 countries. Thus a bare dozen sports journalists working in the offices of these two agencies control the picture of international sport for millions of people.

A way out of this "information imperialism" (which is how this situation was characterised by the former Finnish State President, Urho Kekkonen) is offered by the International Programme of Communication Development (IPCD) which, in accordance with UNO resolution 34/182 (34th General Assembly), pursues the aim "to promote the establishment of a new, more just and more effective world information and communication order intended to strengthen peace and international understanding and based on the free circulation and wider and better balanced dissemination of information".

Large international sporting events - especially the Olympic Games - play an important part in the development of the international sporting press. But here too it is becoming more obvious that the burst of costs considerably reduces the free dissemination of information. The fees for TV transmission rights are astronomical, and a dangerous precedent has been set by the Los Angeles Olympic Organising Committee in selling the broadcasting rights for the 1984 Olympic Games. Furthermore, technical costs, telephone and telegraph fees, and the costs of hotel accommodation and travel are increasing enormously. Hence it follows that purely for economic reasons many countries can no longer send their own reporters and the concentration of sources of information increases instead of decreases. It is perhaps worth mentioning at this point that in December 1981 the ICSPE committee addressed a letter to the IOC President in which it was pointed out that this situation may constitute an infringement of the UNO Charter of Human Rights in respect of free access to information.

Further problems result from the commitment of journalists to the political interests of those circles on which the media in capitalist countries depend economically (for advertising revenue).

Conclusions

1. We believe that co-operation between the governing bodies of sport and the mass media should be increased at both national and international level in the interest of promoting the dissemination of sport, educating the sporting public, and contributing to understanding among nations and to the preservation of peace. Foundations for this are laid in the UNESCO Charter of Sport, in the suggestions made at the XIth Olympic Congress (where 13 speakers dealt positively with this question), in the documents of European sports conferences and in other international material based on consensus.
2. On the basis of the UNESCO Mass Media Declaration and of UNO resolution on the IPCD, the International Programme of Communication Development should also be promoted in the field of physical culture and sport to support, especially in

young developing countries, the training of sports journalists and the development of independent national sporting presses.

3. In co-operation with national federations of sports journalists and on the basis of the existing UNESCO documentation, AIPS and ICSPE should elaborate an international "code of conduct" defining ethical and moral standards for sports journalists and helping to protect their humanistic work.
4. The explosion of costs in the media's work at major international sporting events, especially the Olympic Games, should be countered with the understanding that a just dissemination of information is imperative. Reasonable and adequate working facilities for the media should be part and parcel of athletic competitions organised according to the rules of the international federations.
5. In the field of sports science, more research should be done into the relation between the mass media, sport and international understanding. The ICSPE special committee has given advice in this respect which should be developed further.

In the German Democratic Republic, all institutions in the field of sport and communication - the German Sports and Gymnastics Union as a non-governmental mass organisation, the State Secretariat of Physical Culture and Sport, the GDR National Olympic Committee etc. - will continue to co-operate with the Association of GDR Sports Journalists, the editors' offices of the mass media and all social forces of the country in order to realise the humanistic objectives of physical culture and sport in respect of the well-being of people and the furtherance of peace.

References

Abschlußdokument der V. Europäischen Sportkonferenz in Warschau von 8.-12. Dezember 1982. DDR-Sport 3:IV-V

ICSPE (1979) Committee of Mass Media, Sport and International Understanding. Report to UNESCO. How sports journalists can contribute to international understanding?

ICSPE, Committee of Mass Media, Sport and International Understanding. Terms of references, principles and aims approved in London, November 5th-6th, 1981

UNESCO (1978) International Charter of Physical Education and Sport. Article 8. UNESCO, Paris

UNESCO (1980) Mass media, sport and international understanding. A summary of a review of literature and research. UNESCO, Paris, p 2

2. Co-operation with Developing Countries

Co-operation Between Developing Countries and Advanced Countries in Respect of Sport

M. O. Ajisafe

Introduction

The continent of Africa is vast and heterogenous; moreover it contains more developing countries than any other continent. Therefore, in writing about co-operation with developing countries, one is actually writing about the co-operation that should exist on the one hand between African countries themselves and on the other hand between African countries and the developed countries.

John F. Coghlan, Secretary-General of the International Council of Sport and Physical Education, is right in saying that there are clear similarities in the problems experienced by each African nation but that the nations which comprise Africa vary considerably in wealth, tradition, historical circumstance, socioeconomic development, cultural awareness and political outlook (Coghlan 1980). He further states that there are common problems but no universal needs, and that the needs and priorities of each country in this complex situation vary according to particular local conditions.

Attempts to promote co-operation with developing countries must involve consideration of (a) the current problems of developing countries, (b) possible areas of co-operation between countries, and (c) proposals for co-operation between the developing and the developed countries in areas where action is urgently needed.

Current Problems of Developing Countries

Failure to Accept Physical Education

Article 1 of the UNESCO International Charter of Physical Education and Sports says:

> Every human being has a fundamental right of access to Physical Education and Sport, which are essential for the full development of his personality. The freedom to develop physical, intellectual and moral powers through Physical Education and Sport must be guaranteed both within the educational system and in other aspects of social life.

This Article clearly recognises physical education and sport as integral parts of any educational system. Unfortunately, in most developing countries they are not regarded in this way. According to Ajisafe (1977) some reasons for this are:

1. Ignorance of the benefits that can accrue from physical education and sport
2. Sociocultural impediments
3. Inadequate facilities and equipment
4. Financial constraints in developing countries

Since physical education and sport have not been fully accepted by most developing countries, any money occasionally earmarked for them is usually diverted to the "most urgent needs" of these countries. As a result, it is extremely difficult for developing nations to perform outstandingly well in international sport.

Social, Cultural and Religious Beliefs

Since Africa is not a homogenous region, there are obvious differences in the social, cultural and religious beliefs and practices of the various peoples of the continent. There are some African countries where such beliefs either completely forbid (particularly with reference to the female sex) or discourage participation in physical activities. For instance, in some parts of West Africa, a female person (no matter how young or old) is forbidden from wearing any dress that shows her legs. In other regions, married women (for religious reasons) are placed in *Pudah* - meaning that they cannot come out during the daytime. It is usually very difficult to break down these habits for the sake of participation in physical education and sport.

Colonial Heritage

We are all familiar with the colonial history of Africa and the attendant economic and cultural exploitation of the continent by the colonial masters. Sport, an integral part of culture, did not escape the colonial influence. As in most other areas of African culture, the colonisers succeeded in making Africans develop "complexes" towards their indigenous traditional sporting activities. Consequently, rather than developing and encouraging traditional African sports, which were considered barbaric, the colonisers introduced the "civilised" sports from their own cultures. This was the first area of damage. The second area of damage was associated with the fact that the foreign sports that were introduced were wrongly introduced. Physical education was presented to Africans strictly as an elitist concern. It is therefore not surprising that the majority of Africans, even among the elites, have since considered European sports - which constitute the items of international competitions - to be an unimportant pastime of the privileged educated class. Hence, up until today sport has not been as popular as it should be among Africans. This is reflected in the fact that in most African countries today, physical education and sport are the least favored and the least recognised of all school subjects.

Foreign Sports Encouraged Spectatorship

A corollary to introducing sports as an elitist exercise was that Africans who were natural lovers of sports were alienated and a sporting activity became a curiosity to be watched from afar rather than an event to be intimately involved in. Consequently, most of the games and sports introduced by the colonial masters to Afican countries encouraged more spectatorship and less participation. When, for instance, there is a soccer match in which 22 people are playing, the number of spectators may reach several thousand. In contrast, some African dances can accommodate 100 or more participants at the time; if performed for 15 min such dances will guarantee that the dancers become physically fit.

Physical Fitness

Another major problem of the developing countries is that of physical fitness. This, unfortunately, is not a common attribute of the average African. Ninety percent of the population carry roundworms, hookworms or other intestinal parasites; one in three have malaria parasites swarming in their bloodstream; the food intake of the average African is very low in calories, required for energy, and proteins, used for building up muscles and strength. To get a "fit" African, intestinal and blood parasites must be eleminated, anaemia corrected and adequate diet given.

Factors militating against Africans becoming "fit" are numerous. Prominent among them are: poor environmental sanitation, e.g., impurities of drinking water; lack of or inadequate sewage disposal (with resultant flies causing dysentery, diarrhoea and other infections); mosquitoes ready to re-inject malaria parasites; inadequate ventilation in houses and overcrowding leading to incessant colds and chest infections; bites from gnats and insects; cuts to unprotected feet; and poor roadways. All of these factors make it very difficult for the average African to keep fit.

Areas of Co-operation and Related Factors

Awareness of Background Situation

It is obvious from the foregoing brief summary of the current problems of developing countries that areas of co-operation can be correctly identified only if proper homework has been done and the specific needs of the developing countries in question are understood. In view of the heterogeneity of African countries it is important for each of the co-operating countries to be conscious of the geographical, sociological, cultural and political backgrounds of the country to which help is to be extended. Such awareness provides a solid basis for the development of a co-operative attitude and effective action.

Acceptance of Physical Education as a "Core" Course

Available evidence reveals that nowadays all the developing countries have a strong determination to improve their lot in every aspect of their lives. An important area of co-operation therefore is, as stated by Ajisafe (1976), the commitment to making physical education and sport an integral part of the basic core curricilum in all schools. After all, physical education requires the use of more sense organs in a developing child than does any other school subject. Hence physical education contributes most to the full development of the child.

Provision of Facilities

In most developing countries in Africa, matters of education are the responsibility of ministries of education. Co-operative help should therefore be extented to such ministries of education so as to enable them to adopt a planned policy involving first the provision of physical education and then a gradual increase in facilities for it.

Formulation of a Standardised Curriculum

At present, many developing countries are without a curriculum, while the curricula of others do not meet international standards. Co-operating partners should assist the ministries of education in these countries by providing experts who could formulate a standardised curriculum in physical education.

Training of Adequate Personnel

Developing countries lack experts in the area of teaching. In fact, in most such countries, physical education is not a compulsory subject. For efficient teaching of the subjact, experts should be trained to obtain higher qualifications in the academic and professional aspects of the discipline. Again, the advanced countries can help in this respect.

Retaining Trained Personnel

It is one thing to train experts to teach, it is another thing to retain such trained experts in their teaching jobs. When deciding teachers' salaries, governments should ensure that reasonable enticement is given to qualified teachers in order that they will continue to teach physical education and sport.

Improvisation

Since most African countries cannot afford to purchase all the necessary equipment and facilities, improvisation becomes very essential. Physical education experts should learn how to improvise for each game and sport and put this into practice whenever the need arises.

Developing Games and Sports of African Origin

Games of African origin need to be developed, especially now that Africans have started to emerge from the years of "brain-washing" which made them feel that "African things were bad and foreign things were good". Many countries still rely on foreign content, skills and methods of conducting physical education and sports. This is quite understandable because Africans go abroad to acquire knowledge of these areas of physical education. This is, however, no excuse for remaining limited by these foreign approaches to sports.

With the trend of events in African countries today, there is a need to develop games and sports of African origin with African experts teaching them and using equipment and facilities designed for use in Africa. This would not only boost Africans' ego but would also help them to take the first step towards making significant contributions to the variety of sports and games available to the international community.

Proposals for Co-operation in Areas Where Action Is Urgently Needed

1. *Implementation of the United Nations Charter.* The United Nations Charter, cited earlier in this text, should be made the basis for promoting the acceptance of physical education and sport as an entry requirement in all educational institutions.

2. *Equipment and Facilities.* Those developed countries which manufacture facilities and equipment should design some specifically for African use.

3. *Curriculum.* There should be an International Committee on Curriculum Development for Developing Countries. Such a Committee should formulate an acceptable minimum standardised curriculum of physical education and sport for the developing countries, bearing in mind the individual peculiarities of these countries.

4. *Training of Teachers.* The current practise is for many Africans to travel to the developed countries for training. The unfortunate side of this practise is that since there is a lack of home-based training facilities, those who come back to pass on to others the benefits of their training experience difficulties for obvious reasons. It is therefore important to have African institutions where Africans can be trained to teach Africans. If foreign experts were brought to African-based institutions, greater cost efficiency would be achieved and this would be more beneficial to Africans. In the event that Africans would still have to travel abroad to receive training in physical education and sport, the countries giving the training should do so with the realisation that the final product, i.e., the teacher, is meant to work and stay in Africa. Hence, the training should be biased towards African conditions.

5. *Institutions of Physical Education.* The currently existing departments and institutes of physical education should be properly developed and maintained. Also, all those developing countries yet to establish such departments and institutes should do so as a matter of great importance to the lives of their citizens.

6. *Exchange of Staff.* The spirit with which the Economic Community of West African States (ECOWAS) was established can equally be used to promote among developing African countries the mutual supply and sale of equipment and the exchange of teaching and research staff for physical education and sport.

7. *Publicity.* More people, particularly those without a school education, should be encouraged to participate in native games and sports. These games and sports should also be gradually introduced first to primary and then to secondary schools. A lot of publicity should be given to them via radio, television, and cinema, as well as in churches, market places, parks etc.

8. *Publication.* African physical educationalists have written few textbooks on the subject. It is high time that the long-neglected African games and sports were revived by African specialists in physical education and sport. This revival could only come about through describing them in books. Such books should be made texts for the primary and secondary institutions of education in the developing countries.

9. *Intra-African Competition.* In the view of Oyewusi (1981), indigenous games and sports should be encouraged by establishing intra-African competitions purely involving African games.

10. *Compulsory Educational Requirement.* For the purpose of good health and good human relations, physical education and sport should in every developing country be made examinable and compulsory subject in educational institutions.

11. *Magazines and Journals.* There should be African magazines and journals of physical education that regularly publish information on African physical education and sport; at present, Africa has no international journal or magazine of physical education comparable to the ICHPER magazine.

12. *Establishment of Ministries of Sport.* Instead of adding the responsibility for sports and games to the already heavy workload of the ministries of education, all developing countries should establish ministries of sport to cater more adequately for all aspects of physical education.

13. *Sports-Medicine Associations.* Developing countries should institute Sports-Medicine Associations whose major function would be:

a) to help identify potential sportsmen and women for further coaching
b) to prepare full medical examinations and tests that would identify the sports best suited to these sportsmen
c) to carry out medical examinations that would identify medical problems such as anaemia, malnutrition and parasites which can be treated and elaminated
d) to keep sportsmen and women continually fit by
   - administering preventive drugs such as anti-malarial agents
   - advising on food, water and sanitation
   - ensuring immediate and efficient treatment of injuries and an early return to fitness

Conclusion

If the above suggestions were to be implemented, a foundation would be laid for co-operation in sport not only between developed and developing countries but also among developing countries themselves. The proposals would also help to provide a basis for the growth in the developing world of a population made physically healthy through sport. Finally, they would make a vital contribution to healing the wounds of colonialism by helping the people of the developing countries to regain their dignity through the revival of their neglected cultural traditions in physical education and sport.

References

Ajisafe MO (1976) An indigenous syllabus of physical education for the Nigerian primary schools. Int Physical Ed 13/4:27-33

Ajisafe MO (1977) Problems of physical education in Nigeria. Int Physical Ed. 14/2:40-43

Coghlan JF (1981) Physical education needs in Africa. Bull ICSPE 6:15-19

Oyewusi JA (1981) Sports and physical education in developing countries. Unpublished Paper, Institute of Physical Education, UNICEF

Co-operation with Developing Countries in Matters of Sport

T. Varis

The field of co-operation with developing countries in matters of sport is still a largely unexplored and new area for research. It is a well-known fact that the practise of physical education and sport is not guaranteed everywhere as a fundamental right for all. While 80%–85% of children in developed countries now receive physical education at school, the proportion of those in the developing countries who do *not* receive it is estimated at 80% (UNESCO 1982). This is one rough indicator of the unequal relationships existing in today's world.

According to our recent survey (Hietanen and Varis, this volume) there seems to be extensive co-operation between industrialised countries and developing countries in the flow of sportsmen only in the fields of volleyball, fencing, table tennis, gymnastics and basketball. The exchange of coaches seems to be active between Europe and South America in volleyball, and between Europe and Asia in table tennis and gymnastics.

As described by Varis and Hietanen, there is an encouraging trend of extending the programmes of assistance from federation and association level to club and regional level. However, the basic problem of international relations with developing countries in matters of sport is not only the provision of financial and material aid but also the demand for equity in sports organisations and decision-making bodies. What is needed is co-operation on an equal basis.

General Aspects

The problem can be approached in terms of both principles and practical measures. The process of decolonisation has brought many new nations into the sporting world, and in these countries success in international sport has really meant nation building.

There are no basic documents outlining principles of cultural co-operation between countries of different social system and level of development; by contrast the Final Act of the Conference of Security and Co-operation in Europe (The Final Act 1975) laid just such foundations for sporting relations in the European region, and the United States and Canada were also signatories of this Act.

On the global level, there are only a few universally accepted documents to guide the growing number of intercultural exchanges, including those in the field of sport. One such document is the very constitution of UNESCO which "believes in full and equal opportunities for education for all" and is dedicated to the "purpose of advancing, through the educational and scientific and cultural relations of peoples of the world, the objectives of international peace and of the common welfare of mankind."

At present, this may be the most comprehensive general document regarding the development of equal relations with the developing countries. The participation of new nations in sports organisations has largely taken place on the conditions laid down by the existing international organisations, which are dominated by the industrialised countries. The models of the industrialised world have thus been simultaneously transferred to the new member states.

Although in political disputes the developing countries and teams have in some cases divided according to the East-West division, they have also organised themselves both regionally and politically. The movement of the non-aligned countries has a separate committee for sport and physical education (see, e.g. *Review of International Affairs, August* 5-20, 1978; Granma, September 6, 1981). The oil-rich OPEC countries have shown increasing interest in sports, and there have been attempts to organise regional and international games between the developing countries.

Development aid in the field of sport assumes many forms involving the transferral of people or money. In general, the forms of development aid in sport resemble the forms of any development aid, except that the aid is almost totally bilateral (see, e.g. Kyröläinen and Varis 1981). Not only individual countries but also international organisations like UNESCO, ICSPE, UNICEF and the IOC have shown increasing interest in development aid. In the case of the IOC, the so-called Olympic Solidarity is funded out of the national committee share of the television revenue. As for UNESCO, in the near future it will emphasise the promotion of physical education and sport for those in particular categories (girls and women), age groups (young children) or special situations (the handicapped).

What Kind of "Aid"?

The governments of developing countries have to try to strike a balance between the need to keep in touch with the international sporting movement and the need to deal with the problems of general social development (such problems often appear between mass sports and elite sports). Many developed countries are willing to build stadiums in the developing countries, but great stadiums import new models for sports administration, coaching, organisation and leadership trainig that are inappropriate for mass physical education. The developing countries must find their own indigenous solutions for the latter problem. The key word is "self-reliance", as the non-aligned countries put it.

In North-South relations, and especially in the fight against apartheid, the role of international co-operation in sport has been of a different character from the problems of East-West relations. The orientation has been towards a positive peace, respecting human rights, and here the deliberate use of sports for the goals approved by the United Nations (or inherent in the Olympic ideals themselves) has gathered a wide front of nations.

Some evidence suggests that sports organisations began pressuring South Africa long before the U.N. resolutions were even considered. In the 1950s South Africa was expelled from the international table tennis, boxing and football federations (Lapchick 1975). At present we have the United Nations International Declaration against Apartheid in Sports (UN Resolution 32/105 M) from 1977, and the work continues on drafting a convention against apartheid in sports. The United Nations Centre against Apartheid maintains a Register of Sports Contacts with South Africa (Register 1981) which monitors all kinds of sporting relations with South Africa and its associations.

It is obvious that equal relations with the developing countries can only be strengthened by a strict respect of these documents. The evidence so far tends to confirm the view that there is little awareness of the seriousness of this problem.

References

Granma, 6 September 1981

Kyröläinen H, Varis T (1981) Approaches to the study of sports in international relaions. Curr Res Peac Viol 4:55–88

Lapchick RE (1975) The politics of race and international sport: the case of South Africa. Greenwood, Westport

Register of sports contacts with South Africa. Centre Against Apartheid, Department of Political and Security Council Affairs. Notes and Documents No. 18/1981

The Final Act (1975) Conference on Security and Co-operation in Europe. Helsinki

UNESCO (1982) Draft medium term plan (1984–1989), 4 XC/4, UNESCO, Paris

Report of a Longitudinal Project in Sport Promotion in Brazil as a Means of Fostering International Understanding

L. Diem

The Federal Republic of Germany's programme for the development of sport in Brazil - undertaken in co-operation with the government of Brazil and headed by myself in the name of the Deutsche Sporthochschule Köln - covered about 10 years:

1972–1974: preparatory analysis
1975–1977: part I of project
1978–1980: part II of project
1981–1982: concluding evaluation

Preparatory Analysis, 1972–1974

Background factors included in the analysis were climatic conditions and topography, economic development and structure, social structure, demographic development, educational structure and administration. Discussions with Brazilian representatives covered administration and finance, the possibilities of sport, the regional planning of the 28 federal states, a model plan for sport facilities and analysis of staff requirements. Meetings were held with these representatives at conferences and training colleges in Brazil as well as during their exchange visit to the Federal Republic of Germany.

The following aspects of sport in Brazil were given special attention:

1. Reform of physical education by means of curriculum revision, beginning with elementary education at the kindergarten level and continuing through secondary education. Neglected sports received compensatory emphasis: track and field athletics, apparatus gymnastics, aquatic sports (swimming, water polo, rowing), handball as a newly introduced game, elementary dance and pantomime.
2. The structure of sports studies, particularly teacher training and postgraduate study. The analysis was focussed on pedagogy in general; the humanities and the social sciences (sport pedagogy, sport didactics, sport psychology, motor learning, administration and organisation, sports law, sports sociology and sports philosophy); medicine and the natural sciences (biomechanics, sport physiology, sports medicine and rehabilitation, particularly involving special gymnastics in school and sports for disabled persons). To complement the programme, guidelines were established for the creation of a documentation centre.
3. Information helpful for the recreational sports and the "Sport for All" programmes which already existed in Brazil.
4. Support for sports competition and the top-level sport. Here the accent was placed on the possibility of founding an academy where coaches might continue their

studies, on the organisation of top-level training centres and on the individual care of top-level athletes.
5. Construction of sporting facilities, especially school grounds, playing fields and swimming pools.

The two 3-year sports development programmes were based on the following agreement: for the German experts, the government of the Federal Republic of Germany would cover travel expenses, provide necessary teaching material and pay a daily honorarium of 100 German Marks. The Brazilian contact agencies would pay the costs of interpreters, transportation costs and the expenses of the Brazilian participants. During return visits to the Federal Republic of Germany, a similar arrangement applied to Brazilian representatives.

Parts I and II of the Project, 1975–1980

With the federal state of Brazilia we worked out a pilot programme for the teaching of physical education in kindergartens with the help of educationists and architects; we arranged a visit to the Federal Republic of Germany to inspect and analyse models in cologne, Munich, Berlin and Hamburg. Three kindergartens were at the disposal of reformers in Brasilia; improvements of the equipment in kindergartens and playgrounds were made on the spot with the local educators. This model in Brazilia will now be transferred to other states in Brazil. Special efforts will be made to transform the mostly rigid equipment for children's play and sport into play-stimulating situations especially oriented towards climbing, balancing, ball games and aquatic games. Exemplary new play facilities for all ages were developed (for example in Belo Horizonte).

With regard to *primary and secondary education*, joint seminars developed completely new curricula containing exact educational goals for each level. The Brazilian teachers published new textbooks and translated German textbooks. The previously vague educational goals, wherein sports appeared only under the rubric of "recreation", were now exactly defined for a 6-year period, enabling the teacher to plan, evaluate and control systematically.

The development of postgraduate studies was undertaken in universities selected by the Brazilian Ministry of Education. The university Sao Paulo (a university of the State Sao Paulo) seemed the most appropriate because of its equipment and experts in the faculty, followed by the two universities Santa Maria and Rio de Janeiro (both federal universities). Each university had to work out its own curriculum for postgraduate study in accordance with its capacities. Therefore it was possible, for example, for biomechanics to be developed at Santa Maria because only here was the co-operation of the departments of mechanics, statistics and sport guaranteed. The three universities named above introduced the first master's programme in *Educaçion Fisica* in South America (previously, Spanish- or Portuguese-speaking students had to go abroad for their postgraduate study). Other universities will now follow their example, and the creation of a successful master's and doctoral programme is only a question of time. The development of sports studies was successfully undertaken in all places where faculty members from traditional disciplines agreed to specialise in sports studies, e.g. sports pedagogy, sports didactics, sports philosophy, sports physiology and sports medicine. Up until now the development of the institutes for physical education or sport has been led - as in Europe - by medical experts. The new tendency, however, is for the directors of the scientific institutes to come from the ranks of pedagogues, psychologists and philosophers; again, this parallels the current trend in Europe.

In correspondence with the university credit system, the course of instruction for Brazilian experts in the field of sports studies took place over 2-4 weeks, with three to six lessons a day. Each course was concluded by a graded final examination. The German experts were selected not only from the faculty of the Deutsche Sporthochschule, Cologne, but also from the universities of Heidelberg, Mainz, Karlsruhe etc. in order to secure the best experts with knowledge of the language and experience in foreign countries. In the same programme, interested scholars from Brazilian universities were invited to do research in the Federal Republic of Germany.

The development of *recreational sport in Brazil* was supported by various municipal organisations. Booklets, textbooks, placards and a number of important town plans were published or exhibited. As an example of the action taken, the population of Sao Paulo was invited by citizens' groups from districts free from weekend traffic and industrial work to develop independent recreational activities; the results of this project were excellent. Information on possibilities for recreational sport was distributed by the sports and recreational offices; these officies also dispensed equipment and designated certain streets as "play streets" (*rua de lazer*). In the latter scheme each district could choose those sports most appropriate to its structure and interests. Apart from these play streets, which were meant especially for families, the parking lots of large shopping centres were provided with sports equipment, e.g. baskets for basketball. In this way, employed youths were able to use these areas for sport during evenings and weekends.

In the field of "Sport for All", the co-operation with the German Sports Federation stimulated a number of programmes, including teacher training for recreational activities and the creation of a flexible infrastructure (for regional differences in climate and social life meant that each Brazilian state had to develop its own individualised programme).

The *top-level sports* were promoted with the support of the National Olympic Committee of the Federal Republic of Germany. Apparatus gymnastics, previously neglected, was given a new impetus, as were swimming, rowing, fencing and track and field athletics (where training courses were introduced).

The Federal Institute of Sports Science provided the experts for the development of a *planning programme for sport facilities* and for the *creation of a documentation centre*. In addition to the experts sent by the Federal Republic of Germany to Brazil for short periods to carry out specific missions, one expert was sent for 3 years, which helped assure the positive outcome of the project. This latter expert was responsible for the co-ordination of the different measures and for contact with the Brazilian Ministry of Education and the Secretariat of Sport. On behalf of the Federal Republic of Germany, I supervised the co-ordination of the work of these experts and was responsible for evaluation of results and for regular consultation with our Brazilian partners.

During the follow-up phase in 1981-1982 some teacher training courses and concluding conferences were held.

3. National Measures

International Sport Relations

T. Bedecki

Introduction

In principle, an international relations approach to sport can contribute a great deal towards the development of world citizens. Competitive sport is, by its very nature, universal. International sport is an effective non-lingual medium of communication. As such, its laws are accepted and enforced on a global basis. As a universal language, sport can convey, on a person-to-person basis, through the media to the broader public, an interest shared with other people across political boundaries. These important aspects are often absent in many forms of international communication.

The prospects of increased international co-operation appear more favourable than at any other time. Technology has sparked a revolution in communication and transportation which continually brings increasing numbers of people involved in sport into direct, open and immediate contact. Increasingly, international diplomacy has become a public matter. Many foreign offices no longer confine themselves to speaking with other foreign offices; they help and encourage people to speak for themselves across national boundaries. People-to-people communication has become a dominant force in international relations throughout the world. The geometric increase in citizen involvement in the world affairs has special significance for the diplomat. It is less likely that nations will deal with their differences in absolute terms when their citizens communicate and co-operate with each other freely and frequently.

International Relations and Sport

International sport relations aim at promoting international understanding through the medium of sport by interacting and developing two-way communication. The guiding principle in international relations is to make an effort at reciprocal understanding between countries. It is assumed, even without conclusive evidence, that international sport activities contribute to mutual understanding among people and countries. The relevance of sport is in symbolic communication. People in different cultures have a common understanding of what is taking place.

A new role for sport in the field of international relations has developed during the past decade. For example, the international significance of sport received a new dimension when representatives from Europe, the United States and Canada (under the section entitled co-operation in the humanitarian and other fields) signed an agreement at a conference on security and co-operation in Europe.

Canada's Past and Present Involvement

The role of the Canadian federal government in international exchanges has traditionally been expressed through cultural programmes which fall under artistic and academic exchanges. Little attention has been paid to sport as a factor in cultural relations. The federal government has become much more involved in international cultural programmes in order to provide a national framework for the cultural aspirations and interests of all Canadians.

The federal government, through the Fitness and Amateur Sport Branch, has a recognised role in sport. Part of this role is to enhance the performance level of Canadians, both nationally and internationally. It is, therefore, in the federal government's best interest to help ensure that international exchanges do in fact contribute optimally towards better international relations. Thereby, government acts as a facilitator, aiding the multitude of Canadian sport organisations to carry on their international programmes effectively.

Recently more formal sport exchange programmes have taken place with the USSR, Cuba and China; in these countries sport is a serious endeavour in that they direct impressive resources to sport at many levels. Canada, by maintaining a relatively high profile in sport exchanges with these countries, also serves worthwhile social and political goals. In such closed societies, where conventional information programmes are difficult to carry out, a sport relations event takes on greater significance than it would in other countries.

As international contact continues to increase, so also do the efforts of various international and national agencies to ensure the benefits of sport. The efforts of many of these organisations have become more educational in nature. More attention is being paid to cultural exchanges of personnel, information and co-operative research.

International sport relations is not an issue in the socialist countries, for such relations have an established hierarchy between countries and governments. Too often Western countries rely on non-government agencies for such initiatives.

Despite the growing role of government in this area, government agencies cannot, and should not, replace non-government agencies. There are Western advocates who feel that international relations in sport is not the business of the government and the sport lies outside the scope of official exchanges between nations. It is apparent that international co-operation is a prerequisite for the universal, well-balanced formation of sport. To achieve this, there is need for co-operation between government and non-government agencies.

Implications for Foreign Relations Policy

The principal concern confronting international sport relations is that it has remained a neglected area, this neglect being compounded by absence of an explicit national policy. To date, government sport agencies as well as many non-government sport agencies have paid little attention to developing sport relations internationally.

An effective international sport relations programme means the development of a national policy to encourage and deploy sport in support of Canada's national goals. Such a policy presupposes a recognition of sport as a social influence in numerous aspects of national life - cultural, social and political. Until recently, sport did not benefit from such an awareness or perspective. The guiding principle for exchanges on a private or government basis should be one of mutual benefit and reciprocity. There is a need for a systematic and co-ordinated approach which should be developed with the federal government through External Affairs, the Fitness and Amateur Sport Branch of Secretary of State, and non-government sport organisations.

The underlying objectives for promotion of international understanding in a sport relations programme should be as follows:

1. To support the achievement of the short and long-term goals of the athletes' competitive programmes
2. To reflect internationally the development and scope of Canada's sport scene, and the promotion of mutual aid in this area
3. To facilitate co-operation on international sport problems

The implementation of an international sport relations programme should be threefold. First, Canada's relations with other countries should be improved through the medium of sport by arranging for increased interpersonal contact. The prevailing emphasis is directed towards athletes, coaches, officials and specialists in Canada and abroad. The basic goal should be to maximize the number of opportunities for Canadians to have meaningful people-to-people contacts. Secondly, facilitation and monitoring of international sporting exchanges should occur. The number of opportinities for Canadians to compete abroad is constantly increasing, thereby improving the performance of athletes in their respective sport and providing comparative evaluation. Thirdly, sport should be given greater prominence in international bilateral and multilateral co-operation.

Shaping International Relations in Sport

Where do we go from here to advance our exchange efforts and in managing our international sport relations? One might suggest a study seminar on international sport relations - Strategy for the 1980's. This would allow national and multisport agencies, athletic directors and other people involved in sport to express their views and influence future Canadian strategy.

Such participation might well form the basis of a Joint Canadian Agency/Council to initiate procedures and practices. This would ensure activity and participation by this country in matters of international sport relations. There is a need at this stage to construct channels and institutionalise arrangements. Committed and enthusiastic individuals who can think in complex world terms will continually form the broad base of people able to function in this international environment.

The Joint Council/Agency mandate may well incorporate the following objectives:

- The promotion and development of Canada's international relations through sport
- The development of a clearing-house for volunteers with particular skills and knowledge in this area
- The execution or co-ordination of sport exchange projects when so invited

- The collection and dissemination of current information on sport exchange relations
- The advising of government on exchange programmes to enhance international sport relations

Such a Council/Agency would be a non-profit service organisation and essentially an executive instrument for sports co-operation and furthering international sport relations. Membership, thus, would be open to anyone interested in international sport relations in order to improve cross-cultural communications and promote sport activities. World-wide interest in sport can make an important contribution to the development of this two-way communication. Canada's relations abroad should be the business of Canadian sport at home. For most Canadians there is a reverence or awe about international relations as if it is distant and unreachable.

The major emphasis of this paper is that the mass feelings generated by sport can be used to upgrade contemporary international relations. Sport has contact influence; it is probably that aspect of modern life which is most often encountered throughout the world. It is time to recognise the necessity of encouraging Canadian efforts in the area of international sport relations.

References

AAHPER (1976) Professional preparation: An international relations approach. J Physical Ed Recreation 47 (8):19-22

American Council on International Sports (1977) News Briefs 1 (3)

Centre for International Sports Studies (1978/79) Sports Exchange World 3

Chu EJ (1976) Nature and scope of international amateur sports participation by selected countries and the implications for international relations. Doctoral dissertation, New York University

Council of Europe (1976) Medium-term plan (1976-80): Cooperation in the field of education, culture and sports. Western European Education 8 (3)

Cowley GA (1976) The emergence of culture as a facet of foreign policy. Int Perspectives Sept/Oct:27-32

Dougherty JE, Pflatzgraff RL (1971) Contending theories of international relations. Lippincott, Philadelphia

Heinilä K (1974) Sport and international understanding. FIEP Bull 44 (3):35-38é

Hitchcock WK (1974) Educational exchanges and international relations. Higher Educational Exchange 2:7-8

International Education and Culture. Sports - a Universal Language. Exchange 13(1)

Milshtein OA (1976) Shaping of public opinion regarding sport by the mass media as a factor promoting international understanding. Int Rev Sport Sociol 11 (3):71-84

Mlodzikowski G (1977) International sports relations. Kultura Fizyczna (Physical Culture) 31 (7): 322-327

Reich AA (1974) International understanding through sports. US Dept State Bulletin 70:460-465

Singer RN (ed) (1973) Multidisciplinary Symposium on Sport and the Means of Furthering Mutual International Understanding. United States Department of State Bureau of Educational and Cultural Affairs, Washington D.C., December 4

The Significance of International Co-operation in the Field of Physical Culture Sciences for International Understanding

F. Sýkora

The present paper will deal with the significance, possibilities and forms of development of international scientific co-operation in strengthening the relations and understanding between scientific workers and informing social values in the field of physical culture sciences as well as in sports practice. That scientific co-operation has such a role is evidenced by the participation of Czechoslovakian scientific workers in international co-operation on scientific tasks, in the activities of international societies, and in scientific congresses, conferences and symposia both abroad and in Czechoslovakia, as well as by publications, the education of scientific workers, the mutual exchange of scientific workers, study stays, lectures and other activities.

The conclusions drawn in the paper are that there is room for further improvement of international co-operation and of the themes subjected to research within the framework of international co-operation, as well as for better management of these activities.

In Czechoslovakia physical culture is considered an important part of both our social-political system and the general culture of our population. By means of its individual components, such as physical education, sport, tourism, mobile holiday-making and "mobile recuperation," physical culture significantly contributes towards the improvement of health, the increasing of physical efficiency and the perfection of physical exercise and achievement, as well as towards aims related to the upbringing, education and general development of children, young people and adults.

The highly humanitarian functions of physical culture are, in the main, the same all over the world and in all countries. The general educational aims and the conditions created in this field may differ from country to country, but the basic function of this social activity is common to all: to contribute to the upbringing of healthy, physically efficient, able and happy people. Therefore experts from all parts of the world intending to fulfil this function are interested in acquiring knowledge about the contents, the methods and the possibilities of this educational task in order to increase their abilities to work towards the fulfilling of this function. Research workers in different branches of sciences are also interested in international co-operation in research into the function of physical culture with regard to the way of life of people, their general development and the increase in their capabilities in physical exercise and sport. They are also interested in research into the function of physical culture for the development of society and of mankind.

In Czechoslovakia this co-operation is considered useful not only for fulfilling our tasks in this field with regard to the improvement of our people's physical abilities, but also because it is an important means of both bringing about understanding between nations and contributing to the maintenance of peace in the world (physical culture itself can fulfil its purpose only under the conditions of everlasting peace). The function of physical culture is in fundamental contradiction to any action threatening people's health and physical abilities, and any kind of warefare clearly has the most injurious impact on the health, abilities and lives of individuals, nations and human society.

Since the end of World War II, Czechoslosvakia research workers in the field of the physical culture sciences have been carrying out their research work with great enthusiasm. Their purpose is to contribute in the best possible way towards the fulfilment of the humanistic aims of the physical culture sciences, making all efforts to bring about international co-operation and mutual understanding in cases requiring the solution of problems in this field. They have participated in the activities within the framework of international co-operation on scientific tasks in basic forms such as:

- Participation in the activities of international organisations of research workers
- Active participation in several research activities abroad and in Czechoslovakia
- Participation in international research work dealing with the solution of certain research tasks
- Participation in international exchanges of scientific workers and in study stays
- Publication of the results of scientific works and papers both abroad and in Czechoslovakia

We are able to cite unnumberable examples of how Czechoslovakian scientific workers in the physical culture sciences have been active in all of the above-mentioned ways. At present, for example, 21 Czechoslovakian scientific workers are working in the following international organisations: ICSPE (within the framework of UNESCO), FIEP, ISSP, AISEP, FIMS and others. Both in the past and nowadays, Czechoslovakian scientific workers have held important posts in these organisations. Czechoslovakia is among those countries which have the greatest number of deputies in worldwide and European organs of physical culture and sport as well as in sport federations.

Czechoslovakian scientific workers are taking part in scientific congresses, conferences and symposia every year, and a great number of experts from abroad come to Czechoslovakia to participate in study stays, conferences and lectures concerning many branches of the physical culture sciences.

During the last 10 years international scientific co-operation has successfully been developing, being connected with the solution of several scientific tasks, e.g. research into physical efficiency within the context of the International Biological Year and research into the training of physical culture teachers.

A great number of scientific papers such as reviews and monographs concerning the physical culture sciences are being published in Czechoslovakia (including in foreign languages) and some research results obtained by our scientific workers have been published abroad.

We can, however, see further possibilities for intensifying international co-operation in science and we would like to take part in such possibilities to a greater degree. In particular, the co-ordination of international co-operation in the physical culture sciences requires improvement. Judging by our past experience, we think that the right way to achieve this is to entrust one of several international organisations with the task. We consider ICSPE the most suitable organisation for this purpose, as it is part of UNESCO and has already carried out much useful work in this field.

Another important task which could also be undertaken by an organ of international co-operation is greater stimulation of international co-operation with regard to finding solutions to the most topical contemporary problems. Here I would like to mention some examples: research into concrete methods of international co-operation in the physical culture sciences; research into the physical efficiency of population groups differing in terms of age, sex and state of health; research into the techniques and efficiency of methods of scientific research; and research into the material conditions for physical culture. The conclusions of the Conference on Sport held by the highest representatives of physical culture in Europe also call for such co-operation.

It would be convenient, too, if the co-ordination centre were to provide information about planned conferences and symposia so that those interested would have sufficient time to hand in their application forms and prepare for the events concerned.

Many further problems could be solved on the basis of international co-operation between scientific workers in the field of physical culture all over the world. the conclusions of this conference should stimulate such concrete co-operation, which should be discussed in national and international organisations of workers involved in physical culture science. The next step would be the gradual realisation of these conclusions; in other words, more extensive and useful international co-operation under the peaceful conditions of life in contemprary society. Czechoslovakian scientific workers in the field of physical culture will make every effort to bring about such co-operation.

Sport and Non-alignment: Dilemmas and Prospects

K. Petrovič, M. Žvan and R. Šugman

Sport in International Relations

Sport, which can enrich human life through its elements of play and happiness, is global - it demands an international scene - but at the same time it is also national. Sport both unites and separates: It involves the meeting and the amicable competition of friends, but also the prestige of political formations, nations, races and ideologies - the rivalry of antagonists (enemies). Sport is not an oasis of peace, but a manifestation of the actual relations between the world's nations. Politics uses it as its powerful ally - sometimes to pressure, sometimes to parley - achieving results sometimes impossible by other means.

Sport cannot be the universal panacea for all power confrontations, for the differences between the rich north an the poor south; it is not a new world order, but it can and should be a means towards a happier and a more humane humanity.

Non-alignment and Sport

In order to be able to discuss the significance and role of sport in non-aligned countries, in the so-called Third World, it is necessary, first of all, to understand the basic motivating forces of the non-alignment movement with regard to (1) the position and role of sport in the world in general, and, based on this, (2) what sport can represent, and (3) in what direction it should be developed in non-aligned countries.

The movement of the non-aligned can undoubtedly be regarded as a permanent endeavour of anti-imperialistic revolution by the nations concerned. It has historically been proved that the basic need of individuals and of nations is to become free and equal subjects with their own physiognomy and individuality. The present development of non-alignment cannot be regarded only as a reaction to the bloc division of the world, and as the antithesis of this division. The present role of non-aligned countries and their demands for the rearrangement of the world order refute the opinion that non-alignment is merely a utopian attempt, although it is true that their efforts are evidently a long-term historical process which is not the result of a certain moment in international relations but has its roots in the general contemporary development of economic and political relations. The objectives of non-alignment have all the elements that could be called the prospects of mankind.

We agree with E. Kardelj that

> ...in spite of the crisis through which non-alignment has gone so far, it has not lost any of its significance for progressive mankind as long as the circumstances, powers and processes which lead the

nations into the position of economic and political dependence and inequality, to the domination and hegemony of the world centres of economic and political power of any kind, exist in the world.

In this struggle the Third World is moving in contradictory currents, the two main ones being the emancipation of the nations and the integration of mankind (Kardelj 1975). In the first place, there is the struggle against the forces of international exploitation for political and economic independence and for an adequate place in the process of the distribution of the world's goods, the struggle for the creative freedom of the nations and mankind, including culture and thus also physical culture. On the other hand, there is the opening outwards towards other nations, based on the understanding that nothing is progressive if it does not open outwards. The world process of integration means the approaching and uniting of nations, greater global dependence, and responsibility of nations for an equitable future world. Both processes are actually two sides of the same social process; separately and in interaction, they give rise to a series of contradictions and conflicts of interest.

Non-aligned countries represent an enormous political and moral power, although their narrower interests, their national resources and also their specific political interests are not identical and can, therefore, hardly be characterised irrespective of their long-term and global aims.

An yet sport, which is (only apparently) a moderate factor in international relations and politics, is of real importance for the non-aligned in the process of their emancipation as well as of their integration into the global company of nations (Čop 1981).

Sport - The Extended Arm of World Politics

The boycott of the Olympic Games in Montreal by the African states, the resounding boycott of the Olympic Games in Moscow, the significance attributed to sporting success in some countries, the expression of national identity, the prestige of nations - all this gives sport, in the present world situation, a specific significance which it would not have in a different constellation of world relations and which, by nature, it should not have. In essence, the role of world sport becomes increasingly more important, as well as national, the more planetary it is (Bergant 1981).

Sport in its true sense is the competition of the best with the best. Only in this way can its global significance be developed (Wohl 1977, 1976). At the same time sport is also national. Through sport, human life can acquire the contents which transcend severe exercise and achievement, and reach the level of play and happiness. Both aspects fit into the system of contradictory development of the Third World. Sport as a universal phenomenon has an integrational as well as disintegrational role. Although modern imperialism and other totalitarian systems present sport as an oasis of peace, sport is, nevertheless, the reflection of global national relations. Willingly or unwillingly, sport is becoming a tool for politics (Heinemann 1977).

The boycott of the Moscow Olympic Games and also Mundial 82 have demonstrated the great political impact of sport. It is not rare that through sport nations try in a fictive way to solve mutual conflicts that cannot be resolved at any other level. Consciously or unconsciously, sport is often used to "tranquillize" masses at times of political and economic crises.

Through sport, greater pressure can be exerted internationally than by any other means. And yet, sport is often more successful in promoting peaceful coexistence than are numerous diplomats and conferences.

Sport: What It Should Be, and Often Is Not

Yugoslavia, as one of the founders of non-alignment, has numerous connections with sport associations in non-aligned countries. In accordance with the document from Colombo, Yugoslavia has linitiated a programme of collaboration with other non-aligned countries in the field of sport (Peta konferencija šefova država ili vlada nesavrstanih zemalja u Kolombu 1976; ICSPE 1968). The basic idea is the development of sport as a model of life, play, happiness and relaxation. In sport, small nations and poor nations can become great. It is also clear that in many non-aligned countries sport is a means of searching for and confirming a national identity, the factor of inner integration and of outer affirmation.

By accepting modern sport, the Third World often uncritically accepts the western -capitalistic models and the role of sport that was conceived in terms of the bloc mentality. In future, more attention should be paid to this problem, otherwise very little leeway will be left for the non-aligned in the area of sport. Just as the non-aligned nations struggle for a different economic and political order, for different relations between the poor and the rich, for a different integration of mankind, so they should fight for different sport. The role of sport and its influence on man should not be underestimated. Sport should be given a more human and humane content. In this context the sport policy and activity of the non-aligned should be formulated and carried out in the same way as their struggle for the new economic and political order. Through sport, progressive powers can be engaged, but also the imperialistic mode of thinking can be imposed through it.

The non-aligned should become the promoter of a more humane approach towards top-level sport and achievement, although tis is relatively difficult owing to the universality of sport (Polic 1980). The use of doping, the rearing of champions in retorts and the exploitation of man's potential for self-destruction are approaching absurdity and taking forms similar to those of the arms race and other forms of domination (Coe 1981). In this sense the non-aligned are confronted with an important task: physical culture for large masses, sport for everybody who wants it, absence of elitism, and sport as every man's good, as a component of human life and happiness. Only through such a conception of sport can Yugoslavia see an opportunity to alter the present development of sport in the world, which is ever more rapidly approaching absurdity and self-negation.

Sport is not a universal remedy in the confrontations of blocs; it does not and cannot compensate for inadequate relations in the world; it cannot resolve the problems of the rich North and the poor South; it is not a new world order – but it *can* be a step towards a more humane and happy mankind. One must be extremely sensitive and cautious when analysing the means of achieving various aims: the question should be raised as to whether a certain means (and this goes also for sport), at any level of its development and use, is capable of achieving its objectives. This is the responsibility of the individual and of nations, and finally, also the responsibility of non-alignment.

References

Bergant E (1981) Olimpijske perspektive po Baden Badnu 1981. (Olympic perspectives after Baden-Baden 1981.) Telesna kultura 29:5–6

Coe S (1981) Ansprache beim 11. Olympischen Kongress namens der Athleten. Code V 09, Baden-Baden, 1981-09-11, p 2–6

Čop V (1981) Fizička kultura i sport nesvrstanih. (Physical culture and sport of the non-aligned countries.) Aktuelna politička biblioteka. Borba, Beograd

Heinemann K (1977) Ist ehrenamtliche Mitarbeit noch zeitgemäss. Sportunterricht 26:6

ICSPE (1968) Manifest über den Sport. UNESCO, Paris

Kardelj E (1975) Zodovinske korenine neuvrščenosti. (Historical roots of non-alignment.) Komunist, Ljubljana

Peta konferencija šefova država ili vlada nesavrstanih zemalja u Kolombu 16–19 avgusta 1976 godine (Fifth conference of heads of state or government of the non-aligned countries in Colombo 16–19.8.1976). Dokumenti, prilozi. Komunist, Tanjug, Medunarodna politika, Beograd

Polič B (1980) Fizička kultura u samoupravnom socijalističkom društvu. (Physical culture in a self-managing socialist society.) Institut za fizičku kulturu, Beograd

Wohl A (1976) Sodobne olimpijske igre in vrhunski šport. (Modern Olympic Games and competitive sport.) TK 24:7–11

Wohl A (1977) Humanističke funkcije vrhunskog sporta. (Competitive sport's humanistic function.) Informativni bilten ficzičke kulture 15:46–50

The State as Sponsor of International Sports

H. Klemola

Introduction

Owing to the differences in administration between our countries, as well as the differences in the relations between the administration and the sports organisations, it is not possible to discuss this subject in a general manner. Therfore I will concentrate on the factors that have affected the official sports policy in Finland, particularly the support to international sports. I will begin by recalling some basic facts.

Heads of state have repeatedly stressed the importance of sport in social and international interaction, and even in the relaxation of international tension. In the Final Act of the Conference on Security and Cooperation in Europe it is stated that: "In order to expand existing links and cooperation in the field of sport the participating States will encourage contacts and exchanges of this kind, including sports meetings and competitions of all sorts, on the basis of the established international rules, regulations and practice." It has been said that sportsmen are the goodwill ambassadors of their country, and that they should not neglect the opportunity to act as such. The Charter of the ICSPE from 1968 stresses that sport (a) encourages people to interact in an atmosphere of joy and sincerity, (b) enables people to learn to know others more fully and (c) evokes compassion, a sense of affinity and the will to perform noble and unselfish deeds. Sport thus gives a new dimension to the concept of brotherhood.

The views of the two documents cited above may illustrate the challenging goals that are set out for sport administrators and sportsmen. The tasks of the state as a sponsor of "sport culture" have been pointed out in different contexts; it has been said that a basic sports education should be given in schools, and that the planning and construction of sports facilities should guarantee possibilities for more people to practise sport. But an essential condition for these activites is economic support.

With regard to the future, it is important that UNESCO, as an intergovernmental organisation for the promotion of education and culture, has attached more importance to the universal development of the ethical goals of sport.

Sports Act

During the last few decades in Finland particular attention has been paid to the contacts and co-operation between the sports organisations and the public administration. The division of labour is defined in the 1980 Sports Act as follows: "The creation of general prerequisites for sports activities lies primarily with the State and the municipalities. The sports organisations referred to in this Act are principally responsible for the arrangement of sports activities." In practice this means that the participation of Finland in international competitions is arranged by the sports organisations, usually with state support. The granting of support presupposes systematic planning and co-operation between the sports organisations. The promotion of the official sports policy also demands international contacts on a multilateral and a bilateral level which are separate from the contacts that the sports organisations engage in. The co-operation and division of labour between the organisations and the state have been taken into consideration in the administration of sport in Finland. Thus, before making decisions the Council of State and the Ministry of Education hear evidence and opinions from the State Sports Council and the Council for Physical Education, which both include representatives of the sports organisations.

Two years ago the Ministry of Education and the State Sports Council prepared a "Plan on International Sports Policy and the Participation of the Finnish Public Administration in International Co-operation." In the introduction, reference was made to the objectives of participation in international activities, as presented by the Committee for the Preparation of the Sports Act. The objectives are:

- The promotion of international understanding and peace by means of sports policy
- Education for co-operation and international communication
- The advancement of the international sports policy in accordance with the official foreign policy
- Equality in the participation in international activities
- The inclusion of sports activities in development assistance work

The objectives were based on the view that sport is an important form and means of international co-operation. Our international sporting contacts also relate to the official foreign policy.

International Top-Level and Competitive Sport

As we all know, the most visible form of international sport is top-level competition which follows its own goals and rules as approved by the international organisations. The typical feature of such competitions is that the sportsmen participate in the name of their country, sports society or club. The sports instructors and other experts, for their part, represent their country and organisation at international meetings, congresses and seminars. The principle is clear: the national representative is a kind of ambassador.

Likewise, it has been pointed out that the representatives seek incentives and coaching to raise the level of sport in their own country. Comparisons with other countries and sporting traditions can provide new information and experiences, and the Finnish sportsmen can transmit their knowledge and experiences to the international forum while the sports instructors can promote the general goals of sport.

When examining the prospects for the future, the Committee for the Preparation of the Sports Act emphasised particularly the specific value of international sports competitions. International competitions often result in battles in prestige between countries, but one should also bear in mind that they bring peoples closer to one another and promote the advancement of international understanding. All this means that international sports activities and their goals have to be taken in earnest. The Committee also mentioned that in past years the UNESCO Conference for Ministers Responsible for Sports Affairs, UNESCO's Sports Committee, the European Sports Conference and the Olympic movement haven envisaged an expansion in the tasks of public administration related to sports. It also appears that the increased interest of the states will enhance the status of the organisational work. An overall promotion of sports culture presupposes a more far-reaching planning of sports facilities. Owing to the increased costs, number and size of sports institutes, the community will have to take responsibility for their planning, construction and maintenance. The share of public financing seems to have increased in other respects as well; this is the case in Finland, and emphasises still further the importance of international co-operation.

In Finland the public support for international sports activities is concentrated on economic assistance. The annual state support to the major sports organisations covers from 40% to 70% of their expenses. Thus the state support also affects the participation in international activities. Special training for and participation in the Olympic Games take place mainly with state support. State support is also granted for major international games and events organised in Finland, such as this congress. For international competitions to be sucessful, they naturally require appropriate premises. In Finland these premises have in most cases been constructed, and are maintained, by the municipalities with support from the central administration. The state also grants scholarships to Finnish experts who take part in international congresses and events of special interest for the advancement of sports. In this context it is important to point out that in Finland the state does not concern itself with the selection of sportsmen or teams for competitions. This is done by the sports organisations.

Other Areas of International Co-operation

The international participation of the Finnish state is restricted to sports administration, planning, physical fitness training, physical education and the construction and maintenance of sports facilities. The most important co-operative bodies in which Finland has participated are UNESCO's Sports Committee, the European Sports Conference, the Sport Committee of the Council of Europe (CDDS) and the ICSPE. Finland is engaged in bilateral co-operation with Sweden, Norway, Denmark, Iceland, the Soviet Union, the Federal Republic of Germany, the German Democratic Republic, Hungary, Poland and France. Representatives of the sports organisations take regularly part in the practical implementation of the co-operation, and the Ministry of Education can assign to the State Sports Council and the Council for Physical Education tasks relating to international activities.

In the official sports policy it is important to see that the interests of all citizens are taken into consideration. On the international forum it is important to try to reach the young people and thus to enlarge the scope of international education. In view of this, international youth exchange and friendship activities between towns will be expanded in the future.

In conclusion, one can say that the tasks of the state and the municipalities with regard to the promotion of international activities primarily relate to the creation of economic prerequisites and to the construction and maintenance of appropriate sports facilities. This demands channels of co-operation and participation in international activities, also within the field of public administration.

A favourable attitude on the part of the state is based on the condition that the international and national organisations promote the advancement of sports. Thus the sports culture can maintain the valuable functions that it has endorsed and protected for many decades, as well as maintain mutual confidence between the state and the sports organisations – this is an indispensable condition for the future success of international co-operation.

The Meaning of International Sporting Events to a Small Country (from the Viewpoint of a Sports Leader)

J. Uunila

Finland's Participation in International Sporting Events

Finland has participated in the modern Olympics ever since the games in Athens in 1906. In the Winter Games we have taken part since their beginning, i. e. from the year 1924. In the whole world there are only 11 countries that have participated more often in the Olympics than Finland. We have sent nearly 3000 representatives, competitors and officials to the games. On current trends, this number will increase by 250–300 persons every fourth year, i. e. every time the Olympic Games are held.

Our country has also participated hundreds of times in the World Championships and the European Championships. The development of the international special associations indicates that the number of games at this level is growing all the time, and thus the intercourse in connection with the major sporting events will also increase.

Finland has organised several international sporting events. The highlight for us was the Olympics in Helsinki in 1952. The first World Championships in track and field athletics in Helsinki in 1983 continued our role as an organiser of major sporting events.

The International Olympic Committee and the international special associations were founded to manage the worldwide system of major sporting events. As the activities grew, a world federation of the national olympic committees was founded. Finland participates in the work of all these organisations, and there are now 40 Finns working in different positions.

At present, 151 countries belong to the International Olympic Committee, i. e. the olympic family. Most of them are small. The number of the member countries is growing along with the birth of new states.

Huge sums of money are currently spent on international sports. Organising major sporting events is very expensive, and the costs of the preparations (primarily the training) for the ever mor demanding games as well as of participation itself are high all over the world. For small countries like Finland, the sums in question are really large and are growing all the time. From time to time this fact stirs critical citizens to contemplate what the significance of this kind of activity is for a small nation.

The Olympic Ideology

One of the main goals of organised international sport is to get all nations to participate regardless of race, religion or political views. The rules of, among others, the International Olympic Committee state this explicitly. The Olympic Movement has succeeded very well in its endeavour. As I have mentioned, the International Olympic Committee at present has 151 member countries. The Olympic Movement has existed for almost 100 years. It has been shaken strongly from time to time, and the latest crisis - the boycott of the Moscow Olympics brought about by the most powerful statesmen in the world - put the Olympic Movement in a tight corner. The fact that the Movement was able to withstand the really intense pressure was a great victory for it. It was also promising for the future of the movement. For a small country like Finland the existence and the continuity of a movement of this kind is very important. An activity in which people representing different races, religions and political systems participate serves as an important means of détente, which we should support in every way. The growth of mutual understanding and peaceful co-existence is for the small countries in particular, the basic question of existence.

In the decision making of the international sports organisations, large and small countries are equal. In most organisations the principle of "one man one vote" is followed. No country has the right of veto as, for instance, in the United Nations. This increases the influence of small countries like Finland. In many ways the role of small countries has been to act as bridge builders between the large countries. Particularly in this sense Finland, as a country with notable sporting achievements, has had its own important mission.

The Helsinki Spirit

When a small country is entrusted with organising an important international sporting event, it is always a manifestation of esteem and recognition. The right to organise the Olympics of 1952 was granted to Finland just at the right time. We needed incentive and appreciation after the trying wars. The struggle to organise the Helsinki Olympic Games was not in vain. In a small country, where people are really interested in sports, this could be seen exceptionally clearly. The so-called Helsinki spirit was born, and 30 years later it is still being praised all over the world as something positive and unique. To our joy we sports leaders have been able to experience this on our travels. The fact that Finland managed to organise the games quite successfully strengthened the self-esteem of our people and our belief in the future, and made even the greatest sacrifices worthwhile.

The Mass Media

The continuous development of communication equipment has brought the big international sporting events to homes in all parts of the world. The Olympics as well as the World Championships in the most important disciplines have milliards of TV spectators. The information conveyed by the radio and the press is also significant. There are not often such noticeable events in the world as the Olympic Games. For a small country it is worthwhile taking its share of this kind of publicity by creating, as widely as possible, a positive image of the country and its people. The fact that pictures of Lasse Virén and many other Finnish winners have been conveyed all over the world is something we Finns are proud of. Creating this kind of a positive image is worthwhile for us all.

Sport as a Form of Leisure Activity

In Finland the amount of leisure time has increased continuously. Nowadays a 70-year-old Finnish man has, on average, used about 61 % of his lifetime for studies, work and sleep. Nearly 40 % has been leisure time. How people are using their increased free time is a matter of importance. Idleness has always been the root of all evil. To eliminate the dangers of idleness we need some activity that is useful for both individuals and the whole society. Sport is the most attractive form of leisure activity, and it also improves the citizens' basic abilities, their physical condition and their intellectual alertness. Therefore, to utilise this ample free time, the sports organisations should take really effective measures to stimulate more and more people to practise some kind of sport regularly. Major international sporting events act as a notable source of inspiration in this respect. The success the representatives of small countries gain in international sporting events has a great effect on the general and, let us hope, continuously growing urge for sport. Our membership with full rights in the Olympic family has been important and useful for us. It motivates our best girls and boys to develop their skills and gives them the chance to measure them with the elite of other countries.

For the sports leaders this membership offers a forum where they have the opportunity to contribute to creating a positive, conciliatory and understanding atmosphere between people representing different races, religions and political views. For the common people, especially for the citizens of small countries, major international sporting events offer the possibility "to see the world" in a predominantly positive spirit. If this, furthermore, as I believe, makes an individual pay attention to his personal condition and to exercise sport himself, it really is worthwhile for us to take part in this kind of an activity. Active co-operation in the positive development of major sporting events is in the interest of us all.

Gymnastics as a Subject in Finnish Secondary Schools Between 1843 and 1917

I. Koivusalo (†)

The Background and Aim of the Article

A subject of my interest has, for several years, been physical education as a school subject and as a part of secondary education in Finland. It is my plan to follow the vicissitudes of physical education from the early years to near the present, i. e. to 1970. At that time, a change in the Finnish school system occurred which discontinued the type of school I have been investigating: the comprehensive school system was adopted. As the result of 3 years' work, I have completed the investigation of the first 75 years (1843–1917) of physical education as a school subject (Koivusalo 1982). I will return to this shortly.

The study presents an opportunity to obtain answers to the questions of what physical education used to be, and why physical education was of such and such a nature. In addition, it allows for the comparison of different types of school and different periods of time. The study is related to the research projects dealing with the didactics of physical education launched in the Department of Physical Education of the University of Jyväskylä; to the study of the history of physical activity in Finland, initiated in many universities in this country; and to the studies of the goals of school education, which have aimed at determining the concept of man created by the contemporary school. The relevance of my study is supported by the centenary of the training of physical education teachers, celebrated in Finland this year. The research findings are of use mainly in further studies in the field.

To return to the subject of this paper, it was in 1843 (Suomen Asetuskokoelma) that physical education, then called gymnastics, according to the model of the German philantropist school, was introduced as a subject for the male pupils of the secondary schools established in the same year. The physical education of female pupils was introduced about 30 years later (SA 1873), when the school education of girls became established and the private training of female physical education teachers (Asp and Asp 1872) was started. The 75-year period I am going to discuss is included within the period of autonomy of this country – i.e. 1809–1917 – and thus ends at the same time as the period of autonomy.

Nature of Physical Education in Finnish Secondary Schools During the Period of Autonomy

During the period of autonomy, Finland (then called the Grand Duchy of Finland) experienced unprecedented developments in all walks of life. Finland is said to have been created only around thy year 1860, during the reign of the Russian Czar Alexander II. There was in this country, particularly in the early part of the period of autonomy, a pronouncedly idealistic climate, combined with the nationalistic tendencies typical of that time. The leading philosopher was the German Friedrich Hegel.

According to the prevailing concept of education, physical education should also aim at idealistic goals, such as health, morality, national unity and a harmonic development. As a child of his time, Viktor Heikel, the gymnastics pedagogue known as the founder of Finnish male gymnastics, had acquired an idealistic concept of education (e.g. Heikel 1904). According to Heikel, the goals set for physical education could best be attained by education of the German gymnastics type, emphasising school pedagogy and typically characterised by extended calisthenics and wand drill series followed by a number of apparatus exercises. Boys' gymnastics was faithful to this model of Adolf Spiess and Alfred Maul, with many groups of exercises based on apparatuses, and 9 girls' gymnastics was Spiessian too (Koivusalo 1982, pp 109–117).

Changes in the Content of Physical Education

In the 1880s, realist ideals gained ground in this country. Interest in the sciences increased. People became interested in the ideas of the English philospher Herbert Spencer. When setting goals for physical education in secondary schools, more emphasis was laid on promoting health by strengthening the various vital functions of the human body. A change also occurred in the nature of gymnasics (Koivusalo 1982, pp 17, 109).

From the Gymnastics of the German Type to the Gymnastics of the Swedish Type

Particularly our girls' gymnastics experienced, in the late 1880s, a shift towards the Swedish type of gymnastics founded in the natural sciences. This meant the adoption of the Lingian movement scheme, which was based on the anatomy and physiology of the human body. In the movement scheme, calisthenics and apparatus gymnastics alternated. This change in the type of gymnastics took place through the efforts of the Finnish female gymnastics pedagogues Elin Kallio and Elli Björksten (Koivusalo 1982, pp 58; Kallio 1901; Björksten 1918). Towards the end of the period, Ivar Wilskman, known as an educator and as the founder of Finnish sport, began to endorse a slight shift also of our boys' gymnastics in the direction of the Swedes. By doing this, Wilskman and the female physical educators mentioned wanted to improve the physiological efficiency of school gymnastics (Koivusalo 1982, p 130; Wilskman 1914, 1915, 1917). However, school gymnastics in this country remained essentially German in, for instance its pedagogy.

Towards Outdoor Physical Education

Physical exercise in Finnish secondary schools also experienced another change affecting its contents. At around the turn of the century, modern track and field athletics, basically of an English type, was spreading like a popular movement from alsewhere in Scandinavia to Finland. Voluntary sports activity, which could be observed at some locations in the country ever since the 1870s, became more widespread (the Finnish Central Sports Federation was founded in 1906) (Koivusalo 1982, pp 64–71). Many trained male gymnastics teachers were active participants in the activities of gymnastics and sports clubs, particulary as leaders of extracurricular pupils' clubs (Koivusalo 1982, p 69).

Gradually, sports-like features began to appear also in the physical education classes of secondary schools. Strictly disciplined gymnastics was, at various locations, joined and, occasionally, even rivalled by what must have appeared relatively free field and winter sports activities, and later also by ball games (Koivusalo 1982, pp 122–123; Wilskman 1916). Practising these types of physical activity required that the class move out of doors to the school yard. Although this movement from the often stale air of the confined interior of the gymnasium to the fresh air out of doors was, especially in the opinion of health care professionals, to be greeted with joy, the situation was, from a pedagogic viewpoint, a new one, testing directly the disciplinary skills and pedagogic proficiency of the gymnastics teachers (Wilskman 1916, 1917).

Attitudes Towards Outdoor Physical Education

The confusion caused in many school pedagogues and school authorities by the new types of physical activity in schools was, however, related to educational ideology: Were sport and the ball games any sort of education? (Collan 1911; Koivusalo 1982, pp 130–132) - After all, in the Swedish concept of gymnastics adopted here, there was, in the absence of strictly defined movements, no control of their physiological effects. This being the case, even the underlying symmetry of the Swedish type of gymnastics, the exercise of both sides of the body with identical movements (Koivusalo 1982, p 31; Moberg 1941, p 21; Lindroth 1974), was lacking! When practising the new types of physical exercise, the pupils seemed to forget their outward appearance in terms of a good posture (Koivusalo 19182, pp 132, 139). How could this kind of moving about promote morality, discipline or a harmonic development, they wondered. Considerable headache was also caused by competitive sport, which emphasised measurable achievement and - in stark contrast to the concept of education of that era - individuality, and on which school pedagogues would before long need to take a stand (Koivusalo 1982, p 132).

My review ends with the year 1917. Both sport and ball games as well as competitions in them had by then been incorporated into the curricula of the private secondary schools, most of which were located in the countryside. In the state-run secondary schools, the calisthenics and apparatus gymnastics aiming at qualitatively idealistic goals were continued. True to the heritage of Antiquity, it was the teaching of this type of physical exercise which still attempted to create a both outwardly and inwardly harmonious human beings (Koivusalo 1982, pp 138–139).

School Education as a Factor Uniting Peoples

The above discussion has probably shown that the developmental stages of physical education in Finnish schools have not been individual and isolated occurrences. In keeping with the theme of the congress, I have attempted to touch on physical activity and the mutual understanding between peoples. Admittedly, my viewpoint has been a narrow one. I have mainly referred to the Scandinavian and Middle European countries, and to the concepts of physical education which prevailed in them during the nineteenth century as a background to the physical activity in the secondary schools of this country. Owing to insufficient resources, I was forced to omit from my study such questions as the spreading of the concepts of physical education described above to our easterly neighbour, the Soviet Union, in the nineteenth century.

Common Features in Teaching

It is known that the Engligthenment was a factor which contributed towards the unity of the European peoples, including with respect to education. The demand for equality created popular education. Secondary schools opened their doors to increasing numbers of pupils and to both sexes. A well-rounded human development required physical education of a type which would also improve the physical fitness of the population and even develop military skills. Interest in the sciences and in development had focused attention on the child and his learning ability. Teaching should proceed not only progressively but also from part to whole, and from easy to difficult things. It was further argued that teaching should be based on sensory perception. These pedagogic principles recommended by Amos Comenius in the seventeenth century appeared frequently in the physical education in different countries during the nineteenth century and still do so even today (Koivusalo 1982, pp 32–33).

Common Features in the Didactics of Physical Education

As a further example of a widely accepted feature of mass physical education in different countries, witness the column gymnastics initiated by Pestalozzi (Netorp 1926; Meusel 1973). In outward form, this teaching took place either as a group the size of a class being taught by the teacher - especially in German (Maul 1876) - or as pupil-directed file gymnastics - especially in Sweden (Ling 1853). The apparatus reform made by Hj. Ling in the 1850s in Sweden for the purposes of mass physical education (Moberg 1941, pp 94–101) may also be widely known.

In line with the doctrine of Rousseau, the main purpose of the physical education of school pupils was seen as the promotion of health and the experience of the joy of life and recreation. These, as well as the other goals set for physical education in schools, were parallel with the general goals of secondary education. The main objective everywhere seems to have been to increasingly educate young people into peace-like circumstances, although this goal was not realised. Today, the promotion of health, the experience of the joy of life and recreation, and the striving towards peace-like circumstances are still goals of youth education common to and appreciated by all peoples.

References

Asp G, Asp M (1872) Redogörelse för flickgymnastiken vid Gymnastiska Privat Instutet under läsåren 1868–1869, 1869–1870, 1870–1871. (Report of female pupils gymnastics in private gymnastic institutes during the years 1868–1869, 1869–1870, 1870–1871.) Pedagogisk Tidskrift 1872:238–239

Björksten E (1918) Kvinnogymnastik I. (Female gymnastics I.) Holger Schildts, Helsingfors, pp 250, 252
Collan A (1911) Voimistelu kasvatuskeinona. (Physical education as an educational means.) Kasvatusopillinen Aikakauskirja. Pedagogisk Tidskrift: 29
Heikel V (1874) Praktisk handbok i skolgymnastik för gossar. (Practical handbook of male pupils gymnastics.) Edlunds, Helsingfors
Heikel V (1904) Gymnastikens teori. (IThe theory of gymnastics.) Frenckellska Tryckeri-Aktiebolaget, Helsingfors, pp 161-165
Kallio E (1901) Naisvoimistelun käsikirja. (The handbook of female gymnastics.) Otava, Helsinki, pp II-III
Koivusalo I (1982) Voimistelu maamme oppikoulujen oppiaineena vuosina 1843-1917.(Gymnastics as a subject in Finnish secondary schools, 1843-1917) Liikuntatieteellisen Seuran julkaisu, nro 83 (with English summary). Etelä-Saimaa, Lappeenranta
Lindroth J (1974) Idrottens väg till fokrörelse. (How sports became a mass movement.) Studien i svensk idrottsrörelse till 1915. (Diss.) Studia historica upsaliensia, nr 60 Uppsala
Ling P H (1853) Reglemente för gymnastik (Regulations of gymnastics), 2nd edn. Philip and Meyer, Stockholm
Maul A (1876) Anleitung für den Turnunterricht in Knabenschulen I. Der Lehrverfahren in Turnunterricht, 2nd edn., Karlsruhe, pp 6-7
Meusel H (1973) Johann Heinrich Pestalozzi über Körperbildung. Studientexte zur Leibeserziehung 10. Limpert, Frankfurt, p 38
Moberg G (1941) Hjalmar Ling. Hans systematisering av gymnastiken. En modern orientering. (Hjalmar Ling. His systematisation of gymnastics. A modern orientation.) Nya Litografen, Malmö
Natorp P (1926), Pestalozzi, sein Leben und seine Ideen. Leipzig, Berlin, p 126 Suomen Asetuskokoelma 6.11.1843; 2.10.1873, nro 30.
Wilskman I (1911) Suomalaisen poikavoimistelun opetusmetodeista. (Teaching methods in Finnish male schoolgymnastics) Kasvatusopillinen Aikakauskirja (Pedagogisk Tidskrift), pp 114-118
Wilskman I (1914-1917) Tarkastuskertomukset vuosilta 1914, 1915, 1916, 1917. (Revision reports from the years 1914, 1915, 1917.) KHA III, Eh 11, 12, 13, 14. Valtionarkisto Helsinki

International Exchange in Terms of the Recruitment of Star Foreign Players: The Reactions of Sports Clubs in Finnish Basketball

K. Olin

Introduction

From the sociological point of view it seems that interesting developments are taking place in sports institutions, including those involved in top-level sport. Sport has become professionlised[1] and commercialised (Heinilä 1973), and in the process top-level sport has created its own labour markets with its own labour recruitment systems (Noll 1981), both nationally and internationally. Unfortunately, however, there are no cross-cultural studies that compare the sports institutions of various countries in this respect, and only a few efforts have been made to investigate scientifically some specific aspects of the issue (c.f. Lüschen and Sage 1981; Olin and Laitinen 1981, Foreign players in Finnish basketball, unpublished research plan; Talamini and Page 1973; Wohl 1957). One explanation for this may lay in the widely made claim that international exchange in sport promotes international understanding (Heinilä 1970) and therefore has positive effects in general. This has been taken for granted. In addition, the distribution of new branches of sport, of new equipment and facilities, and of new styles in sports clothing has been considered to enrich the physical culture of the recipient country, making it more multi-faceted. However, the following questions arise:

1. What other effects does international exchange, including the recruitment of professional star players, have on the national physical culture of the country concerned?
2. In addition to any positive effects they might have, do certain kinds of exchange influence sports institutions negatively in any way (Olin and Laitinen 1981, Foreign players in Finnish basketball, unpublished research plan)?
3. What are the reactions of sports institutions and their nuclear units towards, for example, the recruitment of paid foreign players? [In many societies one very key unit in competitive and top-level sport is the voluntary sports club (Seppänen 1977)].

Purpose of the Study

The purpose of the present study was to determine the views of Finnish sports clubs which play basketball on the recruitment of star foreign players. Attention was focused on the positive and negative aspects of such recruitment in terms of (a) the other

1 The concepts of the professionalism and professionalization have been dealt more in detail by McIntosh (1981).

players in the team, (b) the coaching and training of the team, (c) the training of younger players, and (d) spectator interest. In addition, an aim was to find out at which league levels the use of foreign players should be allowed or banned. The following questions were therefore put to clubs:

1. Had the team recruited foreign professional players?
2. If it had, had it used the players for a short time (less than 5 years) or for a long time (more than 5 years)?
3. At which league level was the team playing basketball?
4. Was the club involved just in basketball or in other sports as well?
5. Was the club large or small in terms of membership (large: more than 300 members; small: less than 300 members)?
6. Did the club belong to the Finnish Central Sport Federation (SVUL) or the Workers' Sport Federation (TUL)?

Procedure

All clubs ($n = 55$) playing basketball in the three highest leagues for men and in the highest league for women were selected for the study. Data were collected by mail questionnaire in October 1981, the questionnaire being sent to the person acting as a contact for the club with the Finnish Basketball Federation (Finnish Basketball Federation 1981). This person delivered the questionnaire to the leading administrative body of the club or to the body of the club responsible for basketball. Forty-nine clubs (89.1 %) returned the questionnaire, some only after being reminded to do so by phone at the beginning of November. Data were analysed by the cross-tabulation technique. [The methodological procedures have been dealt with in more detail in the research report by Olin (1981)].

Results

By and large, the results provided some interesting but in part unpromising information for discussion on international exchange in top-level sport in terms of the recruitment of star professional foreign players. The results were quite uniform: in spite of clear support for the use of foreign players, straight demands were made for the limitation of their use. This finding was not so clear-cut in the highest league, but was very obvious in the other leagues.

There was greater variation in response in terms of league level (Table 1) and membership of central sports organisations (Table 2) than in terms of the size of the club as measured by the number of members, the nature of the club, or whether the club had already recruited star foreign players. Of the two variables accounting for most differences of opinion, the league level had the greater influence. Thus the study showed that the use of foreign players in top Finnish basketball is primarily an inside issue of the sport itself, and secondarily a sporting political issue between the SVUL and the TUL.

Table 1. Views of clubs in the top three Finnish basketball leagues on the recruitment of star foreign players (%)

"The recruitment of star foreign players should be allowed in…"	League level of respondent								
	Top (SM)			IInd (Ist div)			IIIrd (Suomi)		
	No	Yes	Difficult to say	No	Yes	Difficult to say	No	Yes	Difficult to say
Top league (SM)	33	58	9	56	44	0	25	64	11
IInd league (Ist div)	45	55	0	67	22	11	64	25	11
IIIrd league (Suomi)	82	18	0	78	22	0	93	3	4
IVth league (Maakunta)	91	9	0	89	11	0	96	0	4

Table 2. Views of the clubs belonging to the central sports organisations, SVUL and TUL, on the recruitment of star foreign players at different league levels (%)

"The recruitment of star foreign players should be allowed in…"	Central sports organisation						
	SVUL			TUL			
	No	Yes	Difficult to say	No	Yes	Difficult to say	χ^2
Top league (SM)	24	73	3	50	31	19	8.53
IInd league (Ist div)	47	44	9	88	6	6	7.84
IIIrd league (Suomi)	81	16	3	100	0	0	3.43
IVth league (Maakunta)	91	6	3	100	0	0	1.60

Various reasons could be found for the somehwat dismissive attitudes of the Finnish basketball clubs to the recruitment of foreign star players: Perhaps they are simply not yet ready for this kind of international exchange – readiness here referring mainly to the ability of the clubs to finance the recruitment of such players. Economic circumstances are probably decisive in many clubs in the lower leagues; nevertheless, the results did indicate that even these clubs, which had no experience in the matter, were quite strongly in favour of recruitment. It seems evident, too, that the specific cultural features of Finland, relating to its language and peripheral geographical location, could explain some of the results. Perhaps the leaders of the sports clubs are, to some degree, suspicious and eager to preserve the traditional voluntary nature of top-level sport in Finland in the face of widespread professionalism in sports internationally. One might also ask whether the results of the study reflect reactions of the respondents to the ethnicity of the foreign players. In fact this does not seem to be the case. In the study, views were requested on the use of foreign players from any country, any ethnic background and any citizenship. It is known that most of the foreign players recruited have been black Americans. Observations of the games, interviews with both foreign and Finnish players and coaches, and some statements in newspapers and magazines show that the ethnic background of the foreign players does not seem to play such a role as it does in some other societies and sports institutions. The preliminary results of the larger study (Olin and Laitinen 1982, unpublished work) on recruitment of foreign professional players support this conclusion.

References

Finnish Basketball Federation (1981) Play Session 1981-82. List of the contact persons of the sport clubs. Helsinki

Heinilä K (1970) Notes on the inter-group conflicts in international sport. In: Lüschen G (ed) The cross-cultural analysis of sport and games. Stipes, Champaign, p 174

Heinilä K (1973) Markets of the audience in top sports. In: Heinilä K, Wuolio J (eds) Top sport and society. Jyväskylä, Jyväskylä Art Festivals, pp 115-125

Lüschen G, Sage GH (1981) Sport in sociological perspective. In: Lüschen G, Sage GH (eds) Handbook of social science of sport. Stipes, Champaign, p 14

McIntosh PC (1981) The sociology of sport in the ancient world. In: Lüschen G, Sage GH (eds) Handbook of social science of sport. Stipes, Champaign, pp 39-40

Noll RG (1981) Alternatives in sports policy. In: Lüschen G, Sage GH (eds) Handbook of social science of sport. Stipes, Champaign, pp 331-343

Olin K (1981) The notions of the sport clubs on the use of foreign star-recruit players in Finnish basketball leagues. Finnish Basketball Federation, Research Report, Helsinki, pp 2-3

Seppänen P (1977) On Finnish sport organizations, physical activity and sport life of today 1977. SVUL, Helsinki, p 13

Telamini J, Page CH (1973) Sport and society. An anthology. Little, Brown & Co., Boston, pp 99-100

Wohl A (1957) Once more about amateurs and professionals in sport. Kultura Fizyczna 1:552-560

Some Recreational and Social Sporting Activities of the Mapuche Indians in the South of Chile

C. López von Vriessen

Purpose

The purpose of this work is to report new elements of tribal games and dances in order to enrich the action of "Sports for All".

Introduction

In the sixteenth century the Mapuche lived between latitudes 30°and 43°south, the population fluctuating between one and two millions. They are known today as Araucanians, and are divided into four groups: Picunche (men of the North), Pehuenche (men of the tree *pehuén-Araucaria imbricata*), Mapuche (men of the land) and Huilliche (men of the South). Stuchlik (1974) stated that they live in 3000 reservations and number nearly 500,000 between latitudes 37.5° and 41°south.

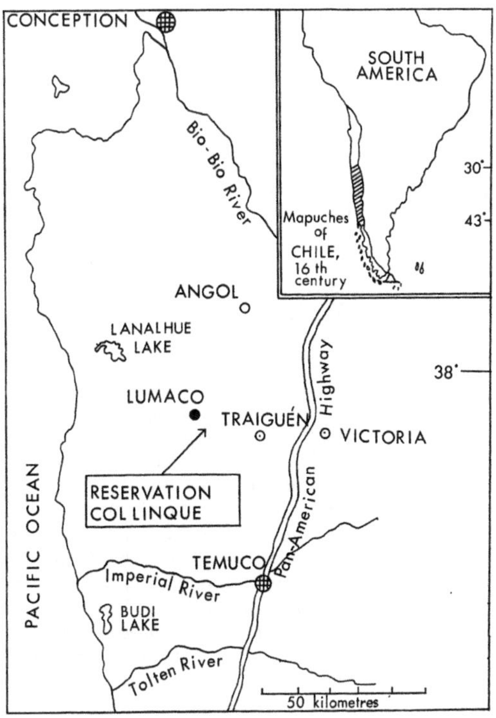

Fig. 1. The Mapuche region of Chile

As to their language, Cooper (1946) reported that Araucanian is an independent linguistic family. Each region and tribal subdivision has its dialect, but these differences are mostly relatively minor. In all dialects there is a more elegant mode of speaking, resorted to especially during meetings of leaders.

The Mapuche were fond of liberty; they were excellent soldiers; and they lived in wooden huts (*ruca*), cultivated the land in a primitive way and did not know of writing. The man's dress was the *chamal*, tied between the legs, and a *poncho*, a woven piece of wool cloth with a slit in the middle for the head, called a *macun*. The woman used the *quipam*, which covered her body, leaving bare one shoulder and her left arm. On her shoulders she wore the *iquilla*, a cape-like garment of chamal shape, pinned at the breast with a wonderful silver brooch, the *tupu* (Moesbach 1959). They did not use shoes, and bathed every day in rivers or lakes. The bark of the tree *Quillaja saponaria* served as a substitute for soap. They were excellent swimmers.

The great feasts, or *cahuin*, lasted several days. One of the most important is still the *nguillatún* (rogation). Faron (1963) reported: "The Nillatun [sic] ceremony is the most elaborate Mapuche ritual in existence today... A number of elements have probably been added to Nillatun rites in the last few generations and others dropped during the recorded history of the Mapuche." Other important feasts were the *machitún*, or initiation of the shaman (Moesbach 1930; Dowling 1973) and the *rucan*, or construction of the dwelling (Moesbach 1930). The feasts included (a) games such as *palín* (hockey game); the *loncotún*, or wrestling by neck; the *linao* (similar to rugby) and the *pillmatún* (ball game) (Manquilef 1914; Matus 1920; Plath 1945) and (b) dances such as the *choikepurún*, or dance of the ostrich, the *loncopurún*, or dance of the head, and the *loncomeu*, or mimic dance (Manquilef 1914). The principal instruments (Fig. 2) are still the *cultrún*, or magic drum of the shaman, the *trutruca*, or large cane

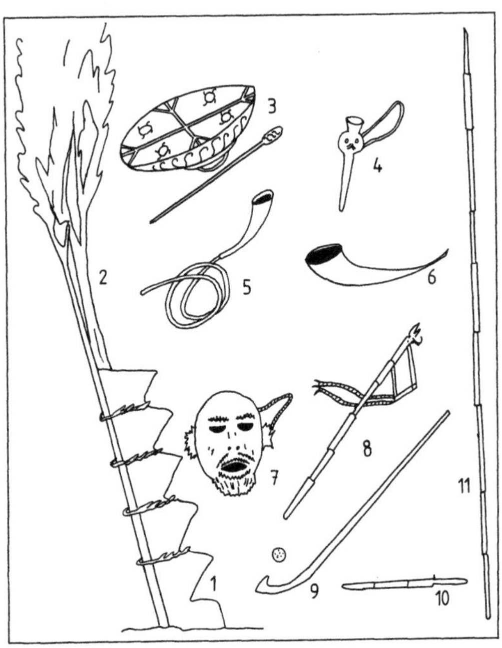

Fig. 2. Some ritual and sporting equipment used by the Mapuche Indians. *1*, Sacred tree of *rehue*. *2*, Branches (*Drimys winteri* and *Aristotelia chilensis*) tied to the *rehue*. *3*, Shaman drum or *cultrun* (magic drum); 39 cm in diameter and made of *Guevina avellana* with a single head of skin; beaten with a small stick. *4*, Wooden flute (*pifilca*), 19 cm long. *5*, Wind instrument (*trutruca*), made of rolled copper tube with a cattle horn at the end. Formerly made of straight cane (3-4 m long) of *Chusquea chumingii*. *6*, Cattle-horn trumpet (*cull-cull*); formerly used in war. *7*, Wooden mask (*collon*) of *Guevina avellana*. *8*, Riding stick used by the assistants of the shaman; made of *Chusquea chumingii* with woollen bridles. *9*, Hockey stick (*uño*) and ball (*pali*) of the *palin* game, both made of wood (*Boldoa fragans* or *Myrtus luma*); 1.20 m long. *10*, Wooden knife of *Chusquea chumingii* used by the assistants of the shaman; 40 cm long. *11*, Stick of *Chusquea chumingii* (4 m long) to chase the evil spirits away.

trumpet (2–4 m), the *pifilca,* or wooden fluete and the *cull-cull* or war trumpet. Orrego-Salas (1966) reported: "... the trutruca and the kultrun can perfectly well be considered as instruments indigenous to this tribe, developed prior to any contact with neighboring cultures." Among the gambling games were the *awarcuden*, or game of beans, the *quechucahüe*, or game of dice, and the *comicán*, a kind of chess (Manquilef 1914; Plath 1945). The Mapuche believed in a Supreme Being or *Ngenechen.* The shaman was at the same time priest and healer. Several of these costumes and beliefs are still found. The most important actual activities are the *nguillatún* (rogation) and the *palín* (hockey game). The woman wears almost the same garment as in the past. The feasts are less frequent, of shorter duration and less concurrent.

Procedure

The information provided below is about a Mapuche feast on the 27th and 28th of March 1981 in the reservation of Collinque (38°lat. south), which I attended at the special invitation of the leader (*cacique*). The first part of the *nguillatún* takes place on the evening before the real feast. The second part commences early on the following morning at 6.30; this is followed by the *palín* (Fig. 3) game, eating, dances and speeches. The feast ground is situated on a hill 50 m high, above the house of the *cacique* and 500 m from it. It covers more than one hectare, and is used several times a year for this purpose. Branch huts of *ramadas* are erected ahead of time as is the *rehue* (sacred tree), a trunk of *Nothofagus obliqua*, 1.60 m high and 40 cm in diameter,

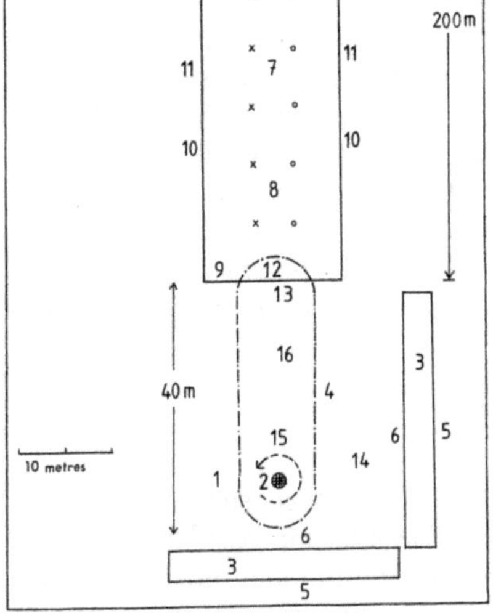

Fig. 3. Place of social, ritual and sporting activities of the Mapuche Indians in the Collinque reservation in the South of Chile, March 1981. *1*, *Nguillatún* rite; *2*, *rehue*; *3*, huts made of branches (*ramadas*); *4*, horsemen's path (*awun*); *5*, ox carriage; *6*, campfire; *7*, playing field for the *palín* game; *8*, initial position of players; *9*, the goal line (*tripalhüe*); *10*, the side line (*cachilhüe*); *11*, spectators' stand; *12*, Chilean flags; *13*, position of the shaman (*machi*) during the play; *14*, eating and drinking area; *15*, dancing area; *16*, area where speeches are made.

containing six steps, cut by axe or saw, and planted in the ground and inclined to the East. Branches of *Drimys winteri* and *Aristotelia chilensis* are tied around it with vegetable cord of *Cissus striata.* The *rehue* is the centre of all actions during the feast.

Nguillatún

The participants begin to arrive at 7 o'clock in the evening with ox carriages. They bring domestic utensils and enough food and drink for one night and one day. The whole family participates. Campfires are prepared, and the ceremony commences at about 9 o'clock in the evening, lasting until midnight. It begins with a procession of about 100 persons, the *cacique*, the shaman and her assistants going ahead, all shouting and dancing around the *rehue* with the purpose that the shaman falls into a trance in order to fulfil her task of establishing contact with the Supreme Being. The group walks and dances anti-clockwise. All contribute with great clamour, accompanied by the sound of their instruments, strokes of sticks and sounds of canes. The sound of the magic drum of the shaman indicates the rhythm. They believe that the evil spirits try to intervene between the shaman and God and must therefore be scared away by chanting, by stroking sticks of *Shusques shumingii* on the ground and by riders who gallop around the people, shouting. The beginning of the trance is noticed when the shaman convulses and becomes rigid. The pages, called *curiches*, who accompany the shaman riding on wooden horses (sticks) give the shaman magic touches with their wooden knives. Only then can she relax. The assistant holds her in his arms; otherwise she would fall. The shaman now begins to fight against the evil spirits. Her voice is tearful and her language unintelligible. The crowd helps her with chants and musical instruments. They kneel on the ground, side by side in one long line looking to the Eastern heaven, where *Ngenechen*, their God, dwells. They call him by his other name, "*Chau*", several times with high voices and beg for a good harvest, rain, good weather, health, peace etc. The *cacique* throws handfuls of seeds toward heaven. The shaman comes to herself. Her assistant informs her what happened while she was in the trance. This ends the first part of the *nguillatún.*

The following day at 6.30 a.m. the second part begins. The actions of the day before are repeated. Nowadays birds are beheaded and their blood is thrown into the air. The shaman again falls into a trance and climbs up the steps of the sacred tree. At the top of the steps she embraces the branches and shakes them violently. She has thus consummated the encounter with the Supreme Being. The shaman descends and is received with great joy by the crowd. She comes to herself, tells of her voyage through heaven and announces that God has heard the wishes of all. The assistant tells her what happened during the trance. This second and final part of the *nguillatún* lasts two hours (Fig. 3).

Palín Game

The invited *palín* team arrives by bus at 8.30 a.m. The players stop at a distance of about 250 m and wait for the hosts to meet them. The latter approach, the *cacique* and the shaman walking ahead to the sound of the magic drum and other instruments. Loud chants are to be heard, as is the stroking of sticks and canes. The riders, holding a

Chilean flag and a large branch of *Drimys winteri*, form an ellipse between the *rehue* and the guests. The chiefs need half an hour to come to terms about the game. The ground measures 200 m in length and 15 m in width. The longitudinal axis lies from east to west, and the playing area is marked with small grooves in the earth. A coin is tossed to decide in which direction the teams will play. The game consists of two 30-min periods, i.e. one hour in all. There are 14 players on each team, and most of them play barefoot, with their trousers tucked up. At the beginning of the game the players face their opponents placed all along the pitch; they shake hands and promise each other a fair game. The wooden ball (4.5-5 cm diameter), called a *pali*, has to pass the goal line, or *tripalhüe* (15 m wide). The play begins with the ball placed in a hole in the middle of the pitch. When the ball passes the lateral lines (*cachilhüe*) the play begins again in the middle of the pitch. Each team has its trainer (*elconafe*) or coach, who is also a player. The shaman of each reservation and the fans stand behind the goal line for the entire game and support their team with music, dances, songs and the sound of the magic drum.

Banquet

Once the match is finished, the guests are welcomed officially by their hosts, and the banquet begins. It consists of turkey in a soup of vegetables, grilled or boiled pork and mutton, bread baked in ashes, and wine and apple or maize must (*muday*).

Dance

People of all ages join hands to dance the *purún*, a very simple dance, around the *rehue* for two hours. The feet are hardly lifted during this time.

Speeches

It is an old custom of the Mapuche to make speeches during the feasts. They take this opportunity to appeal to their people to be more united. They complain of the discrimination they suffer, and thank their friends for the invitation.

Discussion

There were no disturbances or accidents during the *palin* game. The winners received no distinction, and nobody placed bets on the outcome. It served as an excellent opportunity to meet others. The community that made the invitation paid all expenses despite their low income. These feasts are nearly unknown to other Chileans, for the Mapuche distrust those who do not belong to their race. Therefore they invite very few non-Mapuche (*Huincas*) to their feasts.

Sport, in advancing mutual understanding between the inhabitants of a land, may moderate social, religious, political and racial differences and serve as the first step towards international understanding. The Sports for All programme must find a way of integrating such valuable autochthonous games as that described above while at the same time ensuring that they retain their distinctive racial identity.

References

Cooper JM (1946) The Araucanians. In: Steward JH (ed) Handbook of South American Indians, vol 2. Smithsonian Institute, Washington, pp 687-766
Dowling J (1973) Religión chamanismo y mitología Mapuches. Edit. Universitaria, Santiago de Chile, pp 63-112
Faron L (1963) Death and fertility rites of the Mapuche (Araucanian) Indians of Central Chile. Ethnology 2:135-156
Manquilef M (1914) Comentarios del pueblo Araucano II. Rev Folkl Chil 165-190
Matus L (1920) Juegos y ejercicios de los antiguos Araucanos. Bolet Mus Nac 11:162-197
Moesbach EW (1930) Vida y costumbras de los indígenas araucanos en la segunda mitad del siglo XIX. Imprenta Cervantes, Santiago de Chile, pp 331-347 and pp 169-183
Moesbach EW (1959) Voz de Arauco. Imprenta San Francisco, Padre Las Casas, p 255
Orrego-Salas J (1966) Araucanian instruments. Ethnomusicology 10:48-57
Plath O (1945) Juegos, ejercicios y armas araucanos. Bol Educac Fís 12:294-302
Stuchlik M (1974) Rasgos de la sociedad Mapuche contemporánea. Edic. Nueva Universidád, Santiago de Chile, p 16

4. Other Measures

Sports Medicine Training in Kuopio – International Co-operation

J. E. Caldwell

An Idea Is Born

A year ago I was casting about during my mid-life crisis trying to figure out how to meld my seemingly mutually exclusive interests in medicine, science, teaching, sports, travel and financial security. Dropping the last goal temporarily, I decided to try to land a university research-teaching position in sports medicine. Easily enough said, nearly impossible to locate.

Sports medicine in the United States is a labour of love. Nowhere does there exist a truly integrated curriculum which encompasses the breadth of this rapidly evolving speciality. There are excellent rotations and fellowships for orthopaedists and family practitioners and fine exercise physiology programmes for the non-physician. There is an ever-increasing number of continuing education courses for the practising health professional concerning the general and specific problems of athletes and the role of nutrition in sports, and "how-to" clinics for team medical personnel. For coaches, and to a lesser extent for athletes, there are clinics in training methodology. There are, scattered about the country, occasional centres specialising in sports psychology, sports sociology and athletic pharmacology. If exercise medicine can be considered "sports medicine", then we could add the many excellent training programmes for professionals at all levels of expertise in cardiac rehabilitation. Nonetheless, there are simply no integrated programmes for training in sports medicine. The last one in the United States, at the University of Wisconsin-Madison, closed 10 years ago.

So it was to Europe I looked, and because of my interest in Nordic sports, to Scandinavia in particular. I located the names of research centres and individuals to whom to write by reviewing recent issues of several sports medicine journals. I then wrote directly to a dozen of them stating my qualifications, interests and goals. Response was not overwhelmingly positive.

Three and half months later I received a reply from Professor Osmo Hänninen of the University of Kuopio. Formerly the Chairman of the Physiology Department, Hänninen was now writing as Rector of the University. He explained: "We have a number of research projects going on and hands are needed." Except for one other letter 9 months later, this was to be the only positive reply.

During the ensuing 6 months, Professor Hänninen arranged housing for our entire family, schooling for my children (at a Finnish elementary school), a job for my wife (teaching English at the adult evening school) and a source of income for me (teaching medical students). He also pencilled me into a series of research projects in the field of exercise physiology.

The University of Kuopio

The University of Kuopio is now in its 10th year; it has 1500 students, all in one or another field of science, and 200 faculty members, of whom 32 are full professors. Its Department of Physiology is small, with a faculty of nine, and though primarily research-oriented, it does contribute to the broadening of the basic science foundation of the students in most of the graduate disciplines. Its forte is hormone and enzyme research.

The sports medicine faculty consists of those on the various staffs who have an interest or a project in the field of exercise science. Thus it is an ever-changing group with no particular dedication to a teaching programme. The projects in which I had at least temporary involvement included:

1. A study of the effects of dehydration achieved through diuretics, sauna exposure or physical activity on the performance and neuromuscular physiology of power athletes (boxers, wrestlers, judokas and weight-lifters)
2. Evaluation of the anaerobic thresholds of elite swimmers measured during free swimming by blood lactate analysis
3. Observation of training effects on a group of elite motocross drivers following a 3-month interseason training programme
4. Performance evaluations of cross-country and downhill skiers, orienteers, and hockey and soccer players on treadmill or cyclergometer
5. A long-term study of the effects of vigorous training on the health and physiological development of children. This study involves young cross-country skiers from east-central Finland matched against school children from urban areas not involved in skiing competition
6. A study of the effects of non-supervised exercise on the lipoprotein subfractions, lipoprotein lipases and insulin of middle-aged men
7. An ongoing study of the physiological work stress of lumberjacks, and of the total daily energy output of these workers. This is part of a series of studies which have attempted to explain their very high prevalence of cardiovascular disease
8. Clothing physiology and its application to sports medicine - this project was in the early phase of development and equipment acquisition.

Goals of the Training

My goals had been both general and specific, the first being more important:

1. *Basic exercise physiology.* Although I had a smattering of knowledge about this from reading that I had done during my clinical years, I wanted to study it in both depth and breadth; metabolism as it applied to conditioning and training wsas to be my focus.
2. *Research methodology.* Although I had been through a Public Health Master's programme in the United States, I did not feel that I really knew how to approach research problems, and more importantly how to carry out a project from inception to publication/presentation.

My specific goals were more numerous:

1. Exercise stress testing - the nuts and bolts of testing athletes, normal adults and cardiac patients
2. Continue taeaching and expand my teaching repertoire
3. Clinical sports medicine - especially the use of acupuncture in rehabilitation
4. Computer interaction - analysis of data and use of a word processor
5. Establish continuing relationships with those in the European sports medicine community

The Program

My year was divided roughly into thirds, during each of which I concentrated, but did not limit, my activities to one of the three facilities:

September-December:	Kuopio Institute of Exercise Medidine
January-March:	Physiologoy Department
April-August:	Kuopio University Central Hospital

These periods, which were defined more by money availability and accident than by design, were interspersed with travel, some of which (the minority) was partly University sponsored. In assigning job roles at each site, my interests were always carefully weighed before tasks were set (Table 1). Table 2 shows the variety of experiences and skills garnered at each location.

Table 1. Job titles and descriptions, University of Kuopio Sports Medicine Programme, 1981-1982

Department of Physiology
- Instructor and Research Assistant
  - Primary instructor in a weekly sports medicine/physiology seminar for other members of the university faculty and medical students[a]
  - Direct involvement in several ongoing sports medicine research projects in the Department and at the University Hospital

Kuopio Institute of Exercise Medicine
- Exercise Physiologist and Physician Supervisor
  - Responsible for establishing exercise test protocols, supervising tests, analysing and interpreting test results, and ensuring the health and safety of all test subjects[a]

University Central Hospital
- Assistant Physician, Department of Clinical Physiology
  - Cardiopulmonary function analysis, including radio-isotope studies[a]
  - Functional assessment of patients with cardiopulmonary disease[a]
  - Exercise prescription[a]
  - Radiotracer injections[a]

Kuopio Regional Occupational Health Institute
- Consultant

[a] Analysis of field work stress data from lumberjacks by Holter monitoring

Table 2. Components of the University of Kuopio Sports Medicine Programme

Activity	Location[a]
Basic exercise physiology	
Reading	PHYSIO
Teaching	PHYSIO
Applied exercise physiology (field and lab)	
Athletes	KIEM, other[b]
Normal adults	KIEM, KRIOH
Cardiac patients	KYKS
Exercise prescription	KIEM
Research methodology	
Planning	KIEM, PHYSIO
Literature review	PHYSIO, other
Data acquisition	KIEM, other
Data analysis	PHYSIO
Presentation/publication	PHYSIO
Sports and exercise medicine	
Teaching	PHYSIO, KIEM
Specific skills	
Anthropometry	KIEM
Underwater densitometry	Other
Muscle biopsy	KYKS
Radio-isotope analysis	KYKS
Echocardiography	KYKS
Holter monitor analysis	KYKS
Performance testing	PHYSIO, KIEM, other
Exercise electrocardiography	KIEM, KYKS

[a] KIEM = Kuopio Institute of Exercise Medicine
PHYSIO = Department of Physiology, University of Kuopio
KYKS = University Central Hospital
KRIOH = Kuopio Regional Institute of Occupational Health

[b] Specific research projects

The strengths and weaknesses of the programme that Dr. Hänninen and I designed are summarised in Table 3. As is true in most situations, success lay with the people involved, who, given sufficient dedication and interest, overcame most of the built-in shortcomings.

The co-operation of the staff of the small library which was almost devoid of sports medicine literature (I brought with me a larger stock than the library had on its shelves) is an example. Fortunately, much of the applicable applied physiology literature has accrued over just the past 10 years, the period for which the library is current, and the staff was always helpful in finding and acquiring references that were not in stock. This clearly reflects the importance placed by the library staff on information services, rather than inventory.

Table 3. Strengths and Weaknesses of the University of Kuopio Sports Medicine Programmes

Strengths	Weaknesses
Complete office space and all incidentals except typing services provided	Lack of formal appointment to the university staff created a few minor problems
Independence and freedom to pursue subjects of interest at my own speed	Lack of formal teaching programme
Weekly sports medicine seminar	Lack of speakers other than myself
Helpfulness of staff, both professional and personally	Little formal interaction with faculty
Responsibility for performance testing (equipment and protocol)	Performance testing programme not well organised, and range of testing modalities too narrow
Assistance with obtaining financial support and accomodation	Lack of formal ongoing financial support
Co-operation of library staff	Incompleteness of library resources
Computer access and staff assistance	Lack of guidance in statistical analysis
Involvement in research projects at all levels	Inability to complete research of my own design
Encouragement of attendance at international congresses	
Guest lectures usually in English	Almost all meetings, teaching sessions and discussions were in Finnish; many staff members reluctant to speak English

Recommendations and Summary

Based on this experience, and taking into account the requirements of a physician in the field of sports medicine, I would make the following specific suggestions for developing and formalising an international sports medicine programme:

1. The goals of the "student" and the resources of the centre should be clear.
2. A formal teaching programme should exist covering fundamental aspects of exercise physiology as they apply to athletics and exercise. An individualised curriculum can be arranged where no programmes exist, but in this case ongoing faculty supervision and guidance is mandatory.
3. A 40-hour International Federation of Sports Medicine (FIMS) approved course would result in formal recognition of the training programme by making the student eligible for Associate FIMS membership.
4. Faculty members who are comfortable in English (or some other mutually agreeable language) must provide this interaction, and firm goals should be established.
5. Depending on the degree of formalisation and the goals, the programme should last 6-9 months.
6. It would be helpful, though not mandatory if other resources are available, to have a library well-supplied with past and current references in sports medicine.
7. The performance laboratory should be equipped to evaluate accurately strength,

anaerobic power, co-ordination and reaction, and body composition in addition to providing aerobic fitness assessments.

8. It will always be helpful to visiting foreigners to provide either temporary or permanent accommodation. An intensive language acquisition programme may be valuable in some cases.
9. Financial support should be provided or arranged for by the hosting centre, and should include transportation, a stipend and support for attendance at scientific congresses.

In summary, this programme has markedly increased my knowledge of and confidence in the application of basic exercise physiology to both research and clinical situtions. The major drawbacks were the lack of spoken English and the limited formal faculty contact. The freedom to pursue topics of individual interest was most valuable, as was the direct involvement in research activities and performance evaluations.

Structural Variation and Sport Policy: A Comparison of Canadian and British Sport Systems

G. A. Olafson

Introduction

The development of a research protocol to investigate the interorganisational factors related to international sport has received very little attention in the literature. Utilising and adapting research methods from comparative management science, the researcher who is interested in the organisation of international sport has had to evolve a systematic, theoretically sound regime based upon the conscious use of the rules of science (Anderson 1971). As Semotiuk (1980) noted in a recent publication:

> The task of developing explanatory models which would facilitate the systematic analysis of National Government participation in sport has several difficulties. First, the fact that the topic has not been thoroughly researched would lead one to believe that diversities among natioonal systems of sport are not well understood....
>
> Second, the existence of diverse cultural patterns throughout the world presents a problem in arriving at explanatory and analytical tools that are universal in their application.

Thus, the development and advancement of research associated with comparative management specifically related to sport requires a more rigorous use of standard research methods in order to arrive at valid, reliable, objective findings from which conclusions and generalisations can be drawn.

In order to improve upon the present state of such research, Beres and Portwood (1981) concluded "that considerably more work is needed to provide a clear understanding of the nature and extent of sociocultural influences on organizational functioning". As a further refinement of this point, Aldrich (1979) postulated that "a truly open model of organizational change does not take the environment as a given, and does not assume a completely known or uncontrolled internal structure". The internal and external environments of elite sport organisations at the national level have not been examined on a comparative basis. Recognising that there is no one best way to design and conduct research cross-culturally, the outcome of this research may become the catalyst for interorganisational theory to be utilised in sport management research.

This study used the following overall objectives as a general guide for the entire research design:

1. To analyze the development of The Sport Council and Sport Canada/Fitness Canada in order to identify patterns associated with organisational growth
2. To compare and contrast the structural variation as evidenced by statutes and charters

3. To test the proposition that network analysis in concert with the semi-directed focused interview as a valid, reliable method for the comparison of sport delivery systems

Purpose

The main purpose of this study was to formulate a research methodology, based upon the concept of interorganisational theory, which would facilitate the examination of the structural variability and the sport policy of Canada and the United Kingdom.

Procedure

Employing the methods of change agent research (Moriarty et al. 1972) and network analysis (Aldrich 1979; Benson 1975; Stern 1979), an integrative model, entitled Government-Legislative Involvement in the Organisational Structure of Sport Systems (GLI), was developed as a guide for the generation of the Semi-Directed Focused Interview format (SDFI) (see Fig. 1).

Following an exhaustive examination of government documents and associated material in the Sports Information Library at the Sports Council in London, England, and the Sports Information Recource Centre in Ottawa, Ontario, the SDFI was generated to dovetail with the subsets of the GLI model. The data were gathered through personal interviews with the Directors General and selected statt at the Sports Councils of Wales (Cardiff) and Scotland (Edinburgh), The Sports Council (London) and Sport Canada and Fitness Canada (Ottawa). All interviews were taped on an audio recorder and were completed within a 60-min period. A total of 35 hours of interviews was conducted and subsequently analysed employing the method of content analysis (Rummel, 1958; Mouly 1963). The data for each interview were categorised under the following subheadings of the GLI model and summarised in a descriptive format.

Results and Discussion

Because of the space limitations placed upon each author, an abbreviated analysis of data will be presented under the subheadings of the GLI Model.

Administrative Structure

Following an examination of the evolutionary structural changes that have taken place by virtue of Bill C-131 (Canada 1961) and the Charter establishing The Sports Council (United Kingdom 1971), both organisations have evolved an elaborate set of formal structures and attendant bureaucratic interactive networks. The hierarchy of authority is similarly elaborate and extensive, with Canada evolving a National Advisory Council on Fitness and Amateur Sport, and the United Kingdom establishing autonomous councils in Wales and Scotland with a central authority in the Form of the Sports Council in London – the latter with a preciseness of role responsibility not evident in

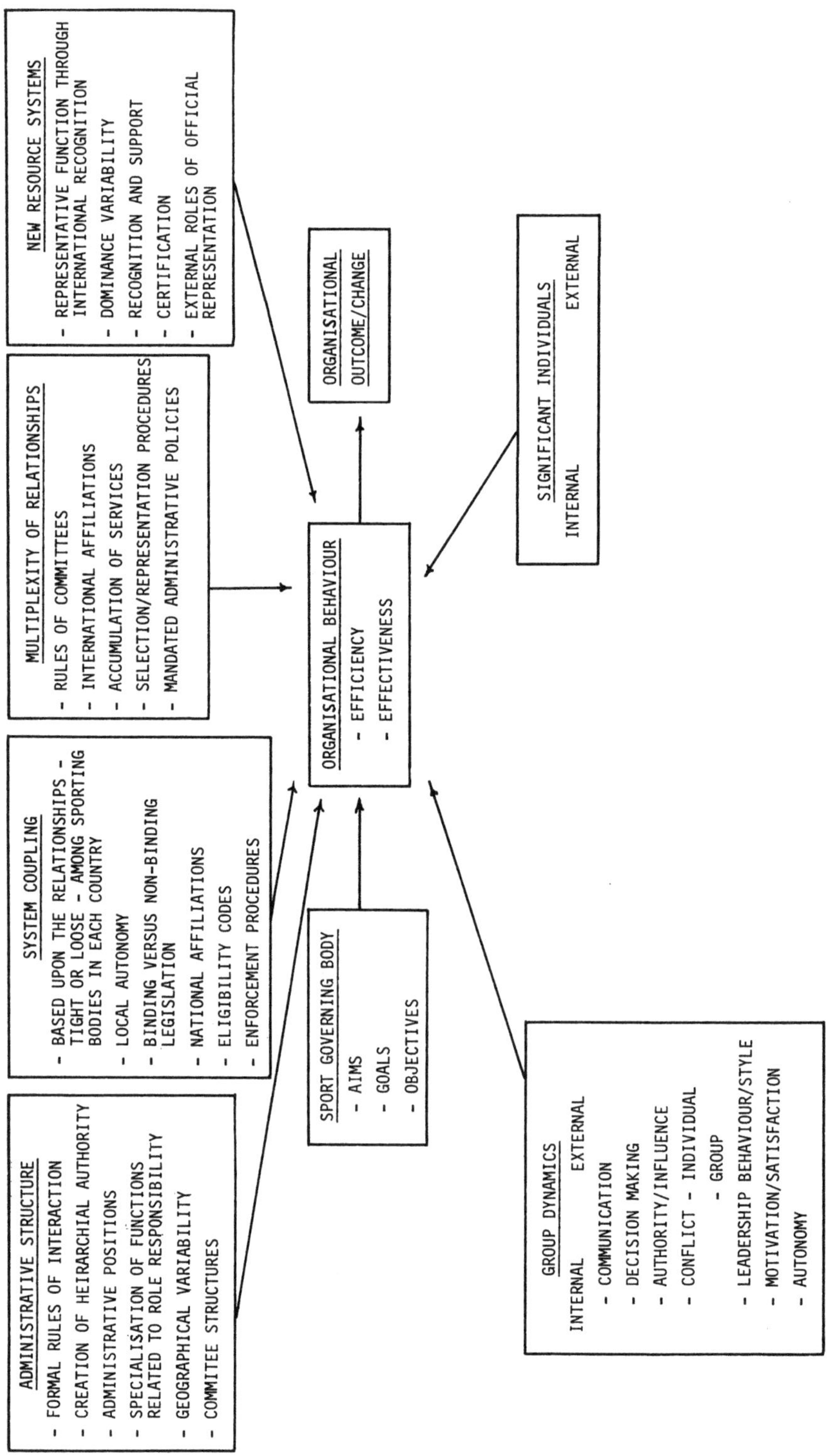

Fig. 1. Government-legislative involvement in the organisational structure of sport systems

the Canadian system. The historical and cultural references are of particular significance in the United Kingdom document.

Organisational accountability is similarly precise: in Canada, a junior minister is directly responsible to a senior minister for this Act; whereas in England, Scotland and Wales, The Sports Council is responsible to a Secretary of State for the Environment. Attendant to this structural variability is the complex set of specialised functions performed by a multitude of committees and specified administrative functions of full-time staff. A notable organisational contrast of the two systems is that Canada, in the past 20 years, has altered the formal structure on numerous occasions (Canada 1969, 1970a, b; 1979a, b), the most recent changes being directed to a wider separation of the sport-for-all concept as contrasted to the pursuit of international excellence. These structural revisions are indicative of the ever-changing sport policy which is reflective of the emergent nature of Canadian objectives for international sport competition as contrasted to the consistency evident in the United Kingdom system which originated in 1935 with the Central Council of Physical Recreation (CCPR). Both organisations recognise the impact of sport internationally and the prestige ascribed to winning.

System Coupling

Closely aligned with the evolution of complex organisations is the necessity to establish relationships in a formal manner. Sport achieves this process by means of the establishment of officially sanctioned levels of autonomy, locally and regionally; binding versus non-binding legislation; the emergence of national affiliations which are generally associated with a specific sport; and eligibility codes, both national and international with attendant enforcement procedures. Thus, regardless of the complexity of the coupling, dependence upon the central system becomes more pronounced. An examination of both systems indicated an increasing reliance upon the central system, namely The Sports Council, Sport Canada, the National Olympic Committees and the national sport governing bodies, for sanctioning, for eligibility and for specified codes of "behaviour" etc. The dominance of these central bodies is primarily focused upon lending stability to the complex environment of domestic and international sport. The apparent movement from a loosely coupled system to a dominant, tightly controlled system needs careful study in terms of the "impact of potentially threatening innovations" (Aldrich 1979) which may result in destrictive adaptations to specific sports.

Multiplexity of Relationships

Upon inspection of the structural composition and the parallel evolution of committees, affiliations (internal and external), selection procedures for representative teams, and other mandated procedures, the two systems have since their inception created a multiplexity of relationships and thereby habe increased the dependence of the sport governing bodies on the central authority. Attendant to this development has been an apparent increase in governmental bureaucratic influence as evidenced by greater fincanical control and expansion of the administrative services.

New Resource Systems

Clearly, this subset of the model represents the visible aspect of the system, since the development of Bill C-131 in Canada and the Charter of 1972 in the United Kingdom, the international function of the Sport Council and Sport Canada coupled with the function of recognition of sport governing bodies that shall represent a country is reflective of the symbiotic relationship between officialdom and a particular sport. The magnitude of exchange of services between the central body and a sport governing body is indicative of the emergence of a new resource coupling modus operandi which gradually becomes the norm expectation for the sport delivery system. Evidence was found to support each of the subsets of this segment of the GLJ model.

The level of external role representatioon was very evident in the United Kingdom as contrasted to Canada - clearly a fact contributing to this difference is the geographical and political nature of international sport in Europe. Thus these important factors enhanced by the highly evolved European sport network necessitate constant interorganisational communication, principally through the Council of Europe and the National Olympic Committees. No such affiliation is necessary for Canada and the United States, mainly due to the reasonably consistent cultural expectations for international sport. Environmental stability, structural formalisation, frequency of interaction and use of a common language contribute to a relatively consistent sport system between these two countries.

Group Dynamics

The central importance of group dynamics in any organisation has long been recognised in management science research. Similarly, the fact that organisational structure and size dictate the manner in which decicion making, communication, organisational conflict etc. are manifest in the system is also widely accepted. Based upon the contrasting sport structures, the historical ties in the United Kingdom, the different political systems and, further, recognising the well-established nature of the United Kingdom system (1935) as contrasted to the recently established Sport Canada/Recreation (1969), the factors of decision making, communication, organisational authority and influence are noteceably different. These should be explored in greater depth in future research in terms of the contributing nature of each related to organisational efficiency and effectiveness.

Conclusion

An interorganisational desgin, using the proposed model, can be used to expand the knowledge and understanding of comparative management science with reference to national and international sport. Network analysis and SDIF in combination with other research methods, such as the modified Delphi system, can be used to improve upon the research findings and thereby contribute to the advancement of understanding in this field.

Acknowledgements. I wish to acknowledge the financial support of the Social Sciences and Humanities Research Council Grant No. 461-820440, and of the University of Windsor Academic

Development Fund. In addition, I gratefully acknowledge the outstanding contribution of Mr. John Coghlan, Deputy-Director General, The Sports Council, for his guidance and assistance in this project.

References

Aldrich H (1977) Visionaires and villains: The politics of designing interorganisational relations. In: Burack EH, Hegandhi AR (eds) Organisational Design: Theoretical perspectives and empirical findings. The Comparative Administration Research Institute, Kent, Ohio, The Kent State University Press, Kent, pp 23–40
Aldrich HE (1979) Organizations and environements. Prentice-Hall, Englewood Cliffs
Anderson BF (1971) The psychology experiment, 2nd edn. Brooks/Cove, Belmont, pp 24–33
Benson JK (1975) The interorganizational network as a political economy. Ad Sc Quart 20:229–250
Beres EM, Portwood JD (1981) Sociocultural influences on organizations: An analysis of recent research. In: England G W, Negandhi A R, Wilbert B (eds) The functioning of complex organizations. Oelschlager, Gunn and Hain, Cambridge, Mass., pp 303-336
Canada (1961) An act to encourage fitness and amateur sport. The House of Commons of Canada, Ottawa, September 25, 1961
Canada (1969) Leisure in Canada. Proceedings of the Montmorency Conference on Leisure, Department of National Health and Welfare. The Queen's Printer, Ottawa
Canada (1970a) Report of the task force on sport for Canadians. The Queen's Printer, Ottawa. pp 1-112
Canada (1970b) Report on physical recreation, fitness and amateur sport in Canada, Part I and II. P. S. Ross, Montreal
Canada (1979a) Toward a national policy on amateur sport. A discussion paper. The Queen's Printer, Ottawa, pp 1-19
Canada (1979b) Partners in the pursuit of excellence. A national policy on amateur sport. The Queen's Printer, Ottawa (1972) pp 1-24
Moriarty MR, Duthie HJ, Olafson AG (1972) Sports Institute for Research. Change Agent Research, The 3M Model. University of Windsor, Windsor, Ontario, Canada
Mouly JG (1963) The science of educational research. American Book, New York, pp 279–284
Negandhi RA, Melcher JA, Schwitter PJ (ed) (1969) Comparative administration and management: Conceptual schemes and research findings. Kent State University Press, Kent, Ohio, pp 1-124
Negandhi RA (ed) (1971) Organization theory in an interorganizational perspective. Kent State University Press, Kent, Ohio, pp 1-104
Negandhi RA (ed) (1972) Modern organizational theory - contextual, environmental, and sociocultural variables. Kent State University Press, Kent, Ohio, pp 1-404
Negandhi RA (1978) Interorganization theory. Kent State Univertsity Press, Kent, Ohio, pp 1-283
Rummel JF (1958) An introduction to research procedures in education. Harper, New York, pp 66–83
Semotiuk MD (1980) Motives for national government involvement in sport. Int Phys 18:23–28
Stern NR (1979) The development of an interorganizational control network: The case of intercollegiate athletics. Ad Sc Quart 24:242-266
The Sports Council (1971) Incorporated by Order of Her Majesty the Queen in Council on 22nd Day of December, 1971
Thompson J (1979) Organizations in action. McGraw-Hill, New York

V

Conclusions

Summary of the Theme "The Role of International Sport in Advancing or Weakening International Co-existence and Understanding" (Section II)

G. Walker

Under this theme a very large number of interesting and well-researched papers were presented, dealing with numerous aspects of the contribution of international sport to international understanding. What conclusions are possible? I would like to suggest that the following are among the more important.

It was agreed that sport is inevitably involved in international understanding (and that international understanding is vital to sport) but there was less agreement on *how* it is: whether it is an inherent factor whether it is, an additional/accidental factor or whether special provision has to be made for it. Some speakers insisted on the importance of general social conditions; others stated that sport as a willing or unwilling factor in international politics contains elements which can promote or hinder international understanding, directly or indirectly. Amongst the ways in which sport may contribute to international understanding, we discussed the role of the Olympic Games, of other competitions, of the sports organisations and, last but not least, of sports science and sports scientists themselves. The shadow of Coubertin haunted the hall. We agreed, I think, that the basis for this understanding lies in the existence of a common code - of fairness, human values, fair play - under the overall banner of the Olympic ideal. Hence, and this was stressed in several contexts, the importance of education, the exchange of educational experiences and material, development etc.

But when it comes to evaluating and understanding the contribution of sport to international understanding, then we encounter more problems. Various analyses, models and metholologies were used. We suffer from a piecemeal approach and we need a commonly agreed overal conceptual framework. The field is wide open! This framework should perhaps distinguish more clearly than hitherto the various *processes* and *levels* of contact in international sport: the sportsmen, the sports organisations, the spectators and the countries. ICSPE's new project aimed at the sportsmen themselves is therefore welcome. The new research also needs to distinguish the *levels of significance* of mutual understanding through sport and thus its possible contribution to international understanding and politics.

Various specific problems were highlighted: violence, the position of developing countries and the need for a greater intercultural understanding, the perceptions of international sports leaders and politicians and the media.

To sum up' there was a general conviction of the need to get to grips with the *"grandeur et servitude sportive"*: for this not only is multidisciplinary work vital, but other social scientists should be urged to pay just attention to the sports phenomenon, its undoubted role in society and international life, and its image.

Summary of the Theme "The Extent and Content of International Co-operation in Sport" (Section III)

M. J. Karvonen

Introduction

The Helsinki Congress on Sport and International Understanding provided the first world-wide forum for the scientific exposition and analysis of a wide spectrum or phenomena of international sports. Duly, the themes of the Congress were introduced from different angles. The competitive sports as a social system have an in-built structure of forces which lead to an escalating recruitment of human and material resources for improving performance and winning, to "totalisation". Competition is a pervasive element in Western societies. The modern sports movement is congruent with the Western culture, with emphasis on competition rather than on co-operation, and hence is also prone to conflicts and crises. For the succesful operation of such a system, strict rules and regulations are necessary. These rules are enacted in a democratic way and their observation rests largely on solidarity. For leaders and competitors, international sports thus offer a school in truly humanistic traditions and values. The spectators, however, may see another picture, appealing to more primitive needs and desires; the presentation of international sports by the media is biased towards the sensational.

Competitive and Top-Level Sport

International sporting competitions are widely regarded as contributing to mutual respect and recognition among the competitors as well as nations. The rapid development of the top performances in the twentieth century has been closely linked with international sport, which motivates training, develops personality and adds to the ethical and moral qualities. The development of athletic performance also has other determinants: at the national level the educational goals, the appreciation of physical culture and sports, the professional standards of coaches and teachers, research in sports sciences and the sports facilities. The main international determinants, on the other hand, are the preservation of peace and respect for the principles of peaceful coexistence. Commercialisation is a severe threat to international competitive sport today: it jeopardises its development, sovereignty and existence and ties the hands of international sports organisations. To exclude unfair means of influencing the athletic performance such as doping, ethical values are to be emphasised and conveyed in education. Increasingly efficient control is expected from medical commissions, whose membership should be politically and geographically balanced.

Competitive sport can promote peace and detente only among nations wanting peace and international understanding. The athletes as well as the sporting public should be exposed to education and mass media in the spirit of the ethical and moral values of sport.

Sport for All

Parallel to but largely separate from competitive sport, sport for all has in recent years shown a spectacular development in several countries. This new mass movement essentially confesses a different ideology. International organisations have lately focussed attention on sport for all, and several aspects have been studied and discussed at international meetings. More psychological, sociological, ecological and health-related research is needed. Documentation and dissemination of information on sport for all is a field fertile for international co-operation. The training of leaders and provision of an increased share for women in the sports organisations are actual challenges.

Sport for Special Groups

Sport for the handicapped may be the noblest contribution of sport to mankind. Even when the purely utilitarian results remain meagre, the quality of life can be improved immensely. Among the disabled, international co-operation is well established, but for the other special groups international contacts remain to be established. Research and pilot projects increasingly supply information on aspects particular to special groups, but wide areas of research are still open for sports sciences and medicine. At the local level special groups need sports services organised on voluntary basis and supported by a core of professionals. Leadership training is an urgent challenge.

Summary of the Theme "Measures Related to International Co-operation in Sport" (Section IV)

A. Koskela and E. Buggel

With regard to the measures related to international co-operation in sport, this congress paid special attention to (1) peaceful and friendly international relations, (2) international mass communication, (3) education for internationalism and (4) co-operation with developing countries.

Peaceful and friendly neighbourly relations between peoples and nations are an important precondition for the development of physical culture and sport in such a way that they will benefit mankind on a national and international level. The international climate is decisive for the development of physical culture and sport. While international sporting contacts were extended and improved by détente in the 1970s, international tension is a danger to its development. Proof of this was the Olympic boycott initiated by the former Carter administration. Attention should be focussed upon the threat to peace (as far as these threats have not yet generally been recognised by all participants in this conference) because the preservation of peace is the first and foremost precondition for sport. There would be no sense in talking about athletic meetings or their value to international understanding after a nuclear war jeopardising the existence of human civilisation!

The lack of research into the relationship of communication, sport and international understanding is evident. Some peculiar features of sport make extrapolation and inference from related research difficult and misleading. Sport has to be classified as both news and entertainment. Coverage by the media emphasises entertainment. It also displays certain tendencies, biases and distortions which may have both positive and negative effects upon international understanding and good-will. Sports scientists should not only develop their own conceptual framework for multidisciplinary research but also ensure that other disciplines include sport when they research international relations and communication systems.

Education for internationalism at schools was considered an important area for developing co-operation as a step towards international understanding. It was felt that in this respect better school curricula are needed in many countries. It was pointed out that competitive sport offers, when correctly used, opportunities for education in internationalism. The other activities in which the educational objectives for international understanding should be remembered are: youth-sport exchanges, tournaments for school teams, mass sporting events and some international programmes.

Co-operation with developing countries can be divided into: (a) current problems of developing countries, (b) areas of co-operation and (c) necessary actions to make co-operation possible. The problems under each topic are numerous and difficult. The need for formulation of a workable programme of co-operation by an International

Committee was stressed. Effective co-operation was considered the best way to build up understanding between countries.

It was felt that the international sports federations should develop their rules and regulations to strengthen co-operation and thus understanding.

When broader measures are to be taken, as they must, one should think in terms of global understanding. Tolerance, patience and enthusiasm must be combined with the potential of a scientific approach. Hopefully, ineffective talk will thereby be replaced by fruitful activity towards a more peaceful world.

Summary of the Congress by the Chairman of the Scientific Committee

P. Vuolle

We have in the course of this congress heard numerous meritorius lectures that have inspired fruitful debate. Seven main lectures, 18 introductory lectures and over 50 free papers have been presented on the four main themes of the congress and subjects closely related to them. We have just heard the summary reports on the various themes. I would like to thank the teams responsible for compiling these reports and the people who presented the summaries.

Summarising the whole congress is no easy task. Analysis of such extensive material calls for thorough deliberation and thus takes a lot of time. The assessment of the congress as a whole and all that it has offered will ultimately be left to each individual participant. Delegates will be assisted in their final assessment by the congress proceedings to be issued later. Without trying to make any sort of summary proper, I should, however, like to take a look at some of the points that clearly came to the fore in the course of the congress.

One observation that was already brought up when the congress was being prepared, and which has here been confirmed, is that there is at the moment very little research material available that is theoretically significant and that covers the problems dealt with during this congress. Many of you have spoken about this, and also about the problems surrounding international research co-operation and the exchange of scientific information on the field. One thing that all these views held in common is that they strongly emphasised the need for multidisciplinary, international research into the future state of sport. A good example of co-operation of the type mentioned was given by Professor Jochheim. He told us about interdisciplinary research in the field of sports for the disabled and a long-term programme based on this, the aim of which is to develop physical activities for various disabled groups in practical situations.

As regards physical exercise and international understanding, the approach of the mass media to sport and the world of values of international competitive sport which they put across has been viewed as another sector in which international research into sport and physical education should be activated. "We need theoretical insights to identify the problems which international communication, sport and international understanding present to us" said Professor McIntosh.

The mass media were not the only subject brought up at the congress; the lectures and reports covered numerous other areas in which international research activities should be increased or begun. Researchers from different fields should, however, be made more seriously interested in co-operation over sport and physical education in particular. Although we support amateur sport, amateur researches are not able to visualise and solve the universal problems of sport to which research must find an answer. On the other hand it is a question of the level of knowledge on sport and physical education, a matter to which the Chairman of ICSPE, Sir Roger Bannister, paid serious attention in his final address at the scientific congress in Tbilisi in 1980.

The potential for expanding international into sport science is good, because, as Professor Hebbelinck pointed out in his lecture, the development of discipline-oriented organisations of sport sciences since the 1960s has been very marked.

The central outcome of the congress is that it threw light, in a very realistic manner, on the position and significance of sport in dealings between nations and peoples. Congress delegates from different parts of the world and other experts on sport agree about the potential of sport for furthering international peace and understanding (Here I would like to mention just the speeches of Professor Sanadze and Professor Ghibu). Doctor Tapio Varis said that it seems possible that in the world of rapid changes, instability and tension, international sport can functions as a stabilising factor. This opinion is reinforced by the fact that, despite political, economic and social differences, modern sport has spread all over the world in what is historically a very short time. The favourable influences are not, however, to be taken as a matter of course, for international sport must be conducted and developed an accordance with certain basic conditions. I refer, for instance, to the paper of Professor Lüschen, which states that abandoning these conditions would mean that instead of reinforcing peace and co-operation, international sport would be a means of accelerating the international arms race serving the objectives of the cold war. There are alarming signs of this in, for example, ultranationalism, racial discrimination, commercialisation and the increasignly violent nature of sport. Such dangers were brought up by, among others, Professor Heinilä in describing competitions between organisations caused by totalised competitive sport in which national and international interests conflict with one another. The danger is obvious in Western countries in particular, as Professor Galtung mentioned, for in them competition, the battle for superiority, is an element firmly anchored in the foundations of the social system and all its main walks of life. The "nothing but victory" principle on the other hand is, according to Professor Niwa, typical of industrial society. Niwa forecasts that during the transfer to post-industrial society sport will again take on its humanistic nature, the preservation of which was stressed by Professors Erbach and Wolanska and others.

International competitive sport and in particular the Olympic Games were well to the fore in discussions of the positive or negative effects of sport. Professor Krüger pointed out that the ideology of peace and international co-operation has always been a marked element of the views and activities of the creators and developers of the Olympic movement, the first presidents of the IOC. Professor Wohl talked about the international functions of competitive and mass sport. As regards international co-operation, competitive sport primarily plays an integrating role, whereas the function of mass sport is evident first and foremost at national and regional level. The future of the Olympic movement is something we all think about. Mr. Tallberg, representing the IOC, stressed that, while preserving its independence, the IOC is seeking co-operation with such organisations as UNESCO. Mr. Tallberg examined the decisions made last year at the Olympic Congress in Baden-Baden and assessed their international significance. These decisions stressed, among other things, that the programmes for future Olympic Games should make allowance for the present trends in sport and be prepared to include forms of sport popular in the developing countries. Along with the increasingly cosmopolitan character of sport, the preservation of national physical cultures was considered by many to be important. A country's national physical culture is part of the national heritage, and special care must be taken to see that it does not become merged with international trends prevailing in sport. On the other hand, interaction between the two may also be fruitful. Professor Erbach said that the more highly developed a national physical culture is, the more it can benefit international physical culture, and vice versa.

This Congress has proved that both international and national sport have a vast potential which, when guided along the right lines, may be of excellent service to international peace and co-operation. Both researchers and those engaged in various tasks in practical sporting activities should on the one hand be clearly aware of the conditions under which favourable development takes place, while on the other they should be able to see the pitfalls which, in the form of distorted developments, may lead to quite the opposite result. If this congress, which was purposely held in the same place as the Helsinki Conference on Security and Co-operation in Europe in 1975, has opened up wider perspectives among the delegates here, it certainly have succeeded in its task.

On behalf of the Organising Committee of the congress and its Scientific Commission I would finally like to express my warmest thanks to the main speakers, those of you who gave introductory lectures, those of you who read free papers, and all those taking part in this congress. Special thanks are due to the congress presidents and the large number of people responsible for the organisation. I further wish to thank the ICSPE and its executive committee for the valuable help we received. My warmest thanks are due to the President, Sir Roger Bannister, to Secretary General John F. Coghlan and especially to Professor Hebbelinck for the irreplaceable help he gave the Scientific Committee. My thanks also go to the other organisations supporting the congress. This congress, in summertime Finland, has been - in my opinion - a success, and the credit for that lies with you all.

Final Statement by the President of the International Council of Sport and Physical Education (ICSPE)

Sir Roger Bannister

No one can doubt the success of this world congress for 300 participants from nearly 30 countries in this beautiful land of a thousand lakes. I measure success in terms of making us think more critically about existing ideas and by our discussion generating new ideas. Some participants may feel they were confused at the beginning. Now they may still be confused, but at a much higher level!

Among the many causes of the lack of peace, one of the most important is misunderstanding. Among the causes of misunderstanding are first, ignorance of other countries and their people, and second, chauvinism, which, as we have heard in this congress, is created sometimes unwittingly but sometimes cynically either by the mass media for profit or by governments for nationalistic purposes.

The best way to counter this misunderstanding is by education. First, education of our young by sports exchanges that have a high social content as well as a competitive content. Second, education of television and the mass media. This congress has stressed the increasing role of television and the media in creating attitudes. Northcliffe, a British baron, was once told that the press bahaved like a harlot, using power without responsibility. We must educate television and the media to use their power more responsibly. Third, we must educate our governments. Sport is probably a more powerful force for good or bad relationships between governments than any other cultural activity. Governments must at all times respect the sportsman's integrity as this is the activity of a free citizen. Excessive concerns for the welfare and success of their sportsmen may lead governments to interfere with the freedom of their citizens in the practice and pursuit of sport. Governments should interfere as little as possible with free exchanges between countries and should give general support in as altruistic a way as possible. Fourth, we must educate the developed world so that it can never forget that at present two-thirds of the world is too malnourished and too poor for sport to have any relevance whatsoever. This congress must never forget that fact, and Mr. Zachariev, the distinguished representative of the Director General of UNESCO, has emphasised this in his speech.

In this congress we have had difficulties in defining terms. Sport can mean so many things. It can mean an aggressive, even violent struggle between a handful of elite athletes in representative national teams. It can mean the sport for all movement involving up to 60% of the population in recreational, non-competitive sports like jogging and long-distance skiing. Sport of such different kinds is governed by utterly different principles.

Sport, like so much else in life, is neither good nor bad in itself but we as human beings can use it for good or bad purposes. We hold no magic wand to turn it into a panacea for peace and understanding but we should not be here unless we all believed it was possible to do better than we have done in the past. We are here to re-dedicate ourselves to harness what remains one of the most powerful potential forces for good in the twentieth century. As the English poet Browning put it "man's vision should exceed his grasp or what is a heaven for".

When speakers here have talked about disasters of misunderstanding and violations of the fair play concept they can do so because we do here all accept a code of fairness, mutual respect, understanding and friendship. There is far more that unites us than separates us. In my 6 years as president of ICSPE with countries from East and West, North and South we have debated many controversial issues. Only once has it been necessary to hold a vote and I cannot now remember clearly the cause!

Reflecting on this congress as a sport scientist, I think we should still more often take the problems of our sport to the parent science, whether sociology, philosophy or psychology. To bud off a separate sport sciences too soon seems to me a mistake.

When we look at the problems of sport it seems to me that the main enemy of understanding is conflict and aggression. I would like to see more attention paid to the psychological factors and an attempt to define and cultivate individual human qualities which tend to be more intellectual and more co-operative as opposed to "herd" qualities which, in defence of the group, are more primitive and more aggressive. This is what civilisation is about. What factors affect the growth of these conflicting aspects of the human personality? One final point concerning research demonstrated by this congress is the need for international research into sport rather than research merely within the frontiers of one country.

In conclusion, in thanking again most warmly our Finnish hosts may I say that they have given us the perfect setting to ask and discuss many questions that are fitting subjects for future research. We can best thank our hosts by our determination to follow these questions to the best of our ability.

Subject Index

Children and Sport

Paediatric Work Physiology

Editors: **J. Ilmarinen, I. Välimäki**

1984. 105 figures, 96 tables. XIX, 274 pages. ISBN 3-540-13044-6

Contents: Growth, Development and Physical Activity. - Physical Working Capacity. - Physical Training and Sports. - Physical Activity and Health. - Subject Index.

This book deals with the safe physiological growth and development of children and adolescents. It includes reports on new findings covering the physical activity required for the psychomotor and mental development of the children, the effects of maturation on maximal aerobic power, children in competitive sports, and the risk factors of coronary heart disease among children. The book provides insight into the experiences of the Tenth Symposium of Paediatric Work Physiology held in Jouta, Finland, regarding the development of a safe and positive sporting life-style for children.

Springer-Verlag
Berlin
Heidelberg
New York
Tokyo

O. Bar-Or

Pediatric Sports Medicine for the Practitioner

From Physiologic Principles to Clinical Applications

1983. 124 figures. XXII, 376 pages. (Comprehensive Manuals in Pediatrics).
ISBN 3-540-90873-0

Pediatric Sports Medicine bridges the gap between recent research in physiology of exercise and your practice. The book emphasizes the effects of growth and maturation of the child on responses to exercise and to physical conditioning. In **Pediatric Sports Medicine,** you will also find a detailed analysis of the relationship between physical activity and diseases, examined from various different perspectives, including that of nutrition and of environmental stress. Three practical appendices have been included to give you concrete tools for clinical use. They are:
Measurements of physical working capacity - norms.
Methodology of exercise testing, including suggested protocols and precautions.
Useful tables and a sample activity questionnaire.

Springer-Verlag
Berlin
Heidelberg
New York
Tokyo

MIX
Papier aus verantwortungsvollen Quellen
Paper from responsible sources
FSC® C105338

If you have any concerns about our products,
you can contact us on
ProductSafety@springernature.com

In case Publisher is established outside the EU,
the EU authorized representative is:
Springer Nature Customer Service Center GmbH
Europaplatz 3, 69115 Heidelberg, Germany

Printed by Libri Plureos GmbH
in Hamburg, Germany